inven

BEAUTY

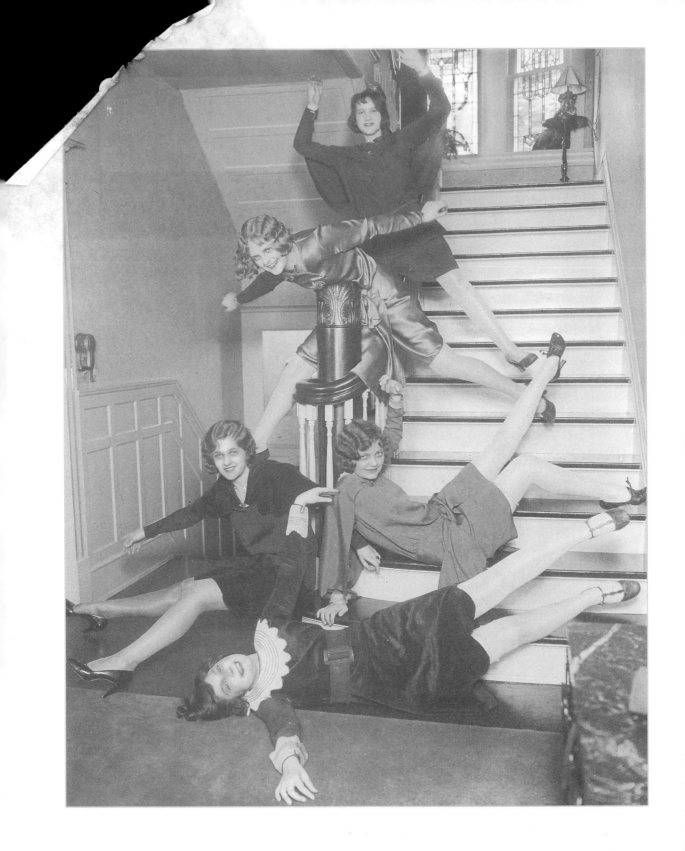

inventing BEAUTY

A history of
the innovations
that have made us
Beautiful

TERESA RIORDAN

BROADWAY BOOKS · NEW YORK

PRINTED IN THE UNITED STATES OF AMERICA

BROADWAY BOOKS and its logo, a letter B bisected on the diagonal, are trademarks of Random House, Inc.

Visit our website at www.broadwaybooks.com
First edition published 2004.

BOOK DESIGN BY DEBORAH KERNER/DANCING BEARS DESIGN

Library of Congress Cataloging-in-Publication Data

Riordan, Teresa.
    Inventing beauty : a history of the innovations that have made us beautiful / Teresa Riordan.—1st ed.
        p.   cm.
    Includes bibliographical references and index.
    ISBN 0-7679-1451-1 (alk. paper)
    1. Beauty, Personal—History.   2. Beauty culture—History.   3. Cosmetics—History.
  4. Clothing and dress—History.   I. Title.
GT499.R56 2004
391.6—dc22

                                                                    2004043876

ISBN 0-7679-1451-1

10 9 8 7 6 5 4 3 2 1

For *Damaris*

and *Lydia*

and the men in our lives,

Elliott

and *Richard*

MONDAY.

TUESDAY.

WEDNESDAY.

THURSDAY.

FRIDAY.

SATURDAY.

SUNDAY.

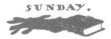

If I were permitted to choose from the rubbish that will be published a hundred years after my death, do you know what I would take? . . .

I would take simply a fashion magazine in order to see how women will dress themselves a century after my death. And their fantasies would tell me more about future humanity than all the philosophers, the novelists, the preachers, or the scientists.

— ANATOLE FRANCE

One cannot take on a new identity by changing trousers.

— SUSAN BROWNMILLER

There are no ugly women, only lazy ones.

— HELENA RUBINSTEIN

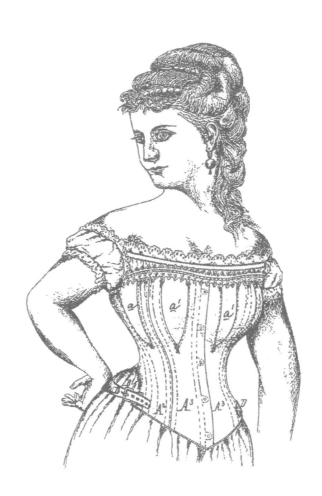

contents

ACKNOWLEDGMENTS • xi

INTRODUCTION • xv

chapter 1 • Eyes • 1

chapter 2 • Lips • 33

chapter 3 • Breasts • 63

chapter 4 • Hair • 115

chapter 5 • Skin • 145

chapter 6 • Waist • 173

chapter 7 • Hands • 203

chapter 8 • Hips • 225

chapter 9 • Derriere • 259

CONCLUSION • 277

NOTES • 279

BIBLIOGRAPHY • 288

ILLUSTRATION CREDITS • 297

INDEX • 301

acknowledgments

Writing this book has been a journey of joyous serendipity, and I received help from many quarters along the way.

The Massachusetts Institute of Technology Knight Science Journalism Program provided me with a yearlong fellowship that transformed this book into a more ambitious effort than it otherwise would have been. Special thanks go to Victor McElheny (whose encyclopedic knowledge of both nineteenth-century steel making and French court life threw me a lifeline one afternoon when I was drowning in hoop skirts), Boyce Rensberger (who engaged in deep philosophical discussions about women's body parts while keeping a straight face), Martha Henry (whose sharp editorial judgment pulled me back from the brink of esoterica), and John Nikolai (a great guy). I also benefited greatly from discussions with my learned fellow fellows: Bari Scott, Seema Singh, Volker Steger, Akin Jimoh, Angela Swafford, Gary Robbins, Sha Hoon Hong, Karen Rafinski, and Sharon Kay.

This book could not have been written without the financial support of the Alfred P. Sloan Foundation, so I extend my undying gratitude to Doron Weber, who made the grant possible. Thanks also to David Rhees, director of the Bakken Library in Minneapolis, who gave me a fellowship at that unique institution. Elizabeth Ihrig served as my intrepid guide during a weeklong romp through the Bakken's unusual collection of electricity-related books and ephemera. A special kiss on the forehead goes to curator Ellen Kuhfeld, who not only patiently showed me the Bakken's collection of electrolysis machines but also reviewed the chapters on hair removal and skin for technical accuracy.

Given that many professional historians loathe attempts by nonprofessionals to popularize history, I am especially indebted to the scholars who generously helped, by varying degrees, with this book. They include Bettyann Holtzmann Kevles, Deborah Jean Warner, Deborah Fitzgerald, Merritt Roe Smith, Gwen Kay, Rachel Maines, Autumn Stanley, Kirsten Gardner, Robert Friedel, Thomas Misa, and John Kenly Smith. Of course, all sins committed here in the name of history are mine alone.

I am indebted to the staff at a number of institutions, including Harvard's Schlesinger Library on the History of Women, the Burndy Library at the Dibner Institute, the National Library of Medicine, the MIT interlibrary loan service, and the interlibrary loan service and the engineering library at the University of Maryland in College Park. Many thanks also to Marjorie Ciarlante at the National Archives; Bob McCoy of the Museum of Questionable Medical Devices; Amy Fischer, Ed Smith, and Lisa Mulvaney at Procter & Gamble; Jim Davie, Ruth Nyblod, and Brigid Quinn at the U.S. Patent and Trademark Office; Laura L. Carroll of the American Medical Association; Susan Rishworth of the American College of Obstetrics and Gynecology; Harry Katz at the Library of Congress; and Deborah Warner, Mimi Minnick, Alison Oswald, Joyce Bedi, Maggie Dennis, Jennifer Snyder, Shelley Foote, and Priscilla Wood at the Smithsonian Institution.

I owe much appreciation to all my colleagues at *The New York Times* business section, with special gratitude to Glenn Kramon, Judith Spindler, Tim Race, Bruce Headlam, and Sabra Chartrand. Other colleagues and friends nudged this project forward in various ways: Barbara Rowley, Debby Baldwin, Irwin Arieff, Isabel Chenoweth, Esther Schwartz-McKinzie, Anne Depue, Alex Heard, Susan Heard, Adam Glenn, Bruce Melzer, Jeff Herr, Barbara Moran, Robert Buderi, and Robert Kanigel. Charles Euchner deserves a bouquet of long-stemmed roses for improving the manuscript with his candid yet gentle editorial advice.

Many thanks also to Elizabeth Haymaker, she of infinite tact, for cheerfully navigating through the never-never land of permissions and illustrations, as well as to the production staff at Broadway Books. Umi Kenyon and Mark Melnick conjured up an eye-catching confection of a book cover. Deborah Kerner's book design is both lovely and inspired. Julia Coblenz and Joanna Pinsker were full of imaginative ideas on how to bring *Inventing Beauty* to readers' attention. Jud Laghi at ICM provided expert advice at crucial moments. Let me give a deep curtsy to the two superlative Krisses: Kris Puopolo at Broadway was the perfect editor—patient, perceptive, and playful. If Kris Dahl of ICM had not graciously taken me under her powerful wing this book would likely have never reached its final destination.

The incomparable Girl Group provided me with sustenance, both emotional and gustatory. Kathleen Currie, Marianne Szegedy-Maszak, Shannon Brownlee, Sheila Kaplan, Mel Hindin, Estelle Campbell, and Amy Cunningham. The Takoma Avenue Provocatives—Jan, Abi, Bev, Bernadette, Nora, Carolyn, and Naomi—challenged my point of view on everything from hair removal to racial politics.

Special thanks go to friends and neighbors who ignored my careless housekeeping, put up with late birthday presents or unreturned e-mails, buoyed my sometimes flagging enthusiasm with their own optimism, or otherwise extended myriad kindnesses during the five years it took me to write this book:

Karen Reinke, Annie Hutchins, Odette Bovenberg, Mata Dova, Yung Lim, Frederique Donovan, Dave Reinke, Beverly Ress, Rick Stack, Elizabeth Becker, Anthony Ruvolo, Hervé Dumez, Jaclin Gilbert, Alicia Wrenn, Peter Sachner, Marejke Taylor, Steve Taylor, Tramell Alexander, Michael Alexander, Sarah Taber, Peter Thomas, Konstanze Greer, Sue Kirchhoff, Jon Lourie, Melissa Houghton, Richard Houghton, Nancy Swenton, Lisa Birchard, Suzie Gurley, John Gurley, Mike Hiestand, Teresa Hiestand, Susie Sivard, Harrison Sohmer, Pat Turner, Hugh Turner, Mairi Morrison, Ellyn McKay, Maggy Sterner, Carter Baldwin, Emory Luce Baldwin, Tashi Bhuti, Gloria Fischer, William Fischer, Michael Robinson, Herschel Gower, Dona Gower, Kitty Chenoweth, Matt Chenoweth, Avery Chenoweth, Alex Roth, Peter Overby, Kurt Wimmer, and Stephanie Wimmer.

Michael Riordan went beyond the familial call of duty with his enthusiasm, ideas, and faith in my abilities. Brian and Quinn Riordan also provided insightful suggestions. (It's not every girl who feels comfortable discussing cleavage with her brothers!) The rest of the extended Riordan clan members deserve a big bear hug for

acknowledgments

their unparalleled warmth, wit, and wisdom: Neil, Renée, Rika, Takuma, Tatiana, Clovis, Chloe, Michaela, Brinn, Tierney, Shirley, Savannah, Alexis, Don—and, especially, Hugh and Jan.

Finally, I owe my husband and children an unrepayable debt for the many hours this enterprise stole from family life. My husband, Richard Chenoweth, a brilliant architect, superb cook, and loving father, managed to wring enough time out of his busy life to help coordinate the illustrations in this book. Our son, Elliott, rescued me innumerable times from digital despair with his computer wizardry. Our daughters, Lydia and Damaris, served as enthusiastic photo researchers and, by inventing their own gorgeously outlandish dress-up outfits, have reminded me again and again that the feminine imagination is boundless.

introduction

When I was in high school, I went to visit my brother's girlfriend at college and stayed at her sorority. Amid this houseful of beauties was a young woman who had recently been catapulted into the highest stratum of femaledom, that of "professional model." But when she shuffled into breakfast in her robe and slippers, the dark swollen half-moons beneath her eyes betraying a late night of carousing at a frat-house beer party, she appeared not only unexceptional but downright dowdy. I looked at her sharply, incredulous that this lump wrapped in dusty pink chenille could be the subject of magazine fashion spreads.

"You have to see her when she's made-up," someone whispered to me. "Then she looks gorgeous."

This book is a history of those inventions that women have used to transform themselves—the gadgets and potions they have used to push, pull, tweeze, squeeze, and spackle themselves in the name of Beauty.

It is perhaps ironic that I should be writing such a book. I buy my bras from discount malls, have never owned nor even coveted a pair of Manolo Blahnik's spike-heeled mules, and have been known to make a $4.69 mascara wand last for three years. I make my living writing about technology, not fashion.

Even more surprising, perhaps, are some of the conclusions I have reached. I tried to approach this project without preconceptions, but I must admit that lurking at the back of my mind was the thought that, surely, these must be tools of oppression foisted by men on an unsuspecting female public. Alas, several years of intensive research failed to confirm—in fact, undermined—this point of view.

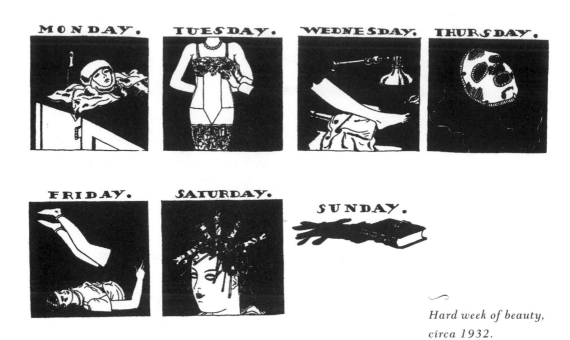

Hard week of beauty, circa 1932.

When it comes to the opposite sex, males from many species are easily deceived. Male fireflies flirt with penlights. Male turkeys become randy at the mere sight of a fake, female turkey head. Male humans find feminine decoys equally beguiling. As Steven Pinker has pointed out, men are aroused by the sight of a nude woman "not only in the flesh but in movies, photographs, drawings, postcards, dolls, and bit-mapped cathode-ray-tube displays."[1]

Women recognize this. And they have shrewdly, cannily, and knowingly deployed artifice in their ceaseless battle to captivate the inherently roving eye of the male. They have painted their lips cherry red, built their breasts into silicone summits, and festooned their buttocks with bustles. As much as it initially galled the feminist inside me to admit this, women have been the driving innovative force behind many of these inventions.

Just take a look at breast-enhancement technology. From the mid-nineteenth to the mid-twentieth century—the period this book covers—women received only about one percent of all patents granted in the United States. Yet when it comes to the category of "gay deceivers" (aka falsies), the number of female inventors takes a dramatic upward leap. Do you have any idea what percentage of false-bosom inventors during this period were women? Go ahead, take a guess. If you guessed fifty percent, you are in the ballpark. Actually, nearly two-thirds of these inventors were women.

I realize the territory of Beauty—even the word *Beauty*—is studded with emotional land mines. Many a hard-boiled feminist probably harbors a visceral pain over having been judged on her appearance for much of her life. I know this because, particularly during my adolescence, I suffered deeply the tyranny of prevailing standards of Beauty. I came of age in the seventies in a Midwestern Babbittland where women seemed to be judged exclusively by appearance. Despite my Irish Catholic name, I have a Mediterranean profile, and I chafed daily at not possessing the blond hair and turned-up nose so highly prized in that time and place.

But having meditated on this subject for several years now, I've come to believe that many women have wielded devices and potions built in the name of Beauty in order to transcend the emphasis that mankind places on Beauty. When successful, the artifice of Beauty is a great leveler. It puts the resourceful and the imaginative on an even playing field with the congenitally beautiful. The scrawny can appear amply endowed. The corpulent can achieve some semblance of a waist. The thin-lipped can look lusciously kissable. The wizened can project a youthful bloom.

This book considers Beauty from the mid-nineteenth to the mid-twentieth century in the United States, roughly from the first Women's Rights Convention, at Seneca Falls, New York, in 1848, to the introduction of the Pill in the 1960s. (The second wave of feminism, post-Pill, brought a righteous and necessary reckoning with standards of beauty and even larger cultural expectations that I do not grapple with here.) Yes, there were huge constraints on women (and still are!). But that doesn't mean that women did not imaginatively, within those boundaries, carve out their own realms of power.

Beauty is one of those realms. In deploying these implements, women have empowered themselves just as surely as did Catherine Beecher, who unlike her father and brother was unable to channel her ambition into religious scholarship during the nineteenth century. So Beecher pioneered a new path to power for women: that of domestic goddess.

I think the stories of inventors and inventions told here will hold great appeal for many Third Wave feminists who appreciate that the long great history of female oppression is a deeply complicated thing. But my point of view will inevitably irk some traditional feminists—some of whom supported the idea of this project enthusiastically at the outset and may be disappointed and even angry at some of the conclusions I ultimately reach.

Sitting in an airport not so long ago I tried explaining to Deborah Jean Warner, an esteemed curator at the Smithsonian's National Museum of American History, that I thought inventions like lipstick, bustles, and stiletto heels were frequently sources of power for women. They actually allow women to put one over on Man as well as Nature, I told her. These inventions transform Beauty, changing it from something that we're born with to something we can impose upon ourselves. She gamely challenged me and said that such a standard of femininity really bothered her. "To me these are feminine," she said, pointing to her white running shoes.

She makes a valid point. What is "feminine" is widely open to interpretation. But despite my own strong personal belief that gender is a continuum rather than an either/or proposition, our society has always drawn bright lines between male and female.

The definition of what is feminine is pretty clear-cut if we take our cues from transsexuals. Makeup, panty hose, high heels, and foundation garments are all things that transsexual women use to better communicate their new gender.

Perhaps the most "feminine" technology, from the transsexual point of view, is hair removal devices. That's because for transsexual women the biggest obstacle to

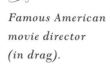

*Famous American
movie director
(in drag).*

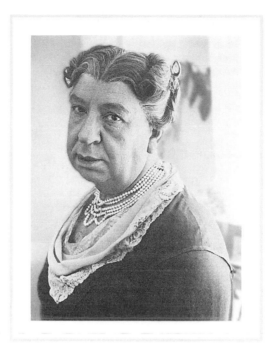

looking womanly is not, as I had originally suspected, switching genitalia but rather getting rid of facial and body hair. In fact, it is the most expensive part of the whole sex-change process! The biggest surprise in researching this book for me was how much of an ordeal depilation is even for women who were born with two X chromosomes. I have plucked my share of chin hairs, but, truly, I had no idea hair removal was such a universal feminine undertaking.

For that reason, hair removal gets a whole chapter here; however, I do admit that the choice of inventions throughout *Inventing Beauty* is to some extent idiosyncratic. I regret the omission of certain inventions, especially nylon stockings and stiletto heels, since they are such stunning examples of how man-made materials can transform our ideas of Beauty. But if I had attempted to cover all such inventions, this book would have taken me twice as long to finish.

It is true that the adornments discussed here can project not just sexuality but also such things as power, status, and tribe affiliation. I have left out certain inventions deliberately—rhinoplasty and skin-whitening creams, for example—because they are so thickly entwined with self-identity and ethnicity, issues better considered elsewhere.

Some critics will surely point to the frauds, some of them hideous, perpetrated in the name of Beauty and demand to know how I can argue that these implements have been empowering for women. At the benign end of the spectrum are antiwrinkle creams that, for a queenly sum, promise the Fountain of Youth. At the malignant end of the spectrum are such products as Lash Lure, a permanent mascara that blinded and disfigured some women in the days before federal regulation. But for every Lash Lure or vanishing cream, there is a cancer-inducing baldness cure or antimasturbation device resembling a tool of torture that is equally ridiculous or appalling. And the targets of those products are unequivocally men.

For the most part, I found that the freewheeling attempts of entrepreneurs, both male and female, to make a buck out of the insecurities and miseries of others were gender-neutral. One of the worst crimes perpetrated against women in the name of Beauty was Koremlu, a depilatory made up essentially of rat poison. Its inventor? A woman. Such entrepreneurs are definitely unscrupulous, but are they trying to oppress women in a conscious way? I have looked for evidence proving that this is so and come up empty-handed.

John Carl Flügel first proposed his theory of shifting erogenous zones in his 1930 book *The Psychology of Clothes,* and the idea was later elaborated by fashion historian James Laver. The theory, basically, is that fashion is the collective shifting of female sexual attention from one body part to another.

The trouble with this theory is that it describes what occurs in fashion at the macro level without explaining why it happens with women individually. In particular, it does not address one of the most vexing questions for fashion mavens and evolutionary theorists alike: Why is it that human females tend to be the flashy dressers when in the rest of the animal kingdom it is the male who sports the vibrant plumage or chandelier antlers?

So now let me boldly claim that I have unraveled this fashion riddle. Charles Darwin's theory of sexual selection goes like this: Women have to be choosy about their mates because mating has such long-term consequences. So females focus on quality; they try to pick the biggest, handsomest, cleverest males available. Males, on the hand, are not at all choosy. Given the chance, they will mate with any and every female they can.

This brings us to a phenomenon known as the Coolidge Effect, named in honor of what is likely an apocryphal story about President Calvin Coolidge and his wife.

One day the president and his wife were given separate tours of a government farm, so the story goes. Mrs. Coolidge, passing the chicken coop, inquired how many times a day the rooster copulated. "Dozens of times," she was told. "Well," Mrs. Coolidge coolly responded to the guide, "please tell that to the president." So the guide mentioned this information to the president as he inspected the chicken coop. "Same hen every time?" the president asked. "Oh no, Mr. President," came the reply, "a different one each time." The president nodded thoughtfully. "Tell that to Mrs. Coolidge."[2]

Dorothy Parker cleverly described the conundrum:

Woman wants monogamy;
Man delights in novelty.
Love is woman's moon and sun;
Man has other forms of fun.
Woman lives but in her lord;
Count to ten, and man is bored.
With this the gist and sum of it,
What earthly good can come of it?[3]

I think women have responded to the male predilection for novelty by using technology to reinvent themselves—to make themselves novel again and again. This works because the male mind tends to equate the part with the whole. Think of Truffaut's classic film *The Man Who Loved Women*. Captivated by a glimpse of a woman's legs while picking up his dry cleaning, actor Charles Denner goes to absurd lengths trying to track the woman down—even though he has never seen her face! By gamely shifting the focus of male attention from the breasts to the hips to the legs to the belly to the face and back again, an individual woman transforms herself from one woman into many women.

Men are clearly clued into the use of artifice. Yet they don't seem to mind. As the old chevalier says in Isak Dinesen's gothic tales, such feminine adornments "made it their object to transform the body which they encircled, and to create a silhouette so far from its real form as to make it a mystery which it was a divine privilege to solve."[4]

Woman may be a work of art, as the old chevalier also said, but she is also a competitive creature. As the evolutionary biologist Sarah Blaffer Hrdy has observed: Woman is out to conquer not just men but her rival females.

Woman has consciously assembled an armamentarium in the battle of love, turning to corsets and bras and girdles and panty hose and electrolysis machines to re-shape and organize and communicate the raw material that Nature gave her. And when she has found that material insufficiently compelling, she has embraced embellishments like falsies and lipstick and bustles. Call it fashion, if you will, but it is no less than an arms race in which the strong relentlessly struggle to acquire better, newer weapons of beauty.

Recently, I was explaining my theory to one feminist historian who gasped, "That sounds like *The Total Woman* all over again!"

This troubled me, so I ordered a used copy of *The Total Woman*, a self-help paperback published in 1973 and written by Marabel Morgan, a conservative Christian and a good friend of Anita Bryant, the Christian singer. Seven years into her marriage, Morgan decided to spice things up. So one night she greeted her husband at the door wearing pink baby-doll pajamas and white go-go boots. He chased her around the dining room table and thus began her lifelong commitment to boudoir costumes and to proselytizing her special gospel: the importance of being a one-woman harem to one's mate.

Quite frankly, as much as I hate to admit it, my theory does sound a little bit like *The Total Woman*. As a committed feminist since adolescence, I can't help but be a bit appalled. However, I'm not saying that this is the way things *should* be but rather the way things have been. This is not all bad news. Indeed, some (male) evolutionary theorists have spent much energy postulating that human creativity evolved from men because men have had to be creative in order to capture the attention of women. Before coming to such conclusions, however, I think they might do well to ponder the imagination it takes for a woman to hold the long-term attention, visual and otherwise, of a male.

"The idea that beauty is unimportant or a cultural construct is the real beauty myth," writes Nancy Etcoff in *Survival of the Prettiest*. "We have to understand beauty, or we will always be enslaved by it."[1]

My book is not a polemic. Most of all, it is a collection of interesting stories that tell us something about the nature of invention itself.

Is a bra a piece of technology? Emphatically yes. Everything in the Beauty arsenal had to be designed and engineered. Hoopskirts, breast implants, and nail polish are not merely articles of fashion but legitimate inventions. Take, for example, the corset. It has been studied by anthropologists, psychologists, feminist theorists, social historians, art historians, and fashion historians. Yet few have looked at the corset as a technological phenomenon. This means that the evolution of the actual design of the corset gets lost during fistfights over whether it constitutes an instrument of repression or one of liberation.

Corsets, though they have been around for centuries, underwent a furious reinventing during the 1800s. And that reinvention, ultimately, explains the near extinction of the corset and, thus, the subsequent rise of the bra—a rather sophisticated piece of engineering whose own ultimate design was by no means inevitable.

This is not to say that invention drives fashion, but it does change what is possible. Many of these inventions constitute early commercial uses of basic innovations in materials. Cheap steel, synthetic rubber, nitrocellulose, and nylon are all innovations that gave rise to inventions that transformed the physical appearance of women—and thereby ultimately redefined what we think of as beautiful.

Where do these inventions spring from? As Richard Rhodes said about a vastly different subject—*The Making of the Atomic Bomb*—ideas spread like viruses. Look at the bra or lipstick. We Americans tend to have a Great Man approach to the history of invention, thinking that Thomas Edison invented the lightbulb, Samuel Morse the telegraph, Alexander Graham Bell the telephone. In fact, invention is a matrix, a zeitgeist phenomenon, with many different inventors coming up with similar ideas at the same time.

Do inventions bubble up from below, from democratic desires? Or do they flow top-down, imposed by the commercial interests of capitalists? The stories here remind us that it is rarely one or the other but rather a constant conversation between consumer and inventor, one that is mediated by businessmen and advertisers. Moreover, as Henry Petroski has pointed out in *The Evolution of Useful Things*, necessity is not the mother of invention, luxury is. Women don't really "need" nail polish, much less fifteen thousand different types of nail polish. Only a culture of abundance can cultivate such a bountiful cornucopia of innovation.

What you will find here are not just the stories of the winning inventions, the ones that have stood the test of time, but also the losers. Much of the historical landscape, as Ruth Schwartz Cowan has so poetically put it, is littered with the remains of abandoned machines: "These are not the junked cars and used refrigerators that people leave along roadsides and in garbage dumps, but the rusting hulks of aborted ideas."[6] Those anonymous rusting hulks, hilarious though they often are, constitute no small part of our history.

Bustles and bras may on the surface seem frivolous inventions. But as Siegfried Giedion, one of the granddaddies of historians of technology, said: "for the historian there are no banal things." "Humble objects," Giedion decreed, have shaken "our mode of living to its very roots." Giedion was not thinking about electrolysis machines when he wrote that line, but he could have been! The inventions you will find in this book tell us not just about who we are but also about who we aspire to be.

Because these inventions cast an illuminating light on our own era, my main hope is that this book will help readers look at the current generation's fashion and beauty customs with a fresh eye. Which of the inventions that we take for granted today—belly rings, fat-blasting electrodes, laser hair removal, Botox—from the distance of a century will look hilarious, dangerous, or simply retro-chic? That is impossible to know but it sure is mind-bendingly fun to guess.

inventing
BEAUTY

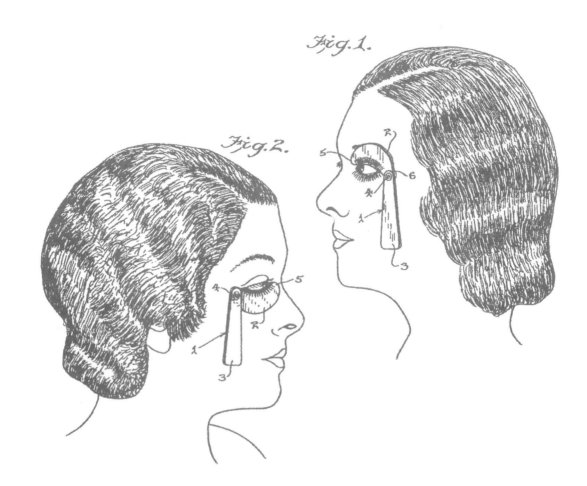

Fig. 1.

Fig. 2.

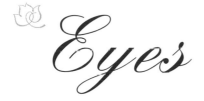

CHAPTER 1

Eyes

*Made-up eyes are by no means desirable, and to many are
singularly displeasing. The same, however, may be said of
made-up faces generally. Nevertheless it is extensively practiced.*

— Mrs. Sarah Jane Pierce, *Homely Girls*, 1890

*As regards cosmetics, the only sin against society seems to be
make-up badly applied. The "Would you brush your teeth in
public?" attitude towards make-up died some time ago.*

— Alice-Leone Moats, *Nice Girls*, 1933

When it comes to flirtation, the eyes can
cast a potent spell. An intense gaze is one of the most effective
ways a woman can broadcast her interest in a man. (Believe it or not,
scientists have actually quantified this.)[1] But how is it that eye makeup,
particularly mascara, became a standard implement in America's cosmetic toolbox?

Mascara became legitimate in the United States only fairly recently in the historic scheme of things. Many a proper Victorian lady, who had no qualms about inflating her breasts with rubber bust enhancers or upholstering her rear end with a bustle, was vociferously opposed to altering her face with any type of cosmetic. Indeed, the late 1800s brought furious catfights over the legitimacy of rouge pots and eyebrow pencils. Were they the province of sophisticated beauties or the downfall of wanton souls?

Charlotte Smith, editor of *The Woman Inventor,* argued against the use of cosmetics while the entrepreneur Madame M. Yale vigorously supported women's right to use them. Both women testified on the subject of cosmetics before the House of Representatives's Agricultural Committee in 1892. Madame Yale—"young and lovely, with masses of blonde hair"—was a successful businesswoman who had built a company worth $500,000 selling cosmetics, soaps, corsets, and a facial steaming machine.[2]

Described by the *Pittsburgh Leader* as a "priestess of the cosmetic art,"[3] Madame Yale lectured on cosmetics at the Chicago Opera House on March 17, 1892, arguing that they should be included among exhibits featuring female inventors. Yale complained volubly about the formidable Bertha Palmer, who, as the head of the board of Lady Managers at the Chicago World's Fair of 1893, decided what did and did not belong in the Woman's Building of that fair.

The logic of Madame Yale's pro-cosmetics argument to feminists was inspired: "Training and skills being equal, the woman who looks better will get the job, so why not make the most of your appearance?"[4] Mrs. Palmer was unswayed. She decreed that such nonsense was not worthy of the Woman's Building.

Harriet Hubbard Ayer also took up the pro-cosmetics mantle in a lengthy screed in her 1899 beauty book.

"I am always a bit amused when anathemas are hurled at the present use of cosmetics, particularly when a hopelessly-soured and pitilessly-unattractive female or a blatant, tobacco-smoking, spirituously-odorous male addresses me on the subject," she fairly sputtered.[5]

Cosmetics were a neutral force, Ayer argued. "As a matter of actual fact, whatever one's opinion may be as to the moral of the question, cosmetics have been used both by good and bad women as far back as we can learn anything of the per-

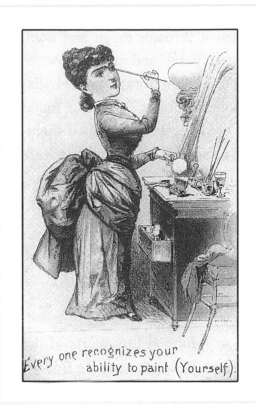

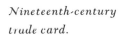

*Nineteenth-century
trade card.*

Every one recognizes your
ability to paint (Yourself).

sonal customs of the sex, just as wine has been drunk by priests and sots, by gentlemen and cads, and will be used and abused so long as men and wine exist."[6]

Women under the age of thirty who used cosmetics, as Ayer saw it, were
painting the lily and gilding gold. But as a woman aged, she warned, "there are times
in a woman's life, when, if she be wise, she will attempt to repair the damage of years
and care."

"When a wife sees a haggard-looking ghost of herself reflected from her mirror, when perhaps she is painfully conscious that the eyes she loves best are turning
from her faded beauty to a less worthy object, then I think she is not only justified in
delicately simulating, by every aid known to cosmetic art, the charms she has lost, but

she is stupid not to do so. It is the plain, unadorned, weary and too natural woman whose husband invariably falls a victim to the wiles of a Delilah, or succumbs to the artificial charms of a Jezebel. The very man who will almost fall in a fit at the sight of toilet powder in his wife's dressing room, will break her heart and waste his substance in the worship of a peroxide or regenerator Titian-red blonde.

"Let a premium be placed on sallow-faced, pale-lipped, dull, thin-haired women in the devotion and loyalty of the other sex, and the trade of the cosmetic artist will soon become a matter of ancient history."[7]

A Mirror with a Memory

As photography steadily became more popular, from 1870 to 1900, so too did cosmetics. An amateur photographer of the time referred to photographs as "permanent mirrors,"[8] while Oliver Wendell Holmes, upon viewing Mathew Brady's photographs of Civil War battlefields, called the camera a "mirror with a memory."[9]

Increasingly, sitters insisted that their images be improved upon for the special occasion of a portrait. Enameling—lacquering the face with white paint—therefore came into vogue. "American women who ordinarily shunned paint requested it at photographers' studios," according to historian Kathy Peiss.[10]

H. J. Rodgers, in his 1872 manual of photography, advised women not just on what clothing was most flattering in a portrait but also provided them with many pages of cosmetic recipes. Clearly, women took advantage of such concoctions, as the photographs themselves attest. In a series of portraits from the 1880s, for example, Baby Doe Tabor, who married a silver magnate in the Colorado town of Leadville, displays eyebrows unapologetically darkened by artificial means. Stage actress Charlotte "Lottie" Mignon Crabtree unabashedly wore kohl on her eyes (and rouge on her lips) in the *carte de visites* she passed out liberally to her fans.

Photographer Henry Peach Robinson lamented the vanity of his clients. "All kinds of powders and cosmetics were brought into play," he said, "until sitters did not think they were being properly treated if their faces and hair were not powdered until they looked like a ghastly mockery of the clown in a pantomime."[11]

Those who did not have the foresight to spackle their faces beforehand often insisted that their portraits be enhanced after the fact by hand-tinting or other sleight of hand.

Around 1870 one New York cosmetics boutique sold thirteen different kinds of powder and twenty types of rouge. Fashionable women carried a Lady's Pocket Companion, or Portable Complection, which discretely held rouge, powder, an eyebrow pencil, and a bottle of india ink. Altman's department store featured a "making-up" department.[12]

In the 1880s cosmetics were beginning to receive celebrity endorsements from the likes of Lillie Langtry, the voluptuous British stage actress who epitomized beauty during that era. By the 1890s ordinary women, not just those who made their living on the stage, were increasingly interested in painting their faces. During that decade the *Baltimore Sun* published more than a dozen letters each week from women seeking answers to beauty questions ranging from how to lighten freckles to how to darken eyebrows.

Certain enhancements were considered legitimate. Pale lashes on natural blonds, for example, were viewed almost as a birth defect. "White lashes and brows are so disagreeably suggestive that one cannot help but pardon their unfortunate possessor for wanting to disguise them by a harmless device," writes Sarah Jane Pierce in *Homely Girls*. "A decoction of walnut hulls should be made in the right season and bottled. Applied to the brows and lashes with a fine hair pencil will turn them to a rich brown, which will harmonize well with fair hair."[13]

Max Beerbohm, then an undergraduate at Oxford, chimed in with his support, albeit facetiously, for the pro-cosmetics brigade. In April 1894 he wrote an article entitled "A Defence of Cosmetics":

"No longer is a lady of fashion blamed if, to escape the outrageous persecution of time, she fly for sanctuary to the toilet-table; and if a damosel, prying in her mirror, be sure that with brush and pigment she can trick herself into more charm, we

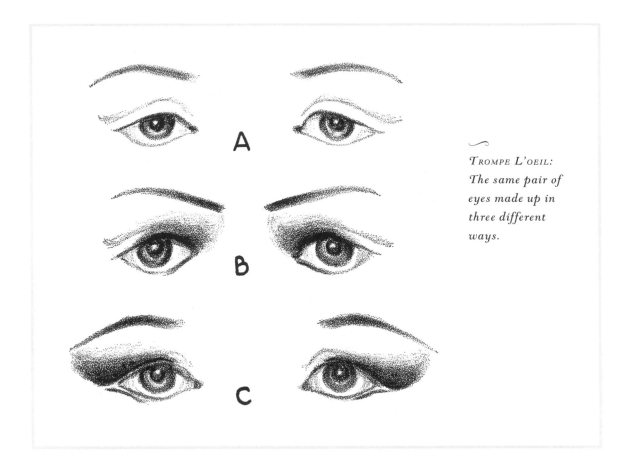

TROMPE L'OEIL:
The same pair of
eyes made up in
three different
ways.

are not angry. Indeed, why should we ever have been? Surely it is laudable, this wish to make fair the ugly and overtop fairness, and no wonder that within the last five years the trade of the makers of cosmetics has increased immoderately—twenty-fold, so one of these makers has said to me."

Many a husband, suddenly realizing that his wife was painted, alleged Beerbohm in his spoof, "bade her sternly, 'Go up and take it all off,' and, on her reappearance, bade her with increasing sternness, 'Go up and put it all on again.'"

The Eyes Have It

While cosmetics had long been made at home or specially ordered from the apothecary and applied on the sly, by the 1910s the tide began to turn in favor of public acceptance of cosmetics.

In Europe, Diaghilev's London ballet production of *Shéhérazade* in 1909 sent sales of mascara and eye shadow rocketing upward. The Russian dancers' dramatic eye makeup stepped up the demand for kohl—at least for the privileged classes—and also started the fad of colored and gilded eye shadows that color-coordinated with daring evening dresses designed by the likes of Paul Poiret, an eccentric French dressmaker who, according to beauty entrepreneur Helena Rubinstein in her autobiography, used to receive his guests with "live panthers chained in the entrance hall, each one attended by a six-foot Negro stripped to the waist, a bejeweled turban wound around his head, and his bare torso oiled and gleaming to resemble statuary."[14]

Dancers had a big influence on American doyennes of beauty like Rubinstein and Elizabeth Arden. Both women recall in their memoirs having been struck by the eye makeup used by the Russian ballerinas and other dancers. Arden and Rubinstein persuaded their wealthy clientele to play with these bold eye cosmetics. "I experimented privately and learned many valuable lessons from stage personalities, which in turn I taught to a few of my more daring clients," Rubinstein wrote in her autobiography. "They spread the word, and I knew that another beauty barrier would soon be toppled."[15] By the end of World War I, "mascaro," the hair dye, had evolved into "mascara," a cosmetic used specifically and routinely by many women—at least in the big metropolises.

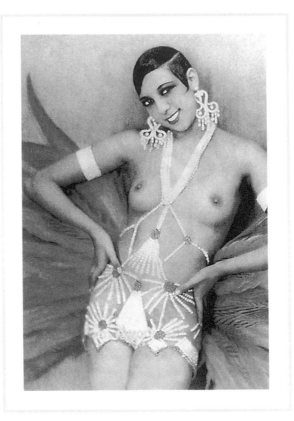

Sticky Lashes

The most daring clientele, and the most influential, were movie actresses. Their expressively painted faces were of paramount importance on the big screen—to the exclusion, at least in the beginning, of breasts or buttocks or legs.

Theda Bara and Pola Negri, smoldering vamps of the silent screen, were especially daring with eye makeup. Rubinstein fashioned a special kohl to dramatize Bara's face, producing her trademark raccoon eyes, which Bara wore not just to work but also about town.

In 1917, when Bara asked Helena Rubinstein to find a way to emphasize her eyes, Rubinstein made the eyes dominate her face. "The effect was tremendously dramatic," wrote Rubinstein later. "It was a sensation reported in every newspaper and magazine—only less of a sensation than when Theda Bara first painted her toenails!"[16]

In the 1920s, Max Factor worked on Theda Bara as well as many other actresses, including Clara Bow. Factor, a Russian émigré who started out as a wigmaker, introduced many innovations as he built a family cosmetics empire in Hollywood. His approach was to "bead" the lashes with his own special concoction. Factor's Cosmetic (pronounced with a French affect, as "cosmetique") was a waxy, waterproof preparation that came in foil-wrapped tubes the shape and size of a roll of breath mints today. The makeup artist or actor would slice off a small chunk and hold it over a flame until it melted. Then he or she would dip an orange stick into the gooey Cosmetic. It could either be applied to the lashes in upward strokes or applied to the tips of two or three lashes, which would be held together until they stuck, giving the lashes a thick appearance.

When Factor first applied his Cosmetic on Clara Bow, according to company lore, she panicked at the end of the day when her lids started sticking together. Someone tracked down Max Factor, who showed Bow how to use cold cream to remove the waxy goo. She reportedly became a "devoted Cosmetic user" thereafter.[17]

Other new weapons were popping up in the eye-enhancement arsenal. Kurlash, the first eyelash curling device, was invented in 1923. It was hard to use, cost a hefty five dollars, and it took ten minutes just to get the lashes of one eye curled. It was a huge success.

The eyebrow pencil really took off in the 1920s, in part because it was technologically superior to what it had been, due to a new ingredient: hydrogenated cottonseed oil (also the key constituent of another wonder product of that era, Crisco Oil). This likely helped the pencil glide more easily and, just as important, kept it from "blooming" with bacteria.

Greta Garbo wielded the eyebrow pencil skillfully and in doing so trans-

Tongs for pressing mascara onto the lashes.

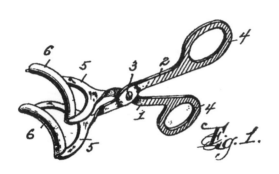

Fig. 1.

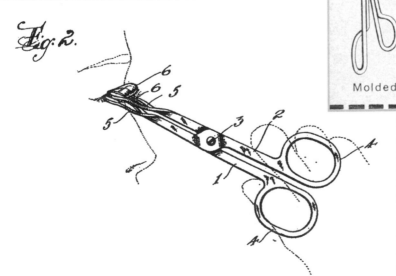

Fig. 2.

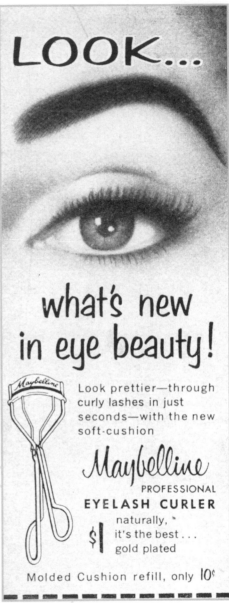

formed the face of America. When she arrived in Hollywood, Garbo was an "unre-touched Swedish dumpling" who had "the shadow of a double chin, frizzy hair, and slightly buck teeth."[18]

Louise Brooks was struck when she met Garbo by "the perfection of her fea-tures and the petal loveliness of her skin"[19] as well as her translucent gray-blue eyes. But these are not features that the audience of her black-and-white screen perfor-mances could appreciate. Moreover, though her real eyelashes were quite lush—Tal-lulah Bankhead reportedly pulled them once to make sure—they were quite blond and thus would have been nearly invisible without mascara.

"If she only knew it, her best disguise would be to use no mascara," said co-star Nils Asther of his famously reclusive friend. "Her eyebrows and eyelashes are al-most white, and without mascara she looks like a different person."[20]

So influential was Garbo's look that other actresses imitated her, prompting *Vogue* to feature a half-dozen photos of popular actresses, noting their Garbo-ization. "Post-Garbo, they wear [what appeared to be] minimal make-up, their hair is straight, their eyebrows thick, their cheeks sucked in, and their expressions uni-formly languorous and inscrutable, as if they were brooding over some abiding sor-row," said John Bainbridge. "Perhaps they are only brooding over their inability to look even more like Garbo."[21] Her use of cosmetics "completely altered the face of the fashionable woman," wrote Cecil Beaton in *The Glass of Fashion*.[22]

Maria Riva, in a biography of her own mother, Marlene Dietrich, beautifully evokes the transformation that actresses underwent in the studio makeup department during that era:

"The smell of greasepaint, fresh coffee, and Danish pastry, the big Make-Up Department all garish light, famous faces naked, devoid of adornment, some tired, half awake, all imperfections showing—terribly human, somehow vulnerable—awaiting the application of their masks of painted perfection. Hair-Dressing, equally lit, equally exposing the normalcy of flat-haired goddesses and some slightly balding gods, the sweet, sticky smell of setting lotion and hair glue replacing the linseed oil of greasepaint, the perfume of coffee and Danish. My mother becoming one of the crowd, an astounding revelation to me, who believed she was unique, the only one of her kind. Watching as she pushed skilled hands away, took over the task of doing her own face, drawing a fine line of lighter shade than her base, down the center of her nose, dipping the rounded end of a thin hairpin into white greasepaint, lining the inside of her lower eyelid. Looking at her in the big bulb-festooned mirror, seeing that suddenly straightened nose, those now oversized eyes, and coming all the way back to my original concept: that yes . . . she was, after all, truly unique."[23]

Actresses who were endowed with great acting talent but not necessarily great beauty remade their faces into glamorous facades. Bette Davis, whose face was less than symmetrical, capitalized, with the help of mascara, on her most attractive feature: her eyes. Jean Harlow's platinum-blond hair made her heavily painted eyes and bright Cupid's bow mouth stand out in deep relief, thereby drawing attention away from her too-broad nose.

The Garbo-ization of America

Millions of American women sought to be unique in the same way, imitating Hollywood goddesses like Garbo and Dietrich (who, according to Jane Gordon's *Technique for Beauty*, never darkened her lower eyelashes in the belief that this cast an unbecoming shadow). Fan magazines, beauty columns featuring makeup tips from stars, as well as actress-endorsed product advertisements cultivated this urge.

Bruce Bliven, writing in *The New Republic* in 1925, reported that the "flapper" was already passé and had been replaced by a new creature, this one completely beholden to cosmetics. "She is frankly heavily made up, not to imitate nature, but for an altogether artificial effect—pallor mortis, poisonously scarlet lips, richly ringed eyes—the latter looking not so much debauched (which is the intention) as diabetic."[24]

Not only was the average woman seeing more and more images of stars she wanted to emulate. She also saw more and more of herself as she really was. Thanks

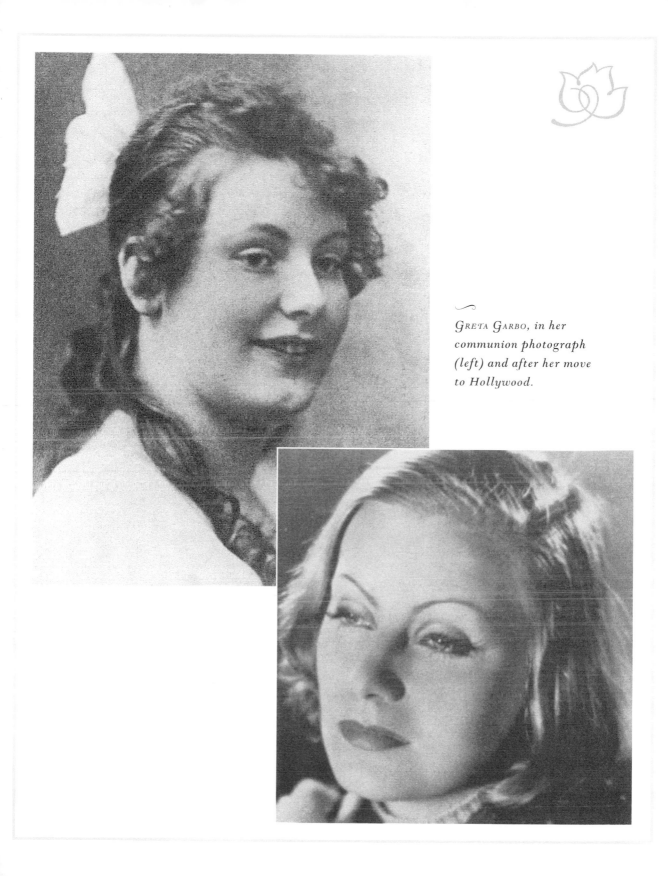

GRETA GARBO, in her communion photograph (left) and after her move to Hollywood.

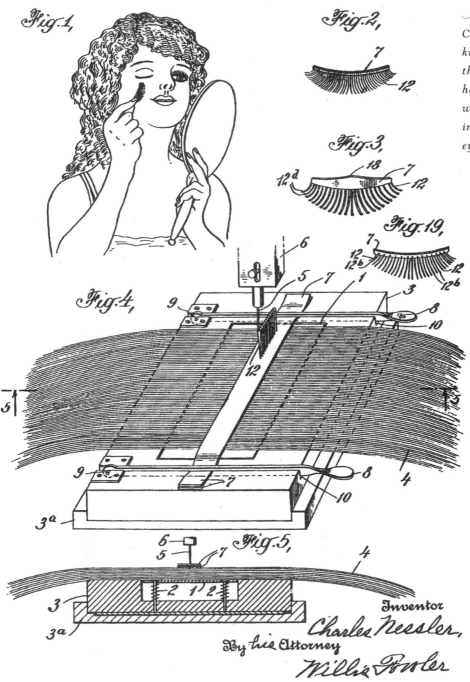

CHARLES NESSLER, best known for inventing the permanent-wave hair-curling machine, was also a lead innovator in false eyelashes.

Fig. 1,

Fig. 2,

Fig. 3,

Fig. 19,

Fig. 4,

Fig. 5,

Inventor

Charles Nessler,

By his Attorney

Willie Fowler

to advances in glass production and silvering processes, mirrors by the turn of the century were becoming increasingly available to the masses.

Businesses gave away oval pocket mirrors to advertise everything from Coca-Cola to cures for indigestion. "Once a luxury of the rich," writes Mark Pendergrast in *Mirror, Mirror,* now "mirrors were everywhere."[25] Women peered into these mirrors on a regular basis, and the mirrors ably assisted them in conjuring their own glamorous facades with cosmetics.

Moreover, the snapshot had become ubiquitous. In 1888, George Eastman had introduced his Kodak "detective camera" (called that because, in contrast to the large, old, unwieldy box cameras, it enabled the photographer to take the picture surreptitiously). Although personal Brownie cameras had been around since 1900, amateur photographers were now documenting everyday life as never before. Candid cameras proliferated.

Picture magazines abounded, "led by the more dignified *Life* and the less dignified *Look.*"[26] Between 1935 and 1937 camera sales went from less than $5 million annually to nearly $12.5 million. Moreover, photographers, whether professionals like Margaret Bourke-White and Dorothea Lange or simply weekend amateurs, now eschewed the blurred, sentimental point of view from earlier decades and instead became clear-eyed chroniclers of social life. Women were seeing more and more of themselves captured in these permanent mirrors and more and more they decided to modify their images with cosmetics.

Crocodile Dung and Asses' Liver

Of course, mascara is essentially a cosmetic that has been used by different cultures for millennia. The substance broadly referred to as kohl, used to darken lashes, lids, and brows, was made from a number of materials. In ancient Egypt, "there was a choice to be made in eyebrow dye," Richard Corson informs us, crocodile earth mixed with honey dissolved in onion water or "asses' liver warmed in oil with opium and made into little balls."[27] But kohl also has been made of malachite, galena, copper, iron, manganese, and lead.

The coloring material was ground with a stone slab or palette and then stored in a container: a shell, a hollow reed, or a small alabaster vase. Then it was probably mixed with fat or oil or applied on top of a base of ointment with a special stick. These handy little sticks—made of ivory, bone, wood, hematite, glass, or bronze—were thick at one end and flat at the other so they could be used not only for mixing the material but also for extracting and applying it.

Even the *Kama Sutra*, the ancient Indian treatise on love and sexual pleasure, offers a recipe for mascara, which sounds like a close cousin to some of those used by nineteenth-century American women.

Lampblack was evidently favored by fashionable but thrifty ladies since it could be made for virtually nothing at home. "By holding a saucer over the flame of a lamp or candle enough 'lamp black' could be collected for applying to the lashes with a camel-hair brush," wrote the anonymous author of an 1834 beauty book, the *Toilette of Health*.[28] Moreover, the book suggested, lampblack was far more suitable for shading the eyebrows than apothecary-shop pencils—those "too voyant aids to beauty," which apparently had an unfortunate tendency to make the hairs fall out.

This exhaustive tome lays out other options for achieving that Cleopatra look: rubbing in coconut oil, dying the lashes with the juice of elderberries, or coating them with burnt cork or cloves. Possibly the best preparations, according to the *Toilette of Health*, employed the black of frankincense, resin, and mastic—apparently a precursor to waterproof mascara. "This black, it is said, will not come off with perspiration." These methods were all recommended over the previous belief that "the length and silkiness of the lashes 'may occasionally be promoted by topping them with a pair of sharp scissors'—a practice most effective when commenced in early childhood."[29]

Mabel's Gift
to the Masses

Although Hollywood cosmetics like Max Factor's Cosmetic were not a reasonable embellishment for the average woman, capitalists responded nimbly to the Hollywood-inspired increase in demand for mascara with standardized products more appropriate for the masses. No longer did a woman have to special order from her apothecary or steam over a candle trying to produce lampblack.

Maybelline trumpeted its mail-order mascara-for-the-masses in movie and confession magazines as well as Sunday newspaper supplements. According to the Maybelline Company, T. L. Williams introduced Maybelline cake mascara in 1917 as the "first modern eye cosmetic produced for everyday use."[30] Williams was inspired by his younger sister Mabel (in whose honor the company was named), who like other young girls used petroleum jelly—which had been used for this purpose virtually ever since it was invented in 1878—to plump up her eyelashes and first gave him the idea for the company. By the 1930s, Maybelline mascara was available at the local five-and-dime store for ten cents a cake.

Men seemed blithely unaware of the modifications. A national survey of undergraduates in 1936 by *Vogue* magazine found that men were disapproving of makeup that was obviously applied. "Practically 100 percent no. How they hate it! They want to be fooled by artificial aids to beauty—never to be made aware of them."[31]

By contrast, a survey that same year of 1,012 female readers by the *Woman's Home Companion* found that sixty-two percent regularly used mascara, with Maybelline being the preferred brand.

While one might expect that the appetite for frivolities dipped during the Depression, quite the opposite was true. This was an era of cheap novelty that spawned

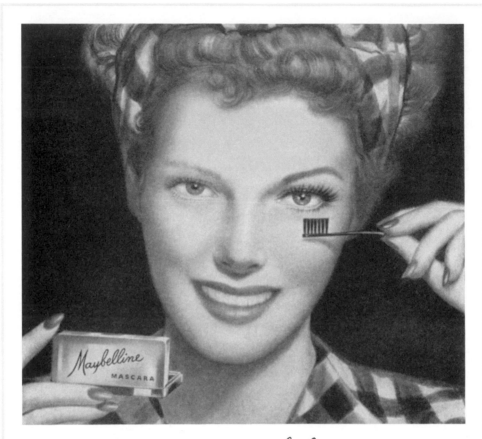

Something *beautiful* happens

...AND IT CAN HAPPEN TO **YOU**

...IN THE TWINKLING OF AN EYE

JUST TRY *Maybelline*

WORLD'S FAVORITE MASCARA AND EYEBROW PENCIL

An ad from the 1930s.

an "utterly fantastic epidemic of tree-sitting"[32] as well as the invention of pinball, bingo, and, for those who could no longer afford the real thing, miniature golf.

Cosmetics were an affordable luxury—or, as some job-seeking women saw it, a necessity. As the Depression deepened, cosmetic sales climbed steadily. "Even in these days of pinch-penny economy women are not running around with wan cheeks and shiny noses," wrote G. W. Vanden in an article entitled "It's Cosmetic Time in America." "WOMEN ARE NOT GOING WITHOUT COSMETICS, even if it takes the last spare change from their pocketbooks to buy. It is up to the beauty shops to get their share of this tremendously profitable business."[33]

Dye-ing to Be Beautiful

The early commercial mascaras, like Maybelline, were simply pressed cakes containing soap and pigments. A woman would dip a tiny brush into hot water, rub the bristles on the cake, remove the excess by rolling the brush onto some blotting paper or a sponge, and then apply the mascara as if her eyelashes were a watercolor canvas.

Next came cream mascara in a tube, one version sold by a company called Tattoo. A little cream would be squeezed onto a brush and then applied to the lashes. This required a more artful hand than the pressed-cake version but some women preferred it because it tended not to dry out lashes. Another popular "cream" mascara was Laleek Longlash, essentially a tinted Vaseline that came in several shades.

Liquid mascara, prized because it did not rub off so easily, could be applied only by those with a truly steady hand. In 1938, Helene Vierthaler Winterstein—a dancer and actress in Vienna, Austria—patented what she claimed to be the first waterproof mascara. Alas, it was fifty percent turpentine, so that while it was fast-drying it stank terribly while being applied and caused allergic reactions in some women.

In any form, however, mascara was an awkward proposition. If a woman ap-

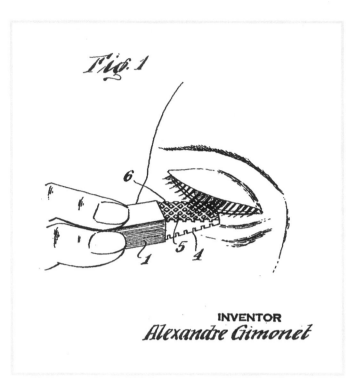

Women were supposed to coat their eyelashes with mascara by batting them against this mascara stick.

plied too much mascara, she would end up with clumpy stalactites dripping from her eyes. Too little and she might as well not have made the effort at all. Clearly, this was an enterprise that could be undertaken only in close proximity to a vanity table. Adding a new coat of mascara while out in public, unlike nose powdering and lipstick freshening, was potentially dangerous to one's beauty.

Given the state of mascara technology, we can sympathize with one socially prominent blue-eyed brunette living in a Midwestern city. On the morning of May 17, 1933, she stopped by Byrd's Beauty Shoppe to get a shampoo and a haircut in anticipation of a banquet that evening, where she was being honored for her volunteer work in the local Parent Teachers Association. Since she wanted to look her best, "Mrs. Brown," as she would later be referred to in a congressional hearing, let herself be talked into having her eyelashes and brows dyed.

The procedure turned out to be a messier, lengthier procedure than Mrs. Brown had anticipated. While Mrs. Brown drove home, her eyes began to sting. It probably did not help matters that she then proceeded to apply a variety of ointments—first boric acid, then a concoction made up fresh for her by her druggist, and then yellow oxide of mercury. Even though she was the guest of honor, her extreme discomfort forced her to leave the banquet early. By the morning, her eyes, which had developed ulcers, were swollen shut and oozing.

Mrs. Brown's eyes were so badly ulcerated that they sloughed off their own corneas. We know this because Mrs. Brown's weekslong nightmare was dryly chronicled at the time in appalling detail by the attending nurse in her notes. "Mrs. Brown's

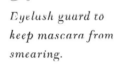

Eyelash guard to keep mascara from smearing.

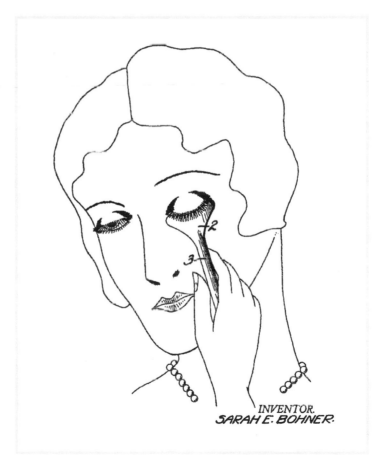

INVENTOR.
SARAH E. BOHNER.

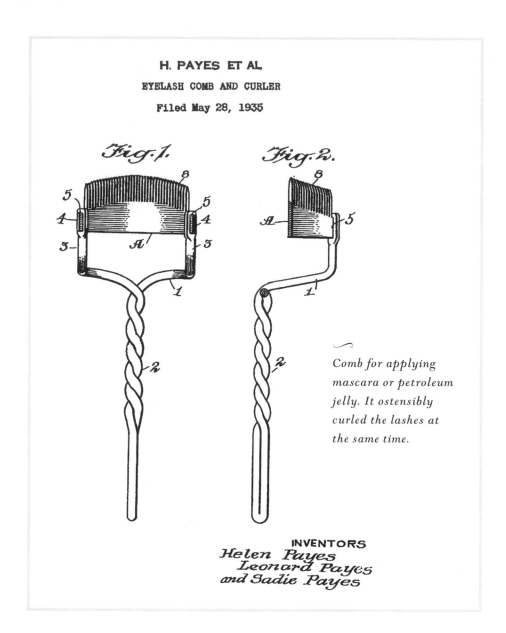

H. PAYES ET AL

EYELASH COMB AND CURLER

Filed May 28, 1935

Fig. 1.

Fig. 2.

Comb for applying mascara or petroleum jelly. It ostensibly curled the lashes at the same time.

INVENTORS
Helen Payes
Leonard Payes
and Sadie Payes

laughing blue eyes have been blinded forever,"[34] Ruth deForest Lamb wrote in her *American Chamber of Horrors*, a 1936 book detailing a number of horrific products consumed by the American public in the name of beauty (including the depilatory Koremlu as well as mercury-based skin "whiteners").

What eyelash dye so devastated Mrs. Brown? Lash Lure, a synthetic aniline dye belonging to the paraphenylenediamine group and produced by the Lash Lure Laboratories, Incorporated, of Los Angeles. Lash Lure was run as a sideline by Sanford M. Kolmetz, an entrepreneur who also ran the National Permanent Wave Company; his brother-in-law, Isaac Dellar, a graduate of the University of Oregon Medical School; and George Eilert, proprietor of the Lilac Beauty Parlor Supply Company. The three pooled together less than $1,000 to start their business. Since there were no Food and Drug Administration (FDA) regulations regarding testing of new cosmetics at that time, the product jumped right into sales.

Lash Lure was not an unreasonable leap, given what was known at the time. Aniline had been used as a commercial dye since the London World Exhibition of 1862, where one exhibitor showed a slab of the stuff that was twenty inches high and nine inches in diameter. The exhibitor boasted that this one small chunk, which had been produced from two thousand tons of coal tar, was sufficient to dye three hundred miles of silk. From the late 1800s, aniline also would be used as a key ingredient

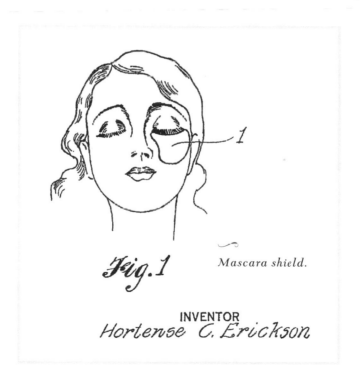

Fig. 1   *Mascara shield.*

INVENTOR
Hortense C. Erickson

in hair dye. While these hair dyes were health-endangering, their effects were not so immediate as were those of Lash Lure. (Indeed, their ill effects would not be truly understood until much later in the twentieth century.) This seems largely due to the fact that Lash Lure was applied near the eyes, certainly the most sensitive external surface of the body.

Congress, urged on by Lamb's book and after numerous chest-thumping congressional hearings, finally acted to regulate cosmetics in 1938. But the controversy over such products as Lash Lure was widely publicized long before then. As early as 1931 and 1932, *The New Republic* published a series of essays on the dangers of unregulated cosmetics. And the American Medical Association published an article identifying fifteen other cases of blindness and one death attributed to Lash Lure.

The mystery is not simply why it took Congress so long to empower the federal government to yank Lash Lure off the market, but also why women continued to use it (as well as several imitators) even when they were being told again and again by the press and consumer advocates that the stuff was potentially disfiguring. Women were not the only targets of such entrepreneurial zest in this paleoregulatory era. Between 1925 and 1930, men quaffed more than 400,000 bottles of Radithor, radium-laced water that was said to restore one's virility. One sip and "immediately the whole body is flooded with billions and billions of Alpha rays that liberate their energy throughout the entire system like floods of sunshine."[35] Eben M. Byers, a millionaire industrialist, drank cases of the stuff, and in 1932—the same year Mrs. Brown was mutilated by Lash Lure—he died a slow, painful, radium-induced death.

Audrey Hepburn and Synthetic Beauty

It is easy to understand why in the 1920s and 1930s many inventors focused their creative efforts on the problem of applying mascara. What is startling from today's

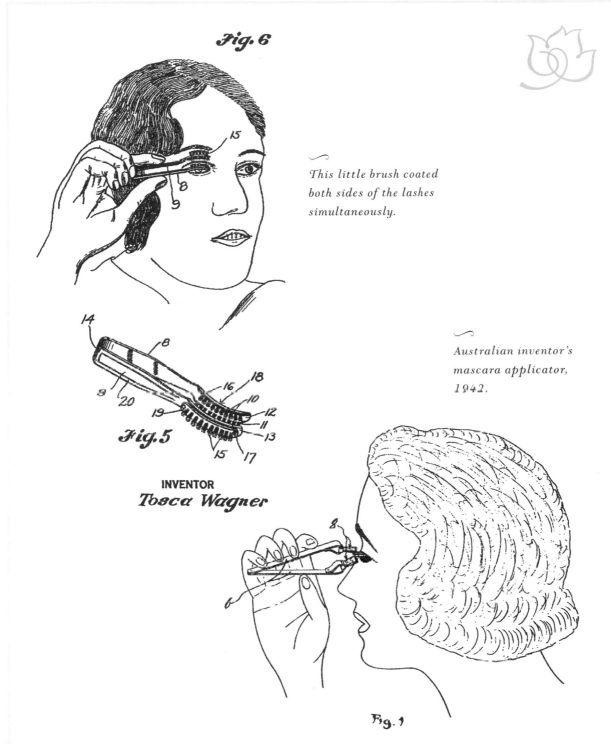

Fig. 6

This little brush coated
both sides of the lashes
simultaneously.

Australian inventor's
mascara applicator,
1942.

14 8
9 20 16 18
19 10
12
11
13
15 17

Fig.5

INVENTOR
Tosca Wagner

8
6

Fig. 1

Inventor
Leslie E. Pithie

S. S. NEWTON.
BLACKING-BOTTLE.

No. 185,693.

Patented Dec. 26, 1876.

Nineteenth-century precedent for the mascara wand: the bootblacking bottle.

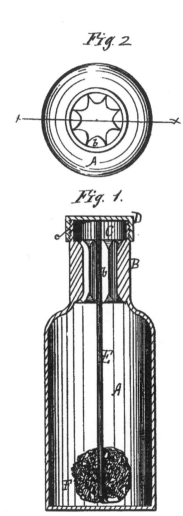

Fig. 2

Fig. 1.

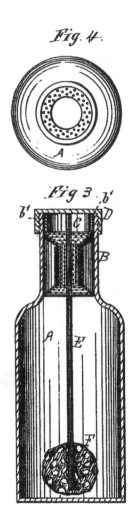

Fig. 4.

Fig 3

Witnesses

Henry Orth

H. H. Bliss

Inventor

Stephen S. Newton

by H. H. Doubleday atty

viewpoint is the wide variety of their solutions, most of which appear absurd from the safe distance of seventy to eighty years.

Many of these inventors, both male and female, lived in New York City or near Hollywood, though there were a few outliers. In 1933, for example, Seattle resident Tosca Wagner (an inventor of operatic ambitions, no doubt) patented a mascara applicator that resembles a tweezers with itty-bitty brushes at the tips.

The tweezers prototype also occurred to other inventors, one of whom

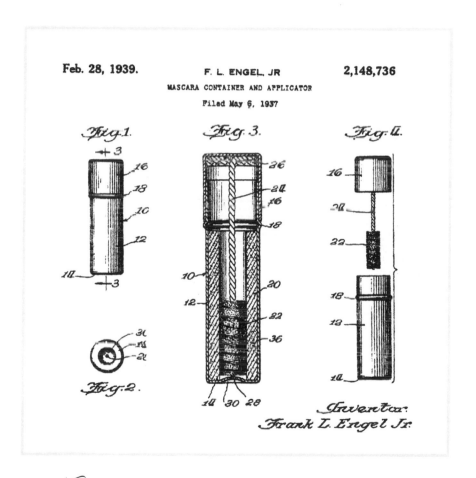

Chemist Frank Engel was about twenty years too early with his idea. The mascara wand didn't take off until the late 1950s.

attached sponges to the end of the device rather than brushes. But none of these inventions caught on for the long-term—and with good reason. None seems much more efficient than the kohl sticks used in ancient Egypt.

One patent, however, bears striking similarity to the modern-day mascara wand. It was granted in 1939 to Frank L. Engel Jr. of Chicago.

If the nail polish bottle had as its precedent the glue pot, the mascara wand's materfamilias is the shoeblacking bottle. The similarity both in function and form is striking. (Another daughter of the shoeblacking bottle is the instrument that gynecologists use to take Pap smear samples, but that's another story altogether.)

The mascara wand did not make it to the commercial market until the late 1950s, more than two decades after Engel received his patent. Why did it take so long if it seemed to solve the problem of applying mascara?

With invention, as with most things, timing is everything. When Engel received his patent, the United States was about to enter World War II—a terribly inauspicious time for an aspiring entrepreneur of eligible draft age. Women had temporarily abandoned their eyes and were instead individually and collectively riffing on other themes: hips, lips, and, especially, breasts.

Until the mid-1950s, that is, when a new musical called *Kismet* opened at the Stoll Theatre in London, reigniting the eye rage. Doretta Morrow, the star of *Kismet*, wore two-inch-long false lashes and dusted her eyelids with ground golden glass. Moreover, she took to wearing such makeup during daytime hours when not on stage. "I feel unfinished without it," she said.[36]

"More space has been devoted to the use of these eye-beauty preparations in women's periodicals in the last three years than to any other single time of the toilet," wrote Neville Williams in 1957. "The wheel of fashion has turned; the eyebrows have become thicker again; there is a steady sale of eyelash curlers, while make-up aims at giving a 'long, gentle-eyed kitten-of-the-Nile look.' "[37]

Cosmetic makers responded nimbly to this surge in demand. In 1958, Helena Rubinstein introduced her Mascaramatic, which dispensed with the old-fashioned block mascara applied by brush and water. The size and shape of a fountain pen, it

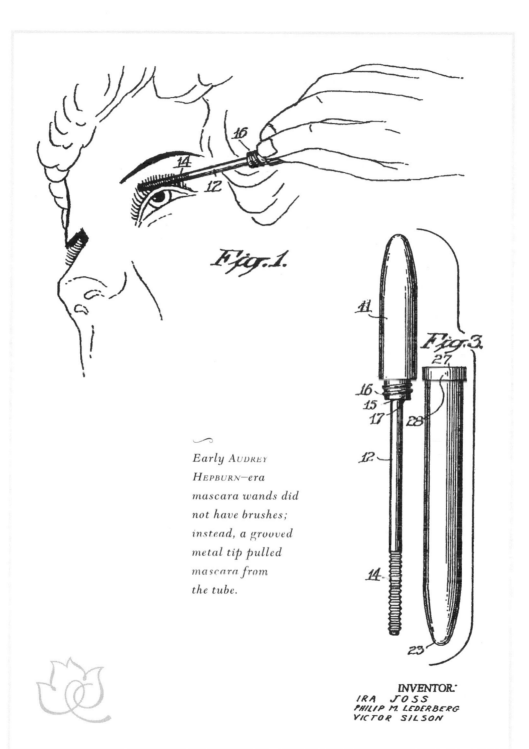

Fig.1.

Fig.3.

Early Audrey Hepburn—era mascara wands did not have brushes; instead, a grooved metal tip pulled mascara from the tube.

INVENTOR:
IRA JOSS
PHILIP M. LEDERBERG
VICTOR SILSON

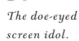
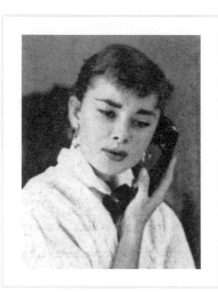

*The doe-eyed
screen idol.*

was immediately popular. (Conveniently, Engel's patent for his very similar device had expired two years earlier.) A viscous liquid mascara pooled in a reservoir at one end of the "pen." A slim applicator, whose tip was grooved metal, fit snugly inside. As the applicator was drawn out, it grabbed just enough mascara to coat the eyelashes without making them gloppy.

From that point on mascara-wand invention was fast and furious. The Italian cosmetics firm Debby and many others jumped into the competition and the technologically sounding Mascaramatic gave way to the more poetic "mascara wand." Soon it featured a little brush at the tip rather than simply grooved metal.

It was not just the mascara dispenser that was new, however; the basic recipe for mascara had changed, making it possible to easily apply the liquid version.

During the boom years of the 1950s and 1960s, industry was transmuting oil into a motherlode of new wonder synthetics. Researchers broke down natural petroleum into its constituent parts and put them back together in sophisticated new combinations that yielded polyesters and acrylics, polyethylenes and polypropylenes.

This hive of experimentation also produced hydrocarbon solvents that ultimately were used in cosmetics. Unlike turpentine, these fast-drying solvents were odorless, seemingly hypoallergenic, and—waterproof. They also gave rise to a liquid version of the eyebrow pencil: eyeliner. In an era when cosmetic formulas were usually guarded as trade secrets, the oil company Esso patented a new mascara made with hydrocarbon solvents.

Of course, this new mascara wand was not without its drawbacks. The wand device itself encouraged fungal growth, and for the careless could result in accidental eye pricks. As for the formula, hydrocarbon solvents would later prove to be not as benign as they initially appeared. Still, by the late 1950s, most American women were experimenting with eye makeup as never before, greatly inspired by Audrey Hepburn's dark doe eyes. In the 1957 *Funny Face*, Hepburn plays a brainiac bookstore employee infatuated with a nutty intellectual movement called Empathicalism. Initially dismissive of "synthetic beauty," she goes on to become a chic Paris model flaunting her trademark Cleopatra eyes.

The wheel of fashion was about to turn again, however. "Hand me my purse, will you, darling?" Hepburn famously said, playing Holly Golightly in the 1961 movie *Breakfast at Tiffany's*. "A girl can't read that sort of thing without her lipstick."[38]

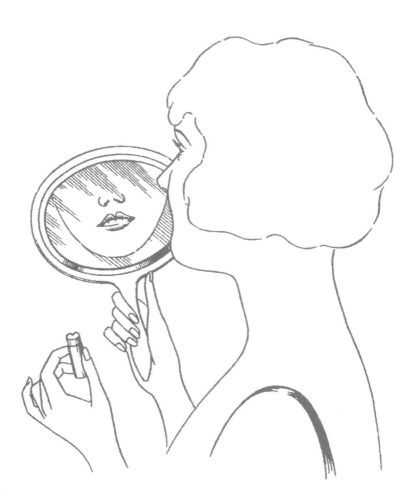

Lips

Lips

Braid the raven hair—
*   Weave the supple tress—*
Deck the maiden fair
*   In her loveliness—*
Paint the pretty face—
*   Dye the coral lip—*
Emphasize the grace
*   Of her ladyship!*
Art and nature, thus allied,
Go to make a pretty bride.

> "Braid the Raven Hair," from *The Mikado*, 1885

Standardization of dress and of taste has reached such a point
that a debutante might look like a thief, and a nice little
murderess . . . looks like a serious young bride on her way to the
market.

> Judge E. R. Wembridge,
> "The Girl-Tribe—An Anthropological Study," 1928

For both men and women, flushed lips signal sexual interest, so it is not surprising that both sexes have throughout the ages enhanced their lip color artificially.

The Greeks brightened their lips and cheeks with the root of a plant called "polderos." The Romans used fucus, a sort of rouge. The Hindus darkened not just their lips but also their teeth with betel. And during the Elizabethan era the lips were painted with a "pencil" made from ground alabaster or plaster of Paris that was mixed, along with a coloring ingredient, into a paste and then rolled into a crayon shape and dried in the sun.

Recipes for rouges, to be used on lips or cheeks, have long been popular in America, despite (or perhaps because of?) the country's puritanical roots and prudish reputation. Handbills, advertisements, and letters from colonial times indicate that women brightened their complexions with various types of rouge, including something billed as "Bavarian Red Liquor"—a versatile distillation that ostensibly would give the cheeks a rosy tint whether patted on the face or quaffed internally.

First Lady Dolley Madison is rumored to have rouged. And when Eleanor Custis Lewis, the granddaughter of George Washington, wanted to give a subtle sheen to her lips, she whipped up a homemade lip concoction out of wax, hogs' lard, spermaceti, almond oil, balsam, alkanet root, raisins, and sugar.

"This was Grandmama's lip salve & I never knew any so good," she wrote in her housekeeping book.[1] Eleanor may have called her ointment a salve—and indeed it may have had therapeutic value for chapped lips—but the alkanet in it, as a beauty book of that era noted, would have given it an unmistakable red tint.

These concoctions were indeed meant for women as well as men. At least they were until the Revolution, when Benjamin Franklin doffed his periwig permanently and American men eschewed the effete affectations of their continental counterparts.

Fashion historians have labeled this the "great masculine renunciation." The trend may have begun with Franklin, but its most pivotal moment was in 1830, during Martin van Buren's bid for a second presidential term. Van Buren's chances for re-election were annihilated when Congressman Charles Ogle, a Whig from Pennsylvania, accused the president of, among other vices, effeminacy. The honorable Mr. Ogle then proceeded to reveal the contents of President van Buren's dressing table, which included Double Extract of Queen Victoria, Corinthian Oil of Cream, Concentrated Persian Essence, and Extract of Eglantine. "Overnight van Buren became the laughing stock of America and his days of political service were over," wrote historian Gilbert Vail in 1947. "From this time the use of cosmetics carried the stigma of unmanliness in America."[2]

This does not mean that men did not exploit entrepreneurial opportunities in cosmetics. In 1860 a businessman in Chicago with the virile name of Sampson American invented a rouge made of alkanet root, oil of turpentine, and oil of roses. "This compound, when applied to the flesh, gives it a beautiful color, similar to that of persons of the fairest complexion when in perfect health," Mr. American wrote. It could be removed, he noted, by a thorough washing with milk.[3]

Many a female career was also built on cosmetics as well, even in the nineteenth century. In 1867, Harriet M. Fish of New York City patented a bolder "rouge pad," which would have been used for both the cheeks and the lips. She colored her pads not with the milder alkanet but with "the best quality of carmine and the juice of the blood-beet, strawberry, and hollyhock root"—a powerfully bright combination.[4]

Look into the Camera and Say "Peas"

Women did not just tint their faces, they also practiced lip calisthenics in an effort to perfect the bee-stung mouth so prized during that era. "The common practice was to repeat in sequence a series of words beginning with p; this would have the effect of rounding and puckering the mouth," according to Lois Banner in her landmark history *American Beauty*. " 'Peas, prunes, and prisms' were the most popular words in the sequence, although 'potatoes' and 'papa' were sometimes added."[5]

Nineteenth-century photographers admonished their subjects not to say "cheese" but rather to say the "p's." Many a belle entered a parlor with the word *prisms* just departing her lips. "Elizabeth Cady Stanton commented that she did not bother to give feminist literature to any woman who had the 'prunes and prisms' expression on her face," Banner writes.[6]

Most making-up, to be sure, was done discreetly at home, with rouge applied to both the lips and the cheeks. But by the late nineteenth century certain stage actresses, whose faces were amply spackled for their theater appearances, started boldly appearing in public wearing makeup. One observer recorded the then-shocking spectacle in the 1880s of Sarah Bernhardt, the kohl-eyed stage idol of the day, extracting a badger-hair brush from her bag and applying carmine dye to her lips while in mid-conversation on the street.

The carmine dye was an extract of cochineal—basically the dried, ground-up remains of pregnant female insects native to Mexico and Central America whose fatty flesh and fertile eggs are a pulsating red.

But at seven thousand insects per pound, cochineal was not cheap. Certain innovations would soon make it cheaper and easier for the average woman to follow the glamorous lead of Bernhardt and, later, screen actresses like Norma Shearer, Jean Harlow, and Madeleine Carroll.

In the years before World War I, for example, there was an important chemical breakthrough: an insoluble, synthetic form of carmine was successfully infused into an oil and wax base. The result was a lip ointment that reportedly gave a much more natural look than previous lip dyes.

This ostensibly "natural" lip rouge lent the act of tarting up one's lips some respectability. "With this opening wedge, public opinion soon swung away from censorship of lip makeup, so that it became respectable, even in conspicuous form, in

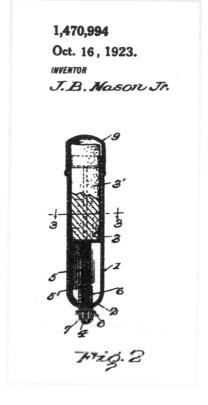

1,470,994
Oct. 16 , 1923.
INVENTOR
J. B. Mason Jr.

Fig. 2

James Bruce Mason Jr. of Nashville, Tennessee, invented this early lipstick dispenser.

most sections of the country," according to *Cosmetics: Science and Beauty,* the bible of cosmetic chemistry. "The well-dressed woman would no longer think of being without several shades of lipstick to provide makeup harmonious with any of her costumes."

Science of Eye Appeal

The other main landmark in the history of lipstick innovation had to do with its packaging. It's not clear who deserves the most credit for the development of the lipstick tube as we know it today. Sometime around 1915, lipstick began to be sold in metal cartridge containers. Theretofore it had been stored in tinted papers or rolled awkwardly in paper tubes that could not be safely carried in a handbag.

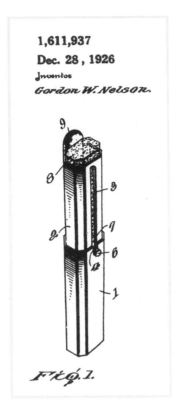

1,611,937
Dec. 28, 1926
Inventor
Gordon W. Nelson.

Fig. 1.

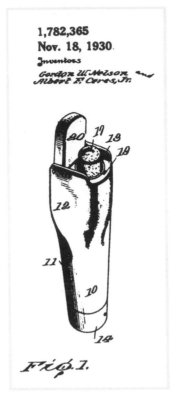

1,782,365
Nov. 18, 1930.
Inventors
Gordon W. Nelson and
Albert F. Ceres, Jr.

Fig. 1.

The push-up lipstick was a popular model before the swivel-up gained momentum.

This case seems to take its inspiration from a streamline train engine.

This was the beginning of a new era in marketing, one in which the package was meant not just to hold the product but to advertise it. "Instead of being packed to be shipped, merchandise was now packaged to sell," historian Daniel Boorstin tells us. Stuff that had been sold in bulk now had its own unique package: the perfume bottle, the matchbook, even the ice cream cone.

"Art is the science of eye-appeal," proclaimed William B. Stout, who designed Union Pacific's first streamline train. "If one builds into a commercial product an appeal to the eye, he establishes the first point of salesmanship, which is impression."[8]

Lipstick was a pioneer in the package-as-advertisement movement. The Scovill Manufacturing Company of Connecticut is credited with manufacturing the first lipstick container, in October 1915, for an American company owned by Maurice

Levy, an importer of French cosmetics. These simple, oval-shaped tubes were about two inches long and had a plain dip-nickel finish. As a woman used up her "lip stick," she could replenish her supply by pushing up a slide lever on the side of the tube. (At the same time, Mr. Levy placed an order for eyebrow pencil holders, which were round, smaller in circumference, and slightly longer than the lipstick containers.)

The first lipstick to swivel out of the tube rather than needing to be pushed straight up appears to have been patented in the United States not by the Scovill Company, but rather by James Bruce Mason Jr. of Nashville, Tennessee, in 1923. To coax the lipstick out of the Mason tube, as it became depleted, a woman turned a decorative screw head at the bottom of the case.

Over the next decade and a half, as lipstick use increased, the United States became an incubator of lipstick innovation. While Freud was everywhere at this

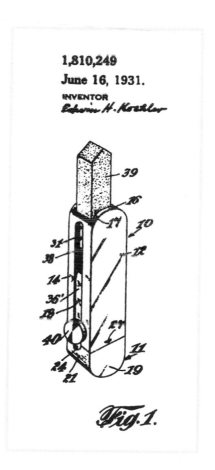

An inexpensive and easily manufactured case.

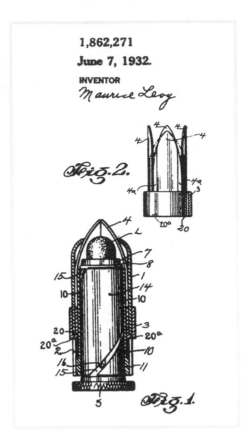

A later, more elaborate case designed by Maurice Levy, who is credited with manufacturing the first metal lipstick dispensers.

time—terms like penis envy and inferiority complex were tossed about lightly at cocktail parties—both the innovators and marketers of these sticks seem largely innocent of the strong Freudian interpretation that lipstick would be invested with decades later.

In the 1920s and 1930s, the U.S. Patent Office issued upwards of a hundred patents for different variations in lipstick shapes and dispensers: obelisk-shaped lipsticks, octagon-shaped lipsticks, streamline moderne lipsticks, lipsticks that looked like a piece of toast popping out of a toaster, lipsticks whose covers rolled back like a rolltop desk, and lipsticks whose four flanges bloomed in a tulip-blossom arrangement to reveal the pistil-like lipstick within. Though the styles of lipstick cases were widely different, their functionality varied little from container to container. Most of them are shafts of lipstick that swivel, twist, or push out of a hollow container.

JOAN CRAWFORD, *in Metro-Goldwyn-Mayer's "ELEGANCE"*

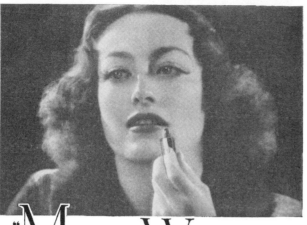

"Most Women
CONCEAL THEIR BEAUTY,"
says Joan Crawford
DO YOU?

LIPSTICK
*"You'll be amazed,"
says Joan Crawford,
"at the alluring color of Max Factor's
Super-Indelible Lipstick. It's moistureproof and may be
applied to the inner
as well as the outer
surface of the lips.*

POWDER
*"and Max Factor's
Powder really enlivens the beauty of
your skin...Matchless in texture, it creates a satin smooth
make-up that clings
for hours. You will
notice the difference instantly.*

ROUGE
*"the exquisite color
harmony shades of
Max Factor's Rouge
impart a fascinating, natural and
lifelike glow to your
cheeks ... Creamysmooth, it blends
delicately and remains perfect for
hours and hours."*

★

*Max Factor's Face
Powder, one dollar;
... Max Factor's
Rouge, fifty cents;
Max Factor's SuperIndelible Lipstick,
one dollar. Featured
by leading stores.*

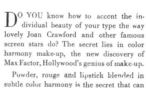

Do YOU know how to accent the individual beauty of your type the way
lovely Joan Crawford and other famous
screen stars do? The secret lies in color
harmony make-up, the new discovery of
Max Factor, Hollywood's genius of make-up.

Powder, rouge and lipstick blended in
subtle color harmony is the secret that can
transform you into a radiant new being. It
doesn't matter if you are a blonde or a
brunette, or if you are twenty or forty...
there is a color harmony make-up that will
bring you new loveliness.

Beautiful women who can choose from
all the world, select Max Factor's make-up because they know they can depend on
it to dramatize their beauty. Now you, too,
can share the magic of color harmony
make-up created originally for the stars of
the screen by Max Factor.

Would you like to have Max Factor
give *you* a personal make-up analysis?
Would you like a sample of your color
harmony make-up? Would you like an
interesting illustrated book on *"The New
Art of Society Make-Up?"* All these will
be sent to you if you will mail the coupon below to Max Factor, Hollywood.
An adventure in loveliness awaits you!

Ladies' Home
Journal *ad, 1936.*

Max Factor ★ Hollywood
SOCIETY MAKE-UP—*Face Powder, Rouge, Lipstick in Color Harmony*

While companies were trying to stimulate demand with their novel, gemlike packages, they were also responding to a spike in demand for such products. Smitten with the highly stylized faces of movie actresses, store clerks and seamstresses and society matrons sought to reinvent their own faces.

Percy Westmore and Max Factor, working their chemical magic in Hollywood, told girls with average looks that they, too, could become beauties and offered a wide range of products to help them do just that. "The lipstick and the eyebrow pencil are even more powerful than the pen," Westmore proclaimed.[9]

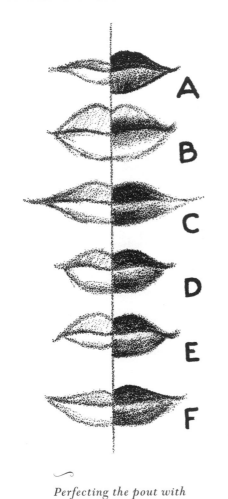

Perfecting the pout with optical illusion.

Factor looked upon starlets as blank canvasses. He created Clara Bow's Cupid's bow mouth seemingly from scratch. After smearing her lips with white makeup, he would then coat his thumb with lipstick and carefully stamp her upper lip with two thumbprints and her lower lip with one thumbprint. For Joan Crawford, Factor suggested "liberally large and broad" lipstick brush strokes to set her apart from other aspiring stars less well-endowed in the mouth department.

Other actresses would go on to create their own trademark mouths with lipstick. Hedy Lamarr created a permanent pout with her lipstick by arching the lips downward at the corners. Lana Turner opted for a "hunters' bow" lipstick shape to offset her broad jawline.

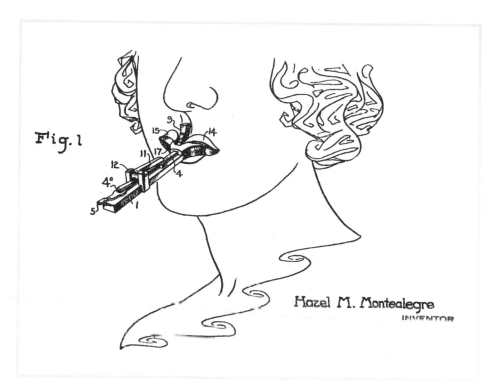

Fig. 1

Hazel M. Montealegre
INVENTOR

Some adventurous inventors sought to produce a more ambitious change than could be achieved with mere cosmetics. Take, for example, contraptions to rearrange a woman's mouth into a more pleasing shape. The Patent Office's role is to grant patents for novel ideas—but the ideas do not necessarily have to be workable. Thus, patents were actually granted for such devices (as well as for myriad other nutty schemes across a wide range of disciplines). Hazel Mann Montealegre of Iola, Kansas, patented a device that allegedly reshaped "the upper lip of a person to conform to what is known as the 'Cupid's bow,' whereby it is unnecessary to resort to a surgical operation to produce this effect."

A Gesture
of the Twentieth Century

Ordinary women, like actresses, experimented to find the lipstick patterns most flattering to them. In 1914 a class of working women at Cooper Union in New York City debated the question of artificial beauty and ended up voting overwhelmingly for it.

By 1920, according to Neville Williams in *Powder and Paint*, it was no longer possible to tell a woman's social position from her appearance: "Even the most cynical of critics could no longer maintain that ladies with lipstick must belong to high society, to the stage, or to the demi-monde. Like wearing short hair, smoking cigarettes, or dancing to ragtime, wearing lipstick and rouge had become classless."[10]

These lipsticked mouths were begging to be kissed, according to F. Scott Fitzgerald. "We find the young woman of 1920 flirting, kissing, viewing life lightly, saying damn without a blush, playing along the danger line in an immature way,"[11] wrote Fitzgerald, who fell in love with Zelda Sayre despite the fact that she had "kissed thousands of men and intends to kiss thousands more."[12]

While not commonly used in the hinterlands, lipstick was increasingly becoming available. *Watkins Timely Suggestions*, a 1920 mail-order catalog published by the J. R. Watkins Company in Winona, Minnesota, endorsed the use of cosmetics—not surprisingly, since it sold them: "It is quite permissible to 'paint the lily' (especially if she be a pale, drooping flower) but let us endeavor to do it as artistically as possible, remember that we are striving to assist, not caricature, Nature."[13]

Not everyone was pleased with this new lipstick mania. Rita Strauss, in her 1924 *Beauty Book*, railed against the trend. "A form of make-up which has become deplorably obvious of late is that of rouging the lips," Strauss wrote. "No effort is made to be sparing with the use of the lipstick. The fashion has come from Paris, of

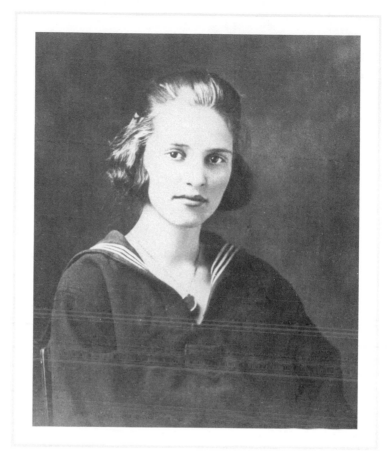

course. It is a pity, because it goes directly against all the canons of successful make-up."[14]

Strauss was, of course, less than prescient. Lipstick became an emblem of the New Woman in the 1920s. Young women shocked their parents by painting their lips (and nails) in increasingly vivid colors thanks to new advances in synthetic dyes. In one 1937 study more than half of the high school girls surveyed said they fought with their families over using lipstick. Immigrant families, straining to retain traditions and morality in a permissive new land, were particularly distressed by their daughters' desires to paint their faces.[15]

The first lipstick many girls used was Tangee, a brand of lipstick that was orange until swiped on the lips, at which point it turned a light red hue. Tangee marketers cultivated the impression that the lipstick changed colors to blend "naturally" with the coloring of each individual girl. This neat little fiction made it easier for parents to accept lipstick. In fact, the degree to which the dye—bromo-acid, a derivative of the synthetic organic dye eosin—changed colors depended upon how alkaline the wearer's lips were.

By 1929, Mme. F. A. LeClair of Milwaukee, in her self-published book on the beauty business, matter-of-factly assumes that her patrons wore lipstick. The act of applying lipstick, *Vogue* proclaimed in its 1933 *Beauty Book*, was one of the most important gestures of the twentieth century.[16] By the late 1930s, women applied lipstick more regularly than they brushed their teeth. And according to Works Progress Administration (WPA) interviews from the era, ladies who lipsticked came from all social, economic, and ethnic categories; they were telegraph workers, department store

Ladies' Home
Journal *ad, 1936.*

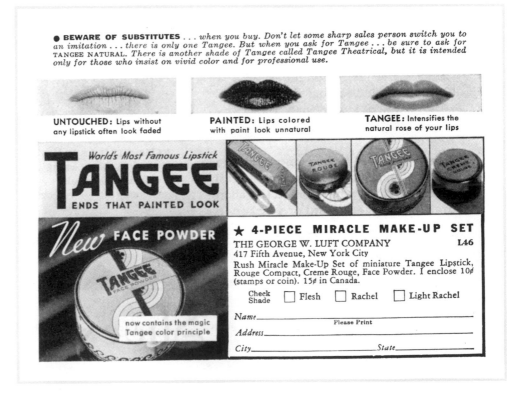

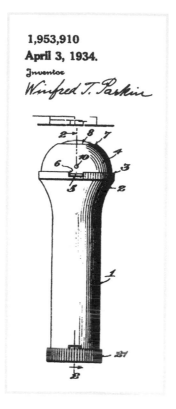

1,953,910
April 3, 1934.
Inventor
Winfred T. Parkin

Winfred T. Parkin, of Providence, Rhode Island, designed a lipstick dispenser that looks like an observatory for stargazers.

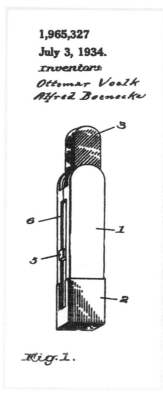

1,965,327
July 3, 1934.
Inventors
Ottomar Voelk
Alfred Boenecke

Fig. 1.

Two German inventors came up with this design, which they claimed also could be used to dispense erasers.

clerks, itinerant trapeze artists, daughters of Southern Baptist preachers, Jewish girls in Brooklyn, African-American butter-and-egg packers in Washington, D.C.

Lipstick Traces

Lipstick also had become a frank symbol of sexuality. "Seems Mr. Parrish came home one night with lipstick on his undershirt," declares one of the gossiping housewives in Clare Booth Luce's 1937 play *The Women*.[17]

In 1938 a cosmetics firm called Volupté brought two new lipsticks to market: Lady and Hussy. Lady, according to *Mademoiselle* magazine, was for "girls who lean toward pale-lacquered nails, quiet smart clothes and tiny strands of pearls." On the other hand, Hussy, which gave the lips a "gleaming luster," was "for the girl who loves exciting clothes, pins a *strass* [paste] pin big as a saucer to her dress, and likes to be just a leetle bit shocking."[18] Hussy was by far the most popular. It outsold Lady five to one.

Things had certainly changed. "Lipstick and rouge would have scandalized a girl in my day," eighty-year-old Ella E. Gooding of Winnsboro, South Carolina, told a WPA interviewer in 1940, noting that the only vanity she was allowed in her youth was a cut-glass, silver-lidded smelling-salts bottle.[19]

Movie magazines featured movie and stage stars who purringly reassured readers that applying makeup was a civilized act. "I think a woman looks more soignée with a hint of lipstick," advised Margaret Bannerman, who was then playing the lead in Edgar Wallace's *The Calendar*.[20]

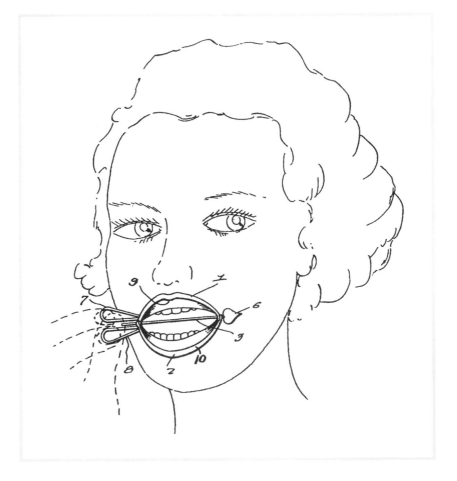

Marie L. Helehan of Butte, Montana, in 1938 patented this stencil to help women apply lipstick symmetrically.

Jack Dawn, the director of the makeup department at MGM, criticized aspiring starlets not for using makeup but for not using it in an original way. In an article entitled "Be Yourself, Girlie!" in a 1942 issue of *Colliers,* the author exhorts readers to "make the most of the face God gave you, instead of trying to look like one of the movie stars."

Dawn facetiously suggests that ordinary women should leave their faces alone "except for a few swipes of foundation cream, powder, rouge, lipstick, mascara, eyeshadow and blueing."

"Main Street anywhere looks half natural and half Hollywood-on-the-loose," he said. "The world is full of Chinese Garbos, Eskimo Ann Rutherfords and Hawaiian Constance Bennetts" or "unreasonable facsimiles thereof." "What the average woman achieves when she sets out to look like her favorite movie glamour girl is not a resemblance, it's a caricature," "a mass production of faces."[21]

By the time war was declared in Europe in 1939, annual sales of cosmetics in America were near $40 million. It seems logical to assume that when the United States entered the war after the bombing of Pearl Harbor, American women would

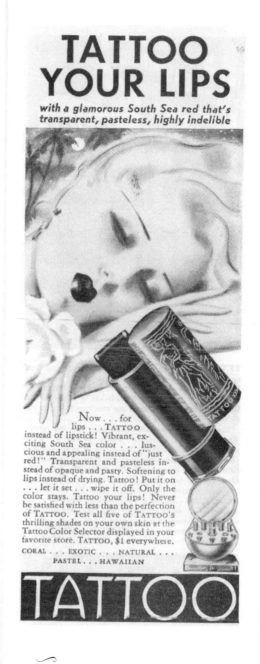

Ladies' Home Journal *ad, 1936.*

have been asked to sacrifice physical adornment so that the raw materials could be put into military goods. And, indeed, metal lipstick cases had to be replaced first with plastic, then with paper. Castor oil, a key component in lipstick, also was hard to come by.

But governments felt that women had an important psychological part to play in the war and that makeup kept up the morale of women as they worked in the munitions factories. Thus, cosmetics were viewed as vital to the war effort. "Lipstick, which little more than a decade before had been regarded as suitable only for fast women, became a priority product," wrote Margaret Allen in *Selling Dreams*. "For a few years the cosmetics companies dropped their competitive thrust against one another and concentrated on supplying lipsticks and other cosmetics cheaply to war workers."[22]

Hazel, the Butter Is Red Again

The next major innovation in lipstick—allegedly, anyway—was introduced by Hazel Bishop in the late 1940s.

The name Hazel Bishop has long faded into obscurity, and the company's place in the annals of lipstick history has gone largely undocumented, but in the mid-twentieth century the name of Hazel Bishop was as well known as that of, say, Lucille Ball (who was just then launching what would become one of America's most enduring television comedies). Indeed, in 1953, Hazel Bishop by one estimate sold half of all lipsticks bought by American women. Hazel Bishop was such a powerful brand name that once when she called on a businessman at his office and identified herself as "Miss Hazel Bishop," he thought she was joking. "Did you bring Mr. Lucky Strike with you?" he quipped.[23]

Bishop had set out not to pioneer new forms of lipstick but rather to become a doctor. In 1929, after graduating from Barnard College with a degree in chemistry, she paid one term's medical school fees at Columbia. The Depression, however, forced her to come up with other career plans. Eventually she became a laboratory assistant to an upscale dermatologist in a plush Park Avenue office.

But then came World War II, and Bishop—like a number of other women in the sciences (for example, Kevlar inventor Stephanie Kwolek, who was enshrined in the inventor's Hall of Fame only in the late 1990s)—finally found entry into the previously sacred male precincts of corporate research labs. In 1942, Bishop became an organic chemist for Esso in petroleum research in the Jersey Meadowland. "My most glamorous research project," she later recalled, "was to determine why a deposit formed in fighter airplanes."[24]

Despite her corporate, career-girl positions, Hazel had an entrepreneurial flair that she inherited from her father, Henry. Henry Bishop had established himself as a "business adventurer maintaining a collection of stores up and down Hoboken's Washington Street," according to *The New Jersey Journal*.[25] His enterprises included a grocery store, a toy store, a pet shop, a candy store, a luggage shop, awning factory, and motion picture theater. Moreover, Henry was the P. T. Barnum of Hoboken, masterminding outrageous stunts guaranteed to garner free publicity photographs in the local press. He once advertised his candy business by parading a Santa Claus atop an elephant on Thanksgiving Day. And his pet shop featured a live alligator in the window.

While suffering from what today's advertisers might call sinusitis, Hazel Bishop got her first moneymaking idea: a mentholated paper handkerchief. And later, when she worked for the dermatologist, she invented a pimple stick. Alas, neither the handkerchief nor the pimple stick made it out of her kitchen laboratory.

Undeterred, the ever-entrepreneurial Miss Bishop eventually settled on another potential product: lipstick.

In 1948, through her mother, Mabel Billington Bishop, Hazel Bishop met Alfred Berg, a lawyer who told her of his fascination with a French indelible lipstick called Rouge Baiser (Red Kiss), which he apparently was hoping to import into the United States. Bishop's mother had bragged to Berg about Hazel, who was now a chemist at Socony Vacuum Laboratories in Brooklyn, and she urged him to seek her daughter's opinion on whether this French lipstick would appeal to American women. At least this is the account of events in Bishop's unpublished memoir, but perhaps it is not unreasonable to conjecture that her mother was hoping most of all to lasso a man for her as-yet unmarried forty-two-year-old daughter.[26]

Whatever the true motivation, Bishop met Berg for lunch when she was on jury duty at Foley Square, near Berg's office. Bishop was frank: The Parisian import that he showed her at lunch, which she subsequently described as having the appearance of dried blood, was a disaster.

"My diagnosis shocked him," Bishop recalled.[27] She then described to him her own concept for a new lipstick. Berg was impressed, and they agreed to moonlight together on the idea while keeping their day jobs. Berg was to raise some venture capital and help to market it, while Bishop was to guide the lipstick from prototype to actual product as well as serve as "the company's authoritative public relations interface with the press."[28]

Over the next two years, Bishop conducted more than three hundred experiments in her kitchen laboratory, pouring her various concoctions into a small mold and then letting the molten mass harden in the refrigerator of the Park Avenue apartment she shared with her mother. Sometimes a drop or two of dye would stray, to dis-

2,219,909
Oct. 29, 1940.
INVENTOR.
Herman C. Kelleher

Fig. 1.

This 1940 design was owned by Clairol. The lipstick snapped open like a switchblade.

astrous effect. "Hazel," her mother would call out at dinnertime, "the butter is red again."[29]

Bishop and Berg made Saturday-morning jaunts over to the Kolmar Laboratories in Port Jervis, New York, which, despite the proliferation of brands on the market, manufactured eighty percent of all lipsticks. These field trips were apparently pleasant, but Hazel's personal archives evince nary a hint of romance. On the contrary, they give important clues as to why Hazel would have had little interest in Berg. Although she was a spinster in the 1950s sense of the word, Hazel did have a relationship lasting much of her adult life with someone named Mike. Her datebooks are filled with tennis dates with Mike. And in 1966, Mike wrote her passionate letters during a trip abroad.

So who was this mysterious Mike? She turns out to have been a classmate of Bishop's at Barnard. Whatever Bishop's ties with Mike, they were personal rather than professional. Mike appears to have been uninvolved in the lipstick adventure.

After perfecting their formula and packaging, Bishop and Berg were ready to find a sales outlet. Their first stop was Lord & Taylor. The answer was no. The next

Josephine A. Rountree, of Foreman, Arkansas, in 1921 invented a device to train the facial muscles to produce a permanent smile.

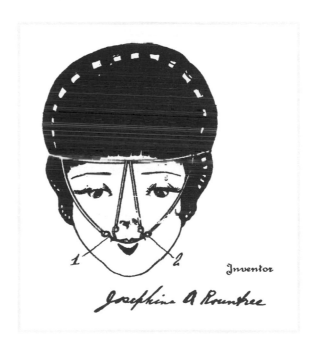

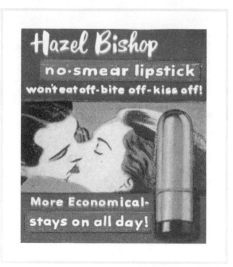

stop was Saks Fifth Avenue. No again. So the duo lowered, but broadened, their sights. Instead of approaching another toney uptown department store, Hazel called upon Stanley Swabach, a friend who was the merchandise manager of Abraham & Straus, a department store in Brooklyn. Swabach agreed to stock the lipstick on the condition that they run a big ad to promote it. On January 15, 1950, a full-page advertisement in the Sunday *New York Times* featured an opened lipstick that stretched from bottom to top. Within an hour after the store had opened, the lipstick demonstrator "was selling the product too fast to have time to ring up sales."[30]

Bishop and Berg moved a bit upscale when they got what Bishop considered, in retrospect, to be their lucky break. The Washington-based Hecht and Company department store decided to carry the line, marketing it as the lipstick that "Stays on you, not on him." This was an unprecedented claim for a lipstick. Restaurants complained about having to pay dearly for heavy-duty laundering of lipstick-stained napkins and table linens. Women themselves, even though newly armed with electric washing machines, had to battle with lipstick stains on their own clothing. Hecht sold six hundred lipsticks in the first day alone.

Within months, however, Bishop and Berg were nearly broke. This is where Raymond Spector stepped into the picture. Spector is perhaps the best and worst thing that ever happened to Hazel Bishop. The Hazel Bishop company could have never succeeded without their partnership, but much like another partnership of this same era—that of Earl Tupper, the inventor of Tupperware, and Brownie Wise, the mastermind behind the Tupperware party—the relationship would prove nasty, brutish, and short.

Laxatives Meet Lipstick

Spector was an ad man with his own small agency in New York City. He claimed to be the marketing genius behind a catchy laxative slogan: "Serutan—Nature Spelled Backwards." Berg had been to call on several big agencies, including J. W. Thompson, Young & Rubicam, and BBD&O. They all expressed interest in the Hazel Bishop account, but only if Bishop and Berg could come up with $50,000 to $100,000 in an advertising budget. At the time, however, they had only a few thousand dollars in the bank.

Spector saw things differently. He saw Hazel Bishop not as a mere ad account but rather as an opportunity to actually own and build a company. Telling Bishop and Berg that they did not have to pay newspapers and other media outlets for sixty days after an ad actually appeared, he offered to take their account in exchange for stock in the company.

The reason Spector was willing to take such a risk, of course, was that in Hazel Bishop he saw fabulous marketing potential. Until that point, cosmetics were sold with a swirl of French adjectives and luxurious packaging. With Hazel Bishop, the product and the person, Spector had a no-nonsense, truly American product and a novel pitch. Hazel Bishop had built the better lipstick. And the reason American women should buy it was not because it was named something like Tiger Lily Passion or because it came wrapped in a pink-chiffon box that cost more than the actual cosmetic but because it actually *worked* better.

"Amazing New Lasting Lipstick Stays On—and On—and On!" the copy read. "Women Go Wild Over Sensational Non-Smear Lipstick That Won't Eat Off—Bite Off—Kiss Off!"[31]

The first post-Spector ad featured a testimonial from Hazel Bishop (the caption identified her as a "famous chemist"). "With this screaming headline and editorial-type copy, Hazel Bishop crashed into the lipstick market with a bang," *Advertising Age* wrote. The ad ran first in the New York *Daily Mirror* and then on the back cover of the *American Weekly* in June 1950, "where it unleashed a flood of more than 162,000 quarters, sent in for a 30-day sample." The response constituted the biggest mail-order response the *Weekly* had ever received, and variations of the ad appeared in newspapers across the country.[32] The Spector campaign was exceedingly successful, as this cooing *Mayfair* article (one can only imagine it being the PR equivalent of a wet dream for Raymond Spector) suggests:

"For years we gals have been slaves to the ritual of re-applying lipstick morning, noon and night, and many times in-between. For years the lipstick makers offered us only new shades to match every color of the rainbow, new scents to rival the flowers of Spring. But the lipstick itself remained unchanged through the year, always leaving telltale marks on cups, cigarettes, teeth—and our boyfriends.

"We complained . . . but we complied always hoping for a miracle. Then it finally happened. One woman, all alone, did more than just hope. And so, for almost four years, noted scientist Hazel Bishop, with a ten-year background of research in cosmetic allergies, delved into her test-tubes for the secret. At long last, Miss Bishop perfected the first great lipstick change in forty years . . . a lipstick in a range of color-true shades of pure-food dyes . . . smooth, creamy, glowing and so long-lasting it would not eat off—smudge off—even kiss off!

"Though Hazel Bishop's formula was guarded with as much secrecy as an atomic bomb, her lipstick, huckstered by a fabulous press, radio and television campaign, became a national by-word for lasting lip allure. Within one short year, the lecturer-chemist who had accomplished what 'couldn't be done' skyrocketed to second place in the country's huge lipstick sales. Her revolutionary 'no-smear' lipstick is apparently here to stay—for everyone in the cosmetic business is climbing on her new-type lipstick bandwagon."[33]

Spector, who shrewdly understood the impact of national penetration on a variety of media fronts, closely followed the example of R. N. Harris and his brother Irving. The Harris brothers had developed a home permanent–wave kit in 1944 and in four years had built it into a $20-million-a-year business with its cross-country "Which Twin Has the Toni?" campaign.

During the same year that Richard Nixon resurrected his career by appealing directly to American voters with his famous televised Checkers speech, the Hazel Bishop company took cosmetics directly to American housewives. The company sponsored the Kate Smith show, where Merv Griffin, then a young singer, pitched the nonsmear brand. Later it was the sponsor of *This Is Your Life*. Bishop saw television advertisements as a sort of a personal one-on-one beauty demonstration, albeit one that was delivered to thousands of customers simultaneously.

The ads demonstrated different lipsticks that rubbed off easily, while (lo and behold) the Bishop brand held fast. Television may have been the salvation of the Hazel Bishop company, but it would also prove its Achilles' heel in the Lipstick Wars to come.

While the relationship between Hazel Bishop and Spector began to founder, Charles Revson was scheming to expand his empire. Though he got his start in the cosmetics business with Revlon nail polish (the blustery Helena Rubinstein always referred to him disdainfully as "the nail man"), he realized the marketing possibilities of color-coordinating lipstick with nail polish. This was not a new idea. Another American company had done something similar several years earlier. And the French haute-couture dress designer Germaine Monteil had began making lipstick to color-coordinate lipstick shades with her clothes.

When Revlon introduced Fatal Apple—"the most tempting color since Eve winked at Adam"—the fashion magazine advertisements were ubiquitous. Bea Castle, Revlon's publicity director, organized a press party to end all press parties. It featured a snake charmer (with snake), a grove of miniature apple trees, a golden apple from Cartier as a door prize, and Maurice the Mindreader (whose presence, though a bit puzzling from the thematic point of view, was clearly a hit).

But Revlon truly pulled out all the stops in the fall of 1952 with its Fire and

Ice shade promotion. The ads peered out of every general-circulation and fashion magazine.

The two-page spread, in a Richard Avedon photograph, showcased the sophisticated beauty of model Suzy Parker's less famous sister Dorian Leigh, dressed in a frosty sequin gown adorned by a brilliant red cape. "Are You Made for Fire and Ice," the copy dared. If so, you could answer yes to eight of the following fifteen questions:

Have you ever danced with your shoes off?

Did you ever wish on a new moon?

Do you blush when you find yourself flirting?

When a recipe calls for one dash of bitters, do you think it's better with two?

Do you secretly hope the next man you meet will be a psychiatrist?

Do you sometimes feel that other women resent you?

Have you ever wanted to wear an ankle bracelet?

Do sables excite you, even on other women?

Do you love to look up at a man?

Do you face crowded parties with panic—then wind up having a wonderful time?

Does gypsy music make you sad?

Do you think any man really understands you?

Would you streak your hair with platinum without consulting your husband?

If tourist flights were running, would you take a trip to Mars?

Do you close your eyes when you're kissed?

The Fire and Ice theme played in nine thousand different store-window displays across the nation. Radio and TV personalities such as Steve Allen, Jimmy Durante, and Arthur Godfrey all managed to work the theme into their shticks. On the *Today Show*, host Dave Garroway gave the Fire and Ice quiz to one of his secretaries.

Such plugs were not serendipitous, as one of Revlon's executives explained to *Business Week* at the time. "What you do is go to see Hope or Skelton or somebody of that nature and tell them about your new product coming out with, oh a couple of million dollars in advertising, and then the scriptwriter writes it in," the executive said. ". . . So that's the way we get it in—sort of inadvertently." The mere thought inspired humorist S. J. Perelman. "The easy negligence of the whole thing is truly captivating," he wrote. "For sheer insouciance, nothing could surpass the spectacle of an incipient Mark Twain grinding out cosmetic yaks with a $2 million pitchfork lightly pinking his bottom."[34]

The Hazel Bishop company was a hive of intrigue. Spector had bought out Berg and was wrestling with Bishop for control of the company. Spector lost a lawsuit to Bishop but retained control of the company. In a gloves-off posttrial interview, Spector called Bishop's lawsuit against him "preposterous." "I was delighted to see Miss Bishop get $310,000 for her stock, even though she never put a penny into the company and even though the formula she allegedly created is not being used by the company," he told *Advertising Age*.[35]

But Spector's bigger problem was Revlon. This was the height of the Cold War, and superpower nations were not the only ones spying on each other. Corporate espionage was pervasive. Suspicious that Revlon kept beating him to market with his own ideas, Spector hired two eavesdropping experts to check his phones. They were indeed tapped. Spector was convinced it was Revlon, though he was never able to prove it.

Whatever the true story behind the wiretapping, the biggest marketing blow for Hazel Bishop was not wiretapping. Rather, it was Revlon's shrewd placement of advertising on the enormously popular TV show *The $64,000 Question*. Within a few years, Revlon would eclipse Hazel Bishop entirely in the lipstick market.

Did Hazel Bishop's new kissproof formula change the course of lipstick history? The answer seems to be yes.

According to *Advertising Age* ultimately about fifty other companies soon brought out competitive lipsticks. But was the formula truly new or even kissproof?

"The claims of Miss Bishop to indelibility are not without foundation," the *Consumers Report* of August 1951 concluded.[36] But Bishop herself claimed that she maintained a healthy skepticism in the face of Berg's initial advertising exuberance. "Only tattooing," she dryly remarked in her unpublished memoirs, "is completely kissproof."[37]

Bishop urgently wanted to be regarded as a serious chemist (she was a card-carrying member of the American Section of the Societé de Chimie Industrielle, the Chemists Club of New York City, and the American Chemical Society). But respect from her fellow (male) chemists proved elusive. When she helped organize the annual American Chemical Society meeting, she was not in charge of organizing a colloquium on cosmetic chemistry but rather had the task of lining up sightseeing excursions for the chemists' wives. Later, when she spoke to the American Chemical Society on "The Philosophy and Science of Cosmetics," she was joined at the podium by a "lariat-spinning sextet of women" who had been bused in from a nearby high school as the entertainment.[38]

Like most cosmetic manufacturers of the time, Bishop never patented her formula. Cosmetics patents proliferated, of course, but mostly for new containers rather than new formulas. This is understandable, given the advice she received from a respected patent attorney—and also given the example of the makers of Toni and the home permanent business, which was embroiled at the time in a massive three-way patent infringement suit.

Nor did she ever disclose the Hazel Bishop formula, although she did publish a paper describing techniques for, essentially, reverse-engineering the contents of lipsticks already on the market. Her lab notebooks are curiously absent from her personal archives, although multiple copies of press clippings of virtually every article written about the Hazel Bishop company have been carefully preserved—constituting, perhaps, the only truly indelible aspect of Hazel Bishop's legacy.

In 1959, according to Kline & Company, Americans spent an estimated $93 million on 62 million lipsticks. None of it was actually smear-proof, as Connie Francis attested in her hit song of that year, "Lipstick on Your Collar."

When you left me all alone at the record hop

Told me you were going out for a soda pop

You were gone for quite a while, half an hour or more

You came back and, man, oh, man, this is what I saw

Lipstick on your collar told a tale on you

Lipstick on your collar said you were untrue

Bet your bottom dollar, you and I are through

Lipstick on your collar told a tale on you

You said it belonged to me, made me stop and think

Then I noticed yours was red, mine was baby pink

Who walked in but Mary Jane, lipstick all a mess

Were you smoochin' my best friend, guess the answer's yes.*

*Lyrics by Edna Lewis and music by George Goehring. Copyright 1959.

Still to be invented: no-smear lipstick.

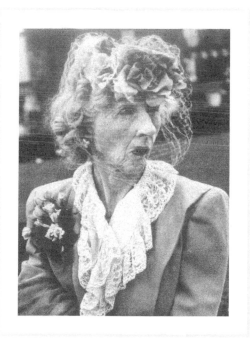

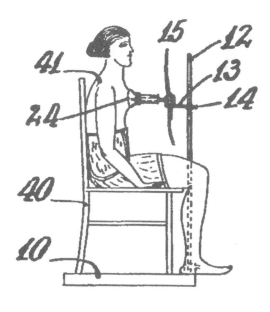

CHAPTER 3

Breasts

Anyone who has ever visited a nudist camp will certainly agree that clothes can sometimes be a help.

— James Laver, 1950.

Certain evolutionary theorists tell us that women's breasts came into being because a perky, prominent bosom served as a sort of built-in advertisement for female humans. Among the Cro-Magnon set, uplifted breasts were the equivalent of a flashing neon sign that said "Hi, I'm a healthy fertile female!"[1]

It may have taken tens of thousands of years for breasts to evolve. But in only two or three millennia, women have managed to manipulate their breasts into myriad new forms that Nature herself has never imagined.

The earliest example of what might be referred to as a push-up bra, according to certain Greek scholars, was reportedly deployed by the Greek goddess Hera. In the *Iliad*, she is described as donning a garment wrought by Athena with "broideries fully many," "brooches of gold," and a "hundred tassels" in order to distract Zeus long enough to keep him from meddling in the Trojan War.[2] Given the controversies engendered by surgical breast implants in the past decade, it is interesting to note that the female impulse to artificially enhance the breasts is ancient. During the past 150 years, however, new technologies have allowed women to transform their breasts at a breathtaking pace.

Titzling and Other Tales

Westerners tend to think of the bra as an essential form of support. But in fact the bra has always been first and foremost a figure shaper, deployed either to draw attention to the breasts in a novel way or to minimize them, thereby accentuating another part of the body.

So who invented the modern bra? First let's dispense with the false histories that gained surprising currency during the twentieth century. The most amusing of these, *Bust-Up,* was written in 1972 by Wallace Reyburn. He recounts the escapades of one Otto Titzling, who, inspired by a buxom aspiring opera singer of Icelandic descent named Swanhilda, is moved to invent a "bust halter" in 1912.

Reyburn provides a detailed description of a legal challenge mounted against Titzling by one Philippe de Brassiere, who ostensibly also claimed credit for the bra's invention. He even features drawings of an upside-down bra for trapeze artists. Would that it were so. Most readers of *Bust-Up* have recognized it as the brilliant parody that it is. But not all. One fairly recent history treats the story as gospel.

More frequently, at least on this side of the Atlantic, a socialite named Caresse Crosby has been given credit for the bra's invention. Crosby is cited in biographical encyclopedias of famous women, in popular press treatments, and even in doctoral dissertations on the history of costume.

In her autobiography, Crosby claimed not only that she was the inventor of the bra, but also that she was the first bona fide Girl Scout and that she set a record for the 220-yard dash, published Ernest Hemingway as an expatriate in Paris, and introduced Salvador Dali to America.

Here is Crosby's version of the invention of the bra: One night, while dressing for a New York debutante ball, the eyelet embroidery of Crosby's corset "kept peeping through the roses around my bosom."[3] So Crosby summoned her maid, Marie, and ordered her to fetch two pocket handkerchiefs, some pink ribbon and a sewing basket.

Caresse Crosby (actually, she was born with the more pedestrian name of Mary Phelps Jacob and reinvented herself as "Caresse" after she married Harry Crosby) pinned the handkerchiefs together and directed Marie to stitch the pink ribbons along the bottom edge. Crosby tied the two ends of the handkerchiefs behind her into a knot. Marie pulled the pink ribbons taut and fastened them to the knot.

Several years later, according to Crosby, a former beau who worked for Warner Corset Company urged her to show her patent to the company, which snapped it up for $1,500. The bra, she claimed, ultimately earned the company $15 million.

It's easy to want to believe the clear narrative of Crosby's story. After all, 1913—the year in which Crosby invented her version of a bra—was a watershed of modernism. That year brought the performance of Igor Stravinsky's ear-blowing *Rite of Spring* in Paris, as well as the scandalous Armory art exhibit in New York City featuring Matisse's *Blue Nude*. It would be nice to point to that exact year as the moment that women cast off their allegedly constricting corsets and donned the ostensibly liberating brassiere.

This, however, turns out to be another good story spoiled by inconvenient facts. As Jane Farrell-Beck and Colleen Gau demonstrate in their amply researched, scholarly history of the bra, there is no evidence whatsoever that Warner even bought Crosby's design, much less produced it.[4]

What Crosby invented was a backless breast flattener for evening dresses. And perhaps it should be considered an early bra, given that it functioned as a form-shaper. Breast flatteners, which had been around since 1900, became fabulously popular by 1920, as women tried to achieve the flat flapper look that allowed their long pearls to swing so freely.

Crosby's was a flapper brassiere, meant to flatten the breasts into the boyish silhouette that reigned in that era (one of the most successful flattener companies was called, not incidentally, Boyshform). Attention was drawn instead to the face, which was highly stylized with cosmetics, or the legs, which were newly exposed.

Crosby's bra and other flatteners lacked the defining features that characterize the modern bra: cups for each breast and shoulder straps that pull the cups upward. Flattening the breasts, it turns out, is a much simpler structural proposition than lifting and supporting them.

Bras and Bridges

Breast uplift presented womankind with a structural challenge that was, arguably, as difficult as what mankind had attempted with the Brooklyn Bridge— the world's longest suspension bridge when it was erected in 1883. The main difference between a corset and a bra is very similar to the difference between a load-bearing bridge and a suspension bridge. Corsets provide support from the hips and waist, thrusting up the breasts from below. In bras, the shoulders bear the load, with straps that grip the breasts from above.

Garments known as "brassieres" first appeared in the United States around 1904, manufactured by Charles DeBevoise. The word itself first showed up in *Vogue* magazine in 1907. By 1911, brassiere business was brisk. In March, Macy's advertised in *The New York Times* that it had just opened a new brassiere department. "This season's low corsets and close-fitting gowns make the Brassiere more indispensable than ever," a Macy's ad advised.[5]

Also known as bust extenders, bust shapers, and bust bodices, most of these brassieres did not resemble the modern bra any more than did flapper flatteners, which came later but were also referred to as brassieres. They were not meant so much to support the breasts as to cover them up or give them shape. By the 1900s the fashionable corset line had dipped just below the nipples, which posed problems for fat women and scrawny women alike, many of whom were trying to achieve the pre-flapper gooselike Gibson girl posture of the time.

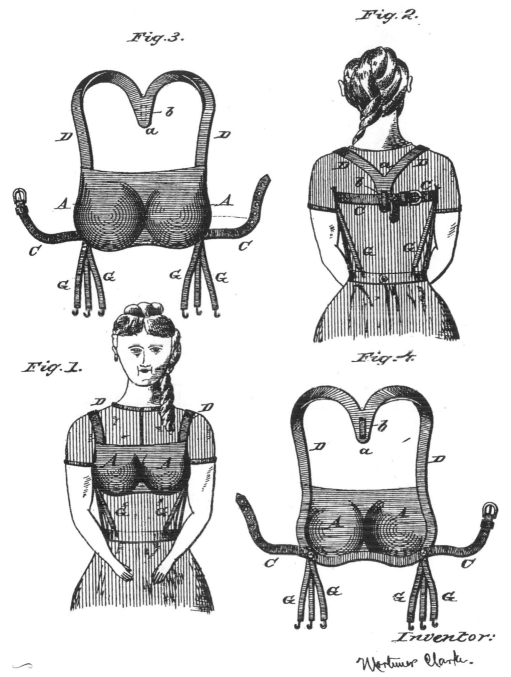

Fig.3.

Fig.2.

Fig.1.

Fig.4.

Inventor:

Mortimer Clarke.

Mortimer Clarke of the District of Columbia came up
with this protobra in 1884. It held up a skirt as well
as the breasts.

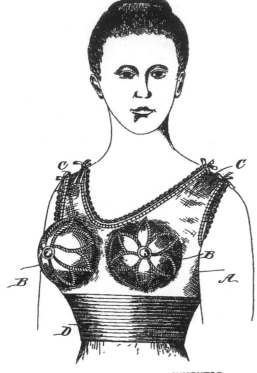

*New York–based Ludwig
Lendry designed this
early bra in 1893. It
could be made out of a
knit fabric or, less
comfortably, rubber.*

INVENTOR

L. Lendry

Fig. 1.

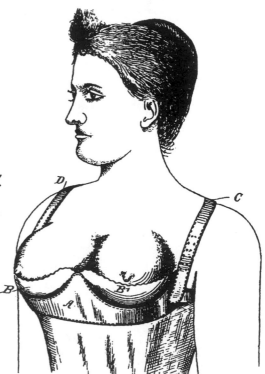

*Marie Tucek's pioneering
push-up bra. It was to be
made of sheet metal or
cardboard and covered
with silk.*

INVENTOR

Marie Tucek

Overweight women used the brassiere to grapple with new bulges created by the lower-cut corsets. Pearl Merwin, author of *The American System of Dressmaking*, published in 1912, described the brassiere as "a positive necessity for a full bust and fleshy forms."[6]

For thin women, gay deceivers—those precursors to falsies—could no longer be inserted into the corsets. "Bust shapers" and "bust extenders" began to provide where nature did not. Caroline Newell's bust supporter, for example, promised "All Deficiency of Development Supplied."[7] Women could make their own by buying patterns for about twenty cents from magazines like *Vogue, Delineator,* and *Ladies' Home Journal.*

But bralike articles appear to have been sold by mail order to no-nonsense Western women as early as the early 1890s. JC Penney, which got its start as the Golden Rule Store in Wyoming, sold its first breast supporter over the counter in 1902. In 1903, Phosa D. Beeman of Minneapolis, Minnesota, patented a bralike garment to be worn over long johns, supporting the breasts "as within a sling" nevertheless permitting "the breast-piece to freely swing outward when the wearer stoops over."[8]

For a long stretch, from the 1860s to the 1930s, dozens and dozens of inventors struggled with the same momentous design challenge: how to free up the waist to give women the ability to move easily while also supporting and shaping their busts.

Madame Herminie Cadolle, a French businesswoman whose company was based in Buenos Aires, made use of a new elastic material in her "breast girdle," which she displayed at the Exposition Universelle of 1889 in Paris. Some historians have proposed that Madame Cadolle should be credited with first inventing the bra. Her 1889 breast girdle, however, is not truly a bra. It's really a corset with the midriff cut out of it, thereby allowing more waist movement. Still, the Cadolle undergarment did have shoulder straps, which normal corsets of the period did not, and in this respect it foreshadowed an important change, for Cadolle's was a hybrid, using both shoulders and hips for support.

Other inventors were dreaming up different solutions for the active woman.

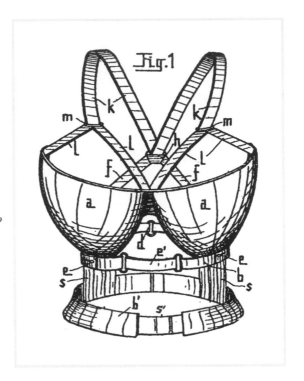

In 1889, Lucy James, an inventor in Pomona, California, patented an ostensibly flexible three-in-one contraption that served as a posture-improver, as suspenders for holding up a skirt, and as a bust form—that is, a protofalsie.

In 1906, Frank Schmitt, a Philadelphia resident of German extraction, patented a remarkable confabulation featuring two half breast cups dangling from a necklace and a tummy flattener suspended from a belt. Fourteen years later, Louise Antoinette Sherry of Carthage, New York, patented a breast supporter that had no band around the torso but which anchored to the wearer's stockings. And in 1936, Roy S. Neal of Kansas City, Kansas, patented a brassiere with three zippers, two in the cups and one in between. It foreshadowed a "rip cord" brassiere designed by self-proclaimed "hubba hubba girl" Evelyn West, a stripper who insured her bosom with Lloyd's of London for $50,000.

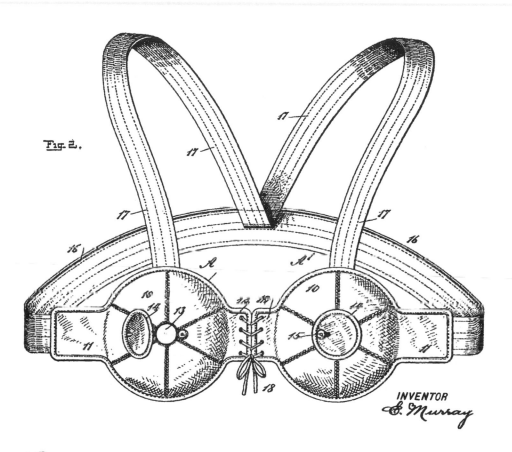

Fig. 2.

INVENTOR
E. Murray

Ebenezer Murray, a resident of the rough and wild gold-mining town of
Deadwood, South Dakota, made big claims for his brassiere: It would build up
the figure "when the tissues of the breast are deficient," aid those with
"pendent breasts," and "enable the milk-ducts to retain their proper position."
The peekaboo nipple caps were ostensibly for nursing babies, but this claim
was likely made tongue-in-cheek.

Breasts of Steel

The last quarter of the nineteenth century was, of course, a period of unsurpassed inventive foment in the United States. Thomas Edison invented the lightbulb. Alexander Graham Bell invented the telephone. Orville and Wilbur Wright were dreaming of human flight. Numerous other inventors directed their energies toward other lofty experimentation: the augmentation of women's breasts.

Many of these inventors were women. Nearly two thirds of all breast enhancements patented between the mid-1850s and the mid-1950s were dreamed up by women—even though, over all, women received only about one percent of all patents during that one-hundred-year stretch.[9] Corsets were designed so that improvements could be easily inserted. The Ideal and The Configurateur featured "regulators" inside the breast gores, allowing the wearer to contract or expand her bust according to her mood.

What appears to be the earliest patent for a false bosom, a contraption of Brunhildean dimensions, was granted to Anne S. McLean of Williamsburg, New York, in 1858. Mrs. McLean invented a steeply inclined cone made of wire that projected perhaps a good four inches from a breast pad inserted into a corset. As for the breast pads themselves, she preferred that they be made of a material "impervious to perspiration, such as bark, grass, curled hair, or any other suitable substance."[10] These pads would have cushioned the breast from the wire cones, but the tips of the cones look as if they could have caused real pain to Mr. McLean or anyone else on the receiving end of a tight embrace.

Mrs. McLean's idea was widely copied and improved upon, given that, due to technical improvements in iron making, wire was plentiful and pliable. Six years later, Eleanor M. Marshall of Hillsdale, New York, for example, envisioned a wire "mammiform breast-protector" that was suspended from shoulder straps and encased the breasts in a wire dome structure. Light and flexible and as "nearly like the natural breasts as possible," Marshall claimed, the springs of her mammiform could be

A. S. McLean.

Corset.

Nº 22443   Patented Dec. 28, 1858.

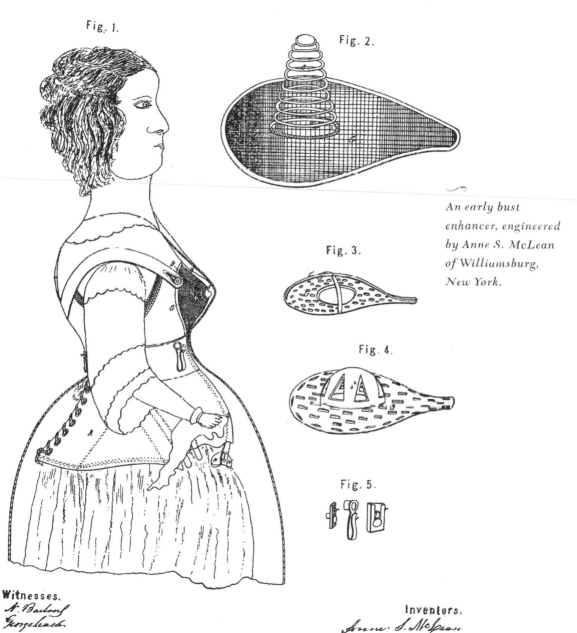

Fig. 1.

Fig. 2.

Fig. 3.

Fig. 4.

Fig. 5.

An early bust enhancer, engineered by Anne S. McLean of Williamsburg, New York.

Witnesses.
N. Barlow
George Leach

Inventors.
Anne S. McLean

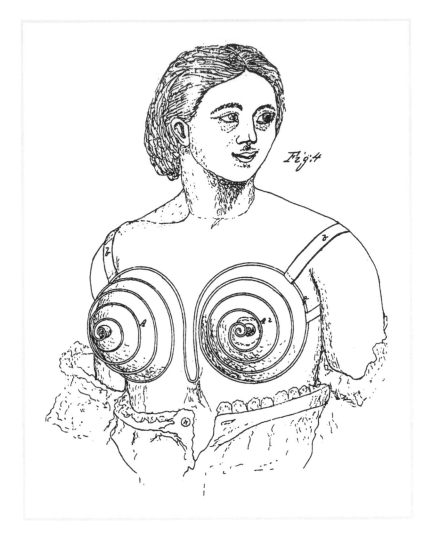

The nation may have been riven by Civil War, but Eleanor M. Marshall's mind was elsewhere. She came up with this variation on the spring-form falsie in 1864.

"pressed together or onto the natural breasts, or in any other direction, and when relieved from such pressure resume their natural position."[11]

Such wire bosom production appears to have been centered largely in New York, but similar designs were also percolating in the imaginations of a number of Midwestern inventors including Elizabeth Leetch of Detroit; Jacob W. Greene of Chillicothe, Missouri; Mary A. Williams of Kansas City; and Chrisie Launer of Arenzville, Illinois.

Some models were quite feminine looking, featuring dainty silk bows tied at the nipple end. Wire may have been springy and firm but, resembling as they did miniature birdcages, they fell far short of resembling actual breasts. So it should not surprise us that women experimented with myriad other materials as well.

Pump Me Up

In the 1840s a new material appeared on the scene that would eventually transform the nature of many everyday objects, from condoms and galoshes to tires and balloons. That material? Vulcanized rubber. Pioneered by Charles Goodyear in America and others elsewhere, vulcanized rubber was immediately seized upon as a viable way to increase the size of women's bosoms. (It took a generation for others to appreciate rubber's versatility; poor Goodyear died a pauper, long before his wonder material really caught on.)

Several decades before John Boyd Dunlop fathomed the idea of rubber bicycle tires, other inventors were already envisioning pneumatic breasts. An early advertisement advised that "the registered bust improver, of an air-proof material" is "an improvement on the pads of wool and cotton hitherto used."[12]

Nevertheless, the use of rubber bust improvers was frequently decried by various doyennes of beauty. Lola Montez, an infamous courtesan, in her 1858 *Arts of Beauty: Secrets of a Lady's Toilet*, dismissed "artificial india-rubber bosoms" as "ridiculous contrivances" that could be ruinous to the beauty of the breast.[13]

A later tome, *The Ugly-Girl Papers*, published by Harper & Brothers in 1874, made the same point. "Of all things, India-rubber pads act most injuriously by constantly sweating the skin, and ruining the bust beyond hope of restoration," wrote Susan C. Power. Rather, Mrs. Power suggested, "flat figures are best dissembled by puffed and shirred blouse-waists, or by corsets with a fine rattan run in the top of the bosom gore, which throws out the fullness sufficiently to look well."[14]

Mary P. R. Tilton of Trenton, New Jersey, in 1870 patented a solution that sounds very close to that recommended in *The Ugly-Girl Papers*. Indeed, hers is an ingenious feat of engineering—undulating whalebone or steel stays covered with a ruffled cambric material. This assemblage extends several inches in front of the real bosom. One drawback to this design, alas, appears to be that anyone much taller than the wearer would, upon looking down, see not a generous décolletage but rather a view of the floor beneath her.

Rubber pads of this era appear to have fallen out of favor not because they were disparaged by the likes of Mrs. Power and Lola Montez, or even because women did not like the sweaty feel of rubber against their breasts. Rather, they were abandoned because they were aesthetic failures. They tended to distend and deflate, rendering the bust uneven or, worse, leaving the putative breasts pointing in improbable directions.

Cork was another popular material during the nineteenth century. An advertisement for the funnel-shaped Cork Bosom Pad in *Demorest's Monthly Magazine* announced, "Graceful—Healthy. This pad being made of cork is light and porous and

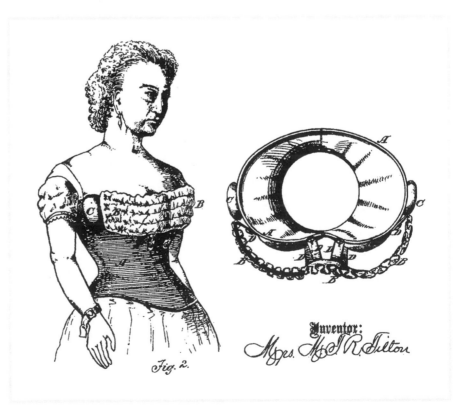

What's behind the ruffles? Mary P. R. Tilton of Trenton, New Jersey, fashioned this flirtatious facade in 1870.

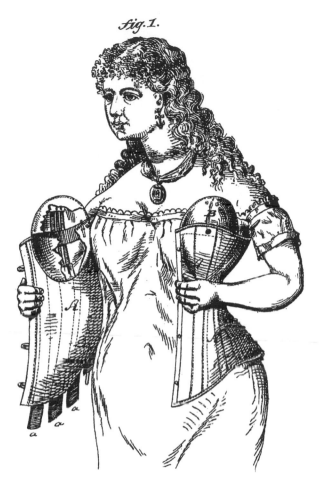

Fig.1.

Inventor.
S. B. Ferris

More bust pads from Sherwood
Ferris. These were easily removable so
that the corset could be worn with or
without enhancement, depending
upon the lady's mood.

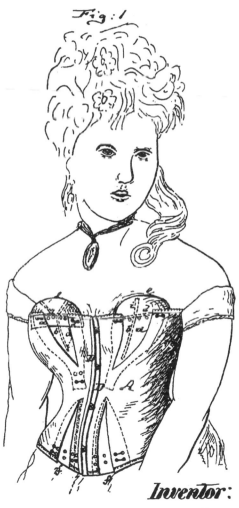

Fig.1

Inventor:
Sherwood B. Ferris

Brooklyn-based Sherwood Ferris's
pads were made of wire or whalebone
and then papier-mâchéd into the
desired shape. They were supposed
to feature either eyelets or
buttonholes so they could be laced or
buttoned into the corset.

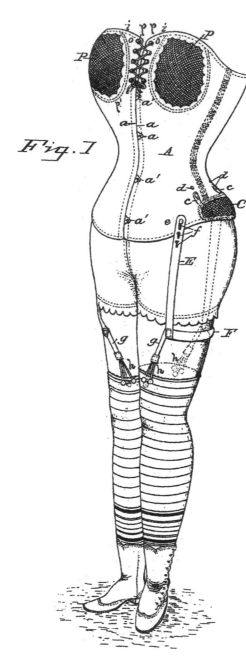

Fig. I

Inventor.
Zénone Lpedóchowski.

Zénone de Lpedóchowski of La Salle, Illinois, constructed a corset with built-in oval-shaped wire-netting breast pads bound with buckskin. The corset provided fullness to the derriere by the same means.

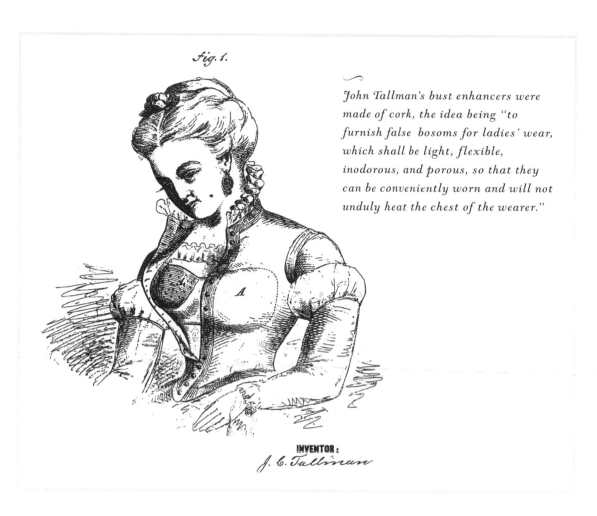

fig. 1.

John Tallman's bust enhancers were made of cork, the idea being "to furnish false bosoms for ladies' wear, which shall be light, flexible, inodorous, and porous, so that they can be conveniently worn and will not unduly heat the chest of the wearer."

INVENTOR:
J. C. Tallman

consequently HEALTHY. It secures a perfect fit in a dress and gives a GRACEFUL shape to the figure. It is neatly covered and neither breaks nor gets out of order."[15]

Elizabeth S. Weldon of New York City in 1876 patented a new type of breast pad whose filling could easily be replaced. Most pads of the time, she complained, became useless after a certain number of wearings "owing to the absorption of perspiration, and the matting or packing together of the filling, which settles into the lower corners of the pockets or sacks, forming a hard lump or knot, which is so extremely uncomfortable to the wearer that the pad has to be discarded, or entirely made over."[16]

Michael A. Bryson, an inventor living in St. Louis, Missouri, brought a frontier sensibility to the bust pad in 1879. He aimed to impart a "natural softness and flesh-like elasticity" to the pads by filling them with the hair of deer, mountain sheep, elk, or antelope. "I am aware that pads have been filled with curled hair of horses, &c., goose-feathers, cotton, granulated cork, wool, or other material, and also have been made of rubber to be inflated, or springs with a suitable covering; but these are either too heavy or too hot, and therefore unhealthy," he wrote.

Bryson, who also produced bustles made of similar material, did acknowledge that elk and antelope hair was not without its drawbacks. Thus, he advised, "to prevent any disagreeable odors, and also to remove any greasy or oily matters contained therein, I prefer to soak the said deer, mountain sheep, elk, or antelope hair for not less than four hours in naphtha, or in a strong solution of alum, which also makes the hair more elastic."[17]

Pneumatic Bliss

The quest for a lifelike rubber breast resumed at the turn of the century when big matronly bosoms came back in style. Dora Harrison of Lansing, Michigan, appears to have staked her career on inflatable rubber bosoms. Her earliest version, from 1898, resembles two large contraceptive pessaries—birth control devices being another early consumer use of synthetic rubber—each fitted with an inflation nozzle and then laced together.

By 1907, Harrison had revised this into a bralike device that was made of "thin, flesh-colored rubber, rendered non-odorous by special treatment" and was meant to be inflated before put on, although it featured nozzles placed "so as to be within convenient reach of the wearer's mouth, in case it is desired to further inflate the pads . . . after they are in place."[18] A cap had to be screwed onto the nozzle to prevent leakage.

Harrison is just one of many inventors who attempted to perfect the art during this second wave of inflatable-breast invention. Oliver G. Dennis of Chicago, for

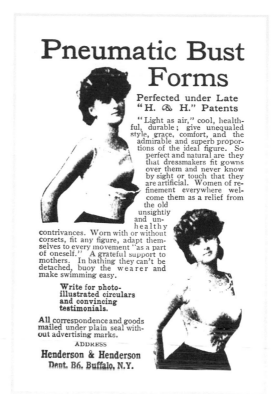

Nineteenth-century newspaper ad.

example, patented something similar in 1912, claiming that his invention gave a more lifelike illusion. "When worn," he said, "they will not have the appearance of lifeless members, but will vibrate responsively to movements of the wearer."[19] This gives, perhaps, new meaning to T. S. Eliot's poem "Whispers of Immortality." "Uncorseted, her friendly bust," Eliot wrote in 1920, "Gives promise of pneumatic bliss."[20]

Mechanical Magic

Women have not only long strapped on or inserted false bosoms, they have also sought to either increase the size of their actual breasts or tried to regain their youthful elasticity by slathering on creams or enlisting machines to work mechanical magic.

Back in the sixteenth century, Jean Liebault, author of *Three Books for the Embellishment of the Human Body*, advised that a woman could keep her breasts small and firm by crushing cumin seeds into a pulp, smearing the paste onto her breasts, and then binding them with vinegar-soaked bandages.[21]

Bust improvement preparations proliferated from the late nineteenth through the early twentieth century, when the federal government began to regulate food and drugs more vigorously. These bust creams are remarkable for their brazen claims, given that it is highly unlikely any of them worked. The American Medical Association, then in its infancy as a professional organization, itemized many such "cures" in its two-volume *Nostrums and Quackery*, published in 1911–12.

The Aurum company of Chicago promised that its potion—not cheap at $1.79 for a month's supply—when used in conjunction with a special exerciser, would en-

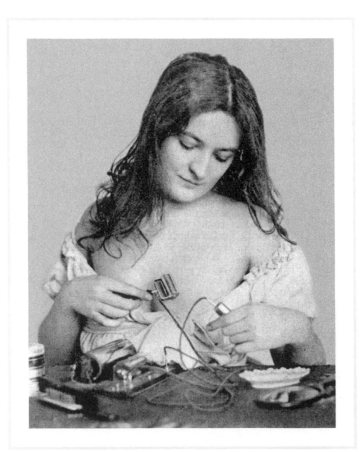

Ladies were assured they could roll their way to larger breasts (the same device would also allegedly eliminate wrinkles and cure lumbago).

large busts a full six inches. Some customers were skeptical that they could achieve such miraculous results. The company wrote to Mrs. E. Huston Haig of Philadelphia, reassuring her: "We are confident if you will use the Vestro carefully according to the directions the result in your case will prove entirely satisfactory."[22]

The Hager Medical Company of North Dakota did a brisk business in Mammary Cell Food, and Dr. Charles Flesh Food not only allegedly developed the bust but also removed wrinkles, crow's feet, pimples, freckles, and sallowness.

Eloise Rae—a company run by several men, none of whom was actually named Eloise or even Ray—promised results for even the most hopeless of cases. The putative Eloise Rae, pictured in a newspaper advertisement sporting a robust décolletage, exhorts: "I don't care how thin you are, how old you are, how fallen and flaccid are the lines of your figure or how flat your chest is. I can give you a full, firm, youthful bust quickly."[23]

In *The Ugly-Girl Papers*, Susan Power admonished women to never touch the breasts "with but the utmost delicacy, as other treatment renders them weak and flaccid, and not unfrequently results in cancer." She went on to advise that "no human being—doctor, nurse, nor the mother herself—on any pretense, save in the case of accident, be allowed to touch a girl's figure."

"It would be unnecessary to say this, were not French and Irish nurses, especially old and experienced ones, sometimes in the habit of stroking the figures of young girls committed to their charge, with the idea of developing them."[24]

Some potions were meant to work from the inside out. Zoe Hamilton, in her "Boudoir Manual," advised women to avoid "any sort of instruments to develop the bust." Rather, she advised ingesting daily Complexion or Attraction wafers from the druggist (one dollar a box) in addition to, every night, taking a coarse towel and rubbing the breasts "as if you wanted to take the skin off."

If you "take them as the directions state, you may be as sure as sure can be that you will very soon see your bust begin to enlarge," assured Hamilton, who was likely commissioned by the manufacturer, Franklin B. Crouch, to write the booklet. A companion booklet explains how the complexion wafers also work wonders for men wanting "to develop the organs," cure their pimples, or reinvigorate themselves after "sexual exhaustion."[25]

Apply Suction and Think Big

The heyday of bust potions coincided with a proliferation of bust-improvement contraptions, most of which operated on some sort of suction principle. Several inventions dating from the Civil War until the turn of the century are for suction devices.

The first U.S. patent to forthrightly acknowledge that its purpose was to increase the size of breasts appears to have been issued in 1889. It was a combination bust developer/bosom form (it was supposed to make the breasts look bigger and simultaneously work to enlarge them).

By 1897 another patented developer (which closely resembles a modern-day toilet plunger) was sold as the Princess Bust Developer through the Sears, Roebuck and Co. catalog. For $1.46 you got not just the developer but also a jar of Bust Cream that was unrivaled in making "a plump, full, rounded bosom, perfect neck and arms, a smooth skin, where before [the flesh] was scrawny, flat and flabby."[26]

The developer, made of nickel and aluminum, was essentially a rod with a large bell-shaped cup stuck on the end of it. The owner was supposed to massage her breast by plunging the cup back and forth. It came in two sizes, either four or five inches in diameter. And if a buyer did not see results after just two weeks, Sears offered a money-back guarantee.

"It is designed to build up and fill out shrunken and undeveloped tissues, form a rounded, plump, perfectly developed bust, producing a beautiful figure," the ad copy for the 1902 catalog reads.[27] A few pages later the catalog also offers another wondrous product: an electric belt that promises to cure male impotence.

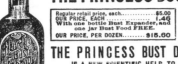

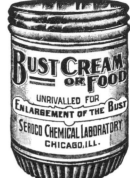

Sears, Roebuck catalog, 1897.

The Health-Culture Company of New York City propagandized its massagers through a book called *Womanly Beauty*. One of these massagers, which consisted of rubber rollers affixed to a handle, was invented by a certain Dr. Forest.

The book instructs thusly: "At night before retiring bathe the breasts lightly with cold water, dry carefully with a soft towel, and over a loose sack or undervest roll with Dr. Forest's Bust Developer from underneath upwards and from the side forward, always toward the centre, throwing the chest well out while doing this; do not do it carelessly or indifferently, but keep your mind on it and feel that you are accomplishing your desire."[28] (This mind-over-matter approach anticipated by several decades the popular seventies tome *Natural Bust Enlargement with Total Mind Power: How to Use the Other 90% of Your Mind to Increase the Size of Your Breasts.*)

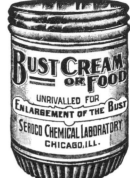

America Goes Dance Mad

With the flat-chested look prevailing in the late teens and early twenties, bust uplift went into eclipse. Women instead racily drew attention to their newly exposed legs and their painted faces while they experimented in wondrous new ways to suppress the breast.

The decade between 1910 and 1920 was, one social commentator intoned, "the period in which America went dance mad."[29] It started with the wildly popular cakewalk, performed by African Americans on the minstrel circuit, who had little chance to do much more than perpetuate racial stereotypes promulgated by white performers. The cakewalk, essentially an exaggerated parody of white ballroom dances, moved from the stage back to the ballroom and in doing so crossed back again, this time from black society back to white society.

By the time William K. Vanderbilt and his wife hired an African-American instructor to teach the new dance at their Fifth Avenue mansion, the cakewalk had come full circle. "The white dancers threw their shoulders back, stuck out their midriffs, and did their stiff-spined best to imitate high-stepping plantation blacks [who in turn had been] parodying stiff-spined white ballroom dancers," Gerald Jonas writes.[30]

The cakewalk opened the way for a whole new dance genre of animal-inspired wriggling, shaking, and twisting: the bunny hug, the camel walk, the chicken scratch, the kangaroo dip, the grizzly bear, and, especially, the turkey trot—the impact of which "was felt at all levels of society."[31]

In 1910, the year the turkey trot was showcased in a hit Broadway show, a group of moral gatekeepers grumbled about its "unwholesome" influence on working-class women. A turkey trotting New Jersey woman was actually sentenced to fifty days in jail. By 1914 the Vatican found it necessary to officially denounce both the turkey trot and the tango, which had arrived in the United States four years earlier from South America. That same year Vernon and Irene Castle opened a school of dancing in New York, smoothing the bouncy athletic moves of the animal dances into a civilized glide.

The Castles' genteel influence notwithstanding, the turkey trot and tango, against the new sound of sultry saxophones, gave way to the signature dances of the 1920s: the "free-kicking Charleston, the butt-slapping Black Bottom."[32]

The corset industry, after decades of denying the trend, finally responded to this "new" athleticism of the New Woman. By 1920, *Bowman's Corset and Brassiere Trade*, a directory of the industry, listed fifty manufacturers who made sports corsets and another fifty who made dancing corsets. So why is it then that young women—who finally had an abundance of ostensibly limber corsets from which to choose—ultimately threw them off in favor of the bra?

One is tempted to conclude that the bra was simply more comfortable than a dancing corset. And in all likelihood it was, at least for the energetic and youthful. But physical comfort was not the only reason young women adopted bras.

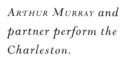

ARTHUR MURRAY *and partner perform the Charleston.*

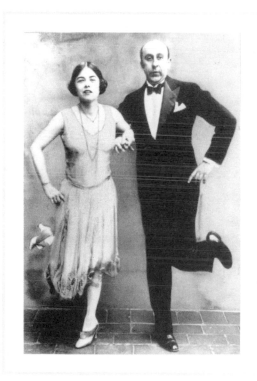

Just consider Clara Bow, the silent-movie siren. Bow is perhaps best remembered for her Cupid's bow smile, which millions of women imitated by stenciling their own lips. But women were taking cues from Bow's breasts as well.

Bow and the Bra

In the 1925 silent movie *The Plastic Age*, Clara Bow plays a hotsy-totsy roadster-driving coed who runs with a fast crowd and nearly leads the star athlete to ruin. In her opening scene she is dancing wildly at a sorority house—and her chest is by no means flattened. Indeed, as we watch her jump up and down, it is difficult to imagine that her youthful, buoyant breasts are restrained by *any* undergarment.

Two years later, appearing in *It*, the movie that would make her reputation, Clara Bow plays a working girl who aspires to marry the scion of a department-store

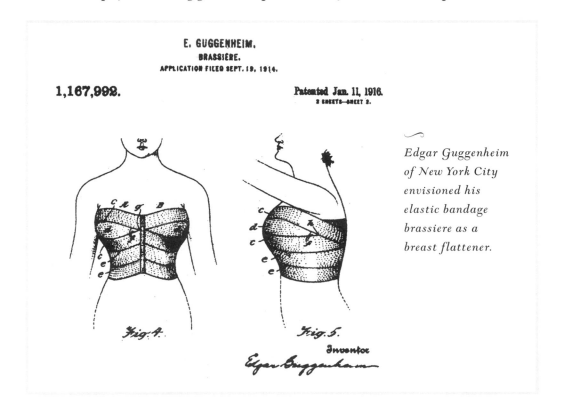

Edgar Guggenheim
of New York City
envisioned his
elastic bandage
brassiere as a
breast flattener.

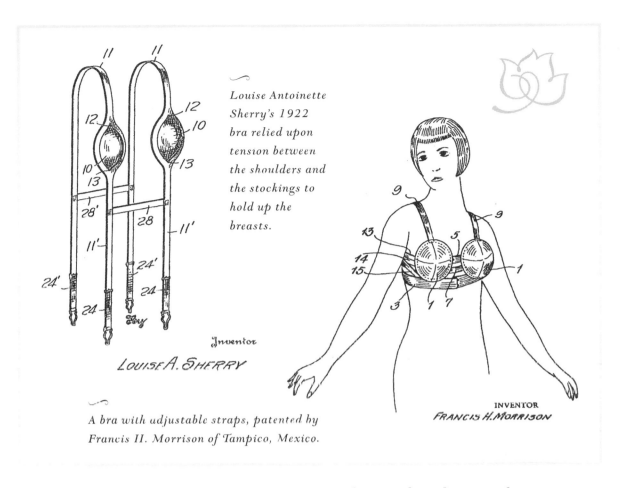

Louise Antoinette Sherry's 1922 bra relied upon tension between the shoulders and the stockings to hold up the breasts.

Inventor

LOUISE A. SHERRY

A bra with adjustable straps, patented by Francis H. Morrison of Tampico, Mexico.

INVENTOR
FRANCIS H. MORRISON

magnate. After accepting an invitation to dine at the Ritz, she grabs a pair of scissors and, in an impulsive, coyly sexual gesture, cuts a décolletage into her day dress. As she transforms her work frock into an evening gown the audience is treated to a clear, lingering look at her foundation garment, which is most definitely a brassiere (similar to one appearing in advertisements of the time for Gossard foundation garments).

In two later scenes in this movie, we see Bow's nipples clearly swelling beneath her silk blouse. "She's top-heavy with 'It,' " one of the male leads winkingly observes, in one of the film's many nods to Freud.[33] Indeed, Mont Westmore, one of the legendary Hollywood makeup artists from the Westmore family, acknowledged that in most of the scenes Miss Bow was not wearing a bra. "By using gauze on the nipples and adhesive plaster across Miss Bow's breasts, instead of a brassiere, he was really

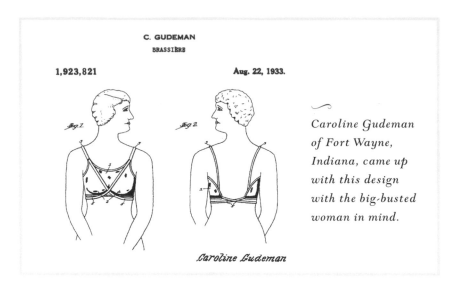

C. GUDEMAN
BRASSIÈRE

1,923,821   Aug. 22, 1933.

Fig.1.   *Fig 2.*

Caroline Gudeman

Caroline Gudeman of Fort Wayne, Indiana, came up with this design with the big-busted woman in mind.

trying to project the effect of nudity beneath a flimsy garment," wrote Mont's brother Frank Westmore in his highly entertaining memoir of the Westmore family.[34]

Sex and Freud were everywhere during the early twentieth century. Sears, Roebuck offered mail-order copies of *Ten Thousand Dreams Interpreted* and *Sex Problems Solved*. The radio crooned tunes like "Hot Lips," "Baby Face," "I Need Lovin'," and "Burning Kisses."

Marquees beckoned moviegoers with picture titles like *Married Flirts, Sinners in Silk*, and *Women Who Give*.[35] A movie called *Flaming Youth* featured "neckers, petters, white kisses, red kisses, pleasure-made daughters, sensation-craving mothers" while *Alimony* promised "brilliant men, beautiful jazz babies, champagne baths, midnight revels, petting parties in the purple dawn, all ending in one terrific smashing climax that makes you gasp."[36]

"Man is the only animal using this function out of season," protested Charlotte Perkins Gilman. "Excessive indulgence in sex-waste has imperiled the life of the race."[37] Gilman was author of the brilliant feminist short story "The Yellow Wallpaper" and a groundbreaking economic analyst of women in society. Nonetheless, on this issue, she was seriously out of step with her American sisters.

While a mere decade earlier the ideal American woman was a demure, curvaceous statue swathed in swirls of fabric and a froth of lace, by 1920 she had bobbed her hair, dyed it black, rolled down the stockings on her pencil-thin legs, and painted her lips cardinal red. The New Woman could smoke, drink, vote, and even hold down a job. Moreover, she was sexually independent as never before.

In 1913, Walter Lippmann introduced Freud's American translator, A. A. Brill, to a group of intellectuals gathered at Mabel Dodge's legendary salon in New York City. In turn, Dodge, who previously had flirted with Christian Science healing, astrology, and theosophy, now embraced Freud, proselytizing his theories to the shopgirls and secretaries who read her widely syndicated newspaper column. Later Brill would lecture on masturbation to the earnest, apparently sober-faced ladies of the Child Study Association, and by 1916, New York City was home to five hundred self-described psychoanalysts. Those stuck in the boondocks could afford themselves of "Psychoanalysis by Mail."

By 1925, Frank Kent, a newspaperman returning from a nationwide tour, remarked that "between the magazines and the movies a lot of these little towns seem literally saturated with sex."[38] "The veriest schoolgirl today knows as much as the midwife of 1885," cracked H. L. Mencken.[39]

And what did the bra provide for the veriest schoolgirl that a corset did not? Easier access during those "petting parties in the purple dawn." During his courtship of Nora, the muse who inspired Molly Bloom, James Joyce wrote her imploring her to jettison her corset: "Please leave off that breastplate," he wrote. "I do not like embracing a letter-box."[40] Back on this side of the Atlantic girls complained that boys would not dance with them if they were wearing a corset.

If Freud was everywhere, so were Fords. And the two had an intimate relationship. Henry Ford established the first moving assembly line in 1914, and was soon producing 100 Model Ts a day. In 1910, nationwide, fewer than 500,000 passenger automobiles were registered in the entire United States. By 1924 that number of "bedrooms on wheels" had roared to 15.5 million.

Middletown, the classic sociological study of a Midwestern town by Robert S. Lynd and Helen Merrell Lynd, found the automobile to be a serious challenge to virginity. "The threat which the automobile presents to some anxious parents," the

Lynds wrote, "is suggested by the fact that of 30 girls brought before the juvenile court in the twelve months preceding September 1, 1924, charged with 'sex crimes,' for whom the place where the offense occurred was given on the records, nineteen were listed as having committed the offense in an automobile."[41]

The Teen Market

By the 1920s, underwear designers collectively abandoned the idea of supporting the torso and the waist with the same garment. Patent Office records indicate that scores of inventors—half of them women—were attempting to free up the waist at the same time. And what a cornucopia of design possibilities they offered! Few of them, however, bore a strong resemblance to what evolved into the modern bra.

Many of the new bra manufacturers marketed heavily to teenagers. "Warner seems to have pioneered the idea that the immature figure required support by a brassiere," write Jane Farrell-Beck and Colleen Gau. "As early as 1917 [Warner] marketed a 'Growing Girl' design, intended for slender women but with a name that invited youthful patronage and may represent the first advertising of brassieres to teenagers."[42] In 1929, saleswomen in foundation departments urged young women to contrast their sweater profiles in a mirror both with and without a brassiere.

By the 1930s many more firms wooed teens and young adults: Foundettes, Hollywood-Maxwell, Bali, Formfit, Maiden Form, Model, Nature's Rival, Vanity Fair, Hickory, Venus Foundations, Carter, Kayer, and Vassarette. But it would be wrong to conclude that these firms were creating an appetite for bras where none had existed before. The marketplace was clearly a two-way conversation between consumer and seller.

Just look at the word *bra*. Until the early 1930s, advertisements always referred to "brassieres." But by 1934, according to a survey of college slang published in *Harper's Bazaar* in 1934, coeds had truncated brassiere to "bra," just as they had abbreviated pajama to "p.j." The brassiere companies responded quickly—by 1935,

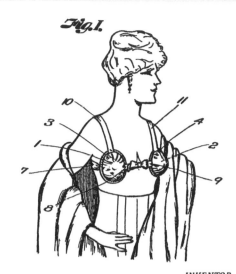

Fig. I.

Kansas City inventor Kaletae Hadley's 1921 bra was fashioned to "prevent the objectionable sagging and hanging of the breasts and at the same time assist the breasts in their natural growth."

INVENTOR
Kaletae Hadley

Warner came out with the A'lure Bra; Carter, Kleinert, and VanRaalte followed with their own "bras" in 1936; and Fay-Miss unveiled its Bali Bra in 1937.[43]

Those companies that did not respond nimbly to the consumer aspirations soon foundered. Virtually all of the manufacturers of paleobrassieres, which did not provide the uplift support that women, especially young women, were seeking, went out of business by the late 1920s.

Boyshform, which successfully produced flapper flatteners, initially seemed a market-savvy firm. Among its successful sales promotions was a giveaway contest held on the Million Dollar Pier in Atlantic City during the second annual Miss America pageant. But by August 1925 it was forced into reorganization. After a failed attempt at marketing flesh-reducing rubber brassieres (Boyshform was not the only firm afflicted with this brainstorm; the perspiration-trapping rubber ensured not only that they were uncomfortable but also that they stank), the firm declared bankruptcy by 1928. Kops Brothers was one of the few protobrassiere companies to make it into the Modern Age. Founded in 1894, Kops did not formally incorporate until thirty years later, in March 1924. At the same time, founders Waldemar and Daniel Kops hired J. Walter Thompson, an innovative market research firm, to take a clear-eyed, nonsentimental look at their product line.

What JWT analysts saw was a stodgy, matronly line of undergarments that, while they had served Kops well during the Gibson girl era, were now seriously out of step with youthful demand. JWT suggested that Kops drop its steel-ribbed corsets altogether and retool its plants to produce elastic corsets and lightweight brassieres.

By 1927, the year of Clara Bow's peekaboo *It* performance, Kops offered an uplift brassiere, featuring cups fitted with darts and a band beneath the breast.

Kops Brothers, which flourished into the late 1960s, was shrewd in other ways as well. Following the lead of winners in other industries, the prime example being Thomas Alva Edison and his electrical empire, the firm patented widely and deeply. Out of approximately two hundred bra patents granted in the United States between 1918 and 1929, Kops received twenty-nine.[44]

Kops also heavily trademarked its brassieres—the Ego, the Lasticurve, Marvel Lace, Little Nemo, Wonderlift—just as it had previously vigorously trademarked

A matronly Kops brassiere design, before the JWT makeover.

all its corsets until then. The Curvmold, the Delta Dip, the Festoon, the Flat-ning, Lasticurve, and Willowshape are some of the dozens of Kops creations.

Equally shrewd was the Maiden Form company, though neither it nor Kops was first on the scene with an uplift bra. The Model Company, for example, showed an "unmistakably contoured brassiere" in the August 1925 *Corset and Underwear Review.*

Although Maiden Form first filed for a patent in 1926, notice of its designs did not appear in *Corset and Underwear Review* until 1927, with its brassiere advertisements coming out a year later, in *Harper's Bazaar.*

The basis of the company was a bandeau-type bra created by two young New York dressmakers, Ida Rosenthal and Enid Bissett. Their design featured breast "pockets"—what today we call cups—that were achieved by stitching a band between the gathered material that covered the breasts. First designed as an integral part of the dresses they designed, the garment emphasized, rather than inhibited, the natural undulations of the breasts.

Maiden Form would later turn out to be on the cutting edge in terms of marketing of bras: In 1932 it boldly hawked bras in New York City bus advertisements. Millions of visitors to the 1939 New York World's Fair were greeted with seventy strategically located neon signs blinking the Maiden Form logo.

Nubbins, Snubbins, and Droopers

With the bra we see a tremendous blurring of the line between "marketing" and "invention." Many of the patented bra inventions are nothing but novelty for novelty's sake. The bra we know today evolved out of lots of designs—most of them silly but some of them sensible. For the central design features of the modern bra did not emerge full blown, like Athena from the brow of Zeus. Rather, they emerged individually over time, as many different inventors groped toward what in the end turned out to be an elegantly simple design solution.

So what are the elements of the modern bra? One of them, certainly, is the idea of individual cups for each breast. Bra inventors faced the intrinsic design challenge of coming up with a uniform design for a wide array of different body types, since breasts come in different shapes and sizes. They can resemble pears, apples, melons, even eggplants or turnips. They can be close together or far apart. Breast tissue can weigh as little as eight ounces in one woman and as much as ten pounds in the next. Buoyant in the young, breasts tend to deflate earthward as they age.[45]

Such observations have been quantified, thanks to some earnest administrator in the Works Projects Administration. The WPA, the Depression-era government agency that employed millions of otherwise unemployable Americans to build such public works as Hoover Dam, also dispatched a team of "gynemetric" measurement takers in the 1930s. Their job? To determine the ideal female figure by measuring a cross section of women—"matron, maid, scrubwoman, show girl"—"in 59 different places"—fifty-nine places on their bodies, that is, as all of the women surveyed lived in New Jersey. The measurement takers' conclusions? That only five percent of women have "ideal" proportions.[46]

Initially, early uplift bra makers appear to have used a stretchy material for the cups to accommodate different breast sizes. The very first firm to identify cup sizes by the letter system (A, B, C, D) was S.H. Camp and Company, based in Jackson, Michigan. Camp prided itself on its "scientific" approach to foundation garments. Indeed, Mr. Camp, president of the company, imported a transparent nude female anatomical model from Germany and sent it on a national tour. Its first stop was the New York Museum of Science and Industry.

Camp's cup system was not, however, meant to address the size of the breast. Rather, it assessed the relative firmness of the breast—A being pert and D being saggy. (Ruth Kapinas, a pioneer in bra design at Munsingwear, devised her own unofficial nomenclature: "nubbins, snubbins, droopers, and super-droopers.")[47] Formfit Company announced a sizing system in October of 1932 that not only offered cups in small, medium, and large but also offered a range of band sizes (34 inch, 36 inch,

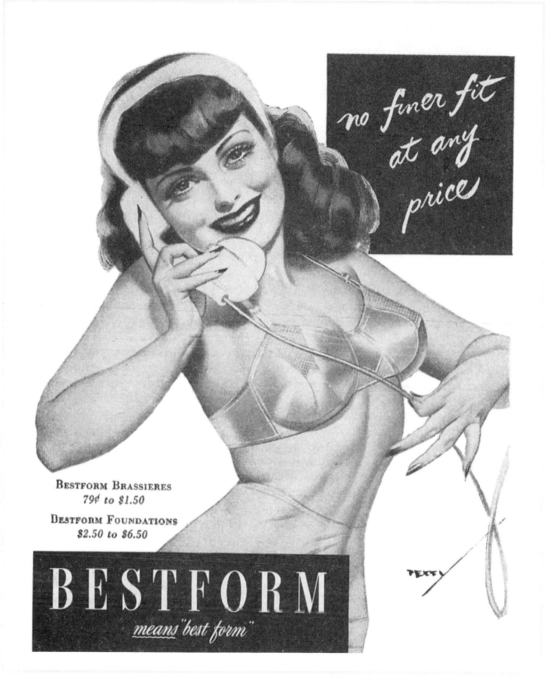

no finer fit at any price

BESTFORM BRASSIERES
79¢ to $1.50

BESTFORM FOUNDATIONS
$2.50 to $6.50

BESTFORM
means "best form"

A 1940s ad.

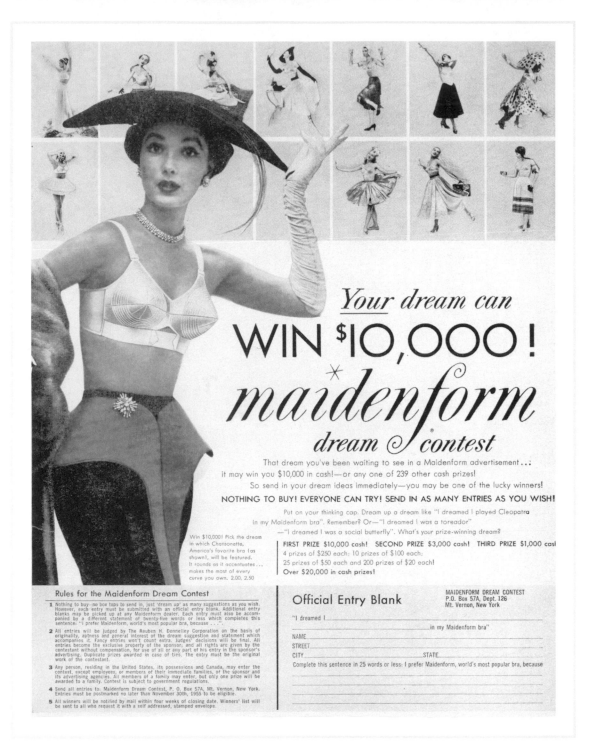

Kickoff ad for the Maidenform "I Dreamed" campaign.

38 inch, for example—a feature that would become another essential element of the modern bra).

Other firms soon borrowed both of these ideas, transforming them into a standardized breast-sizing system. By the late 1930s, Warner, Model, and Fay-Miss all offered cup sizes in A through D. Maiden Form, which had devised its own sizing system, did not give in to standardized sizing until the 1940s.

One of the most important innovations in the evolution of the bra was the invention of Lastex. It came on the market in October 1931 and Depression-weary "foundation manufacturers seized it like a life preserver."[48]

Percy Adamson came up with the material when he worked for the New York–based U.S. Rubber Company. Once it was perfected, he set up a spin-off company, Adamson Brothers, for distribution. Essentially, Lastex was rubber that had been extruded into tiny filaments, each one wrapped in a double cocoon of cotton, rayon, or silk.

Unlike natural rubber, which split easily when sewn on industrial machines and degraded steadily with use, Lastex was light, washable, and resilient. Not overly resilient, however. The Lastex bra wore out more quickly than its ironsided ancestor, the steel-ribbed coutil corset, and thus it offered a quality paramount to modern commerce: built-in obsolescence. True, brassieres were cheaper to begin with, but the trade estimated that a woman might buy four brassieres to every corset that she purchased.

Lastex's two-way stretch helped solve the sizing challenges inherent in designing an intimate, close-fitting garment for women of every shape and size. *Women's Wear Daily* went so far as to claim, in its November 11, 1932, issue that Lastex had "wiped out the depression for the foundation garment industry by raising the unit price with increased profits for manufacturer and retailer."[49] Warner Brothers Company president John Field, whose firm had introduced in 1933 the A'lure line, made of pieced sections of Lastex, went even further, calling the adoption of Lastex "the greatest change in the corset field any of us have ever witnessed."[50]

While not a standard feature, underwires soon became an important option on bras. A precursor to the idea of the underwire is a brassiere patented by Marie Tucek of New York City in 1893. Her entire bra was meant to be constructed of either sheet metal or cardboard and then covered with silk or cotton. Another pioneer in underwire was Leon Hain, a Russian exile living in Philadelphia. Hain's invention was a wide metal band wrapped around the torso with breast pockets made of "some knitted or crocheted material which will conform to the shape of the breast and snugly confine the same."[51]

Neither of these ideas appears to have caught on. But in 1931, Helen Pons patented an underwire scheme that became the first to be mass produced. By 1938, Beautee-Fit Brassiere Company of Los Angeles patented a modern-looking U-shaped wire insertion to "afford greater separation of the breasts and so achieve a more natural contour."[52] These bras, however, were not good enough for Howard Hughes, the aerospace magnate turned moviemaker who was legendary for his personal idiosyncrasies.

Hughes became obsessed with Jane Russell's cleavage when he began filming *The Outlaw* in 1941. "We're not getting enough production out of Jane's breasts," he reportedly lamented.[53] His complaints were made known to the wardrobe mistress, who dryly retorted that she was a designer, not an architect.

So Hughes got out a paper and pencil himself and had a prototype worked up for an aerodynamic bra that got its lift from underwire. Russell, then a va-va-voom receptionist in a chiropodist's office who was getting her first big acting break, claimed she never wore the bra. Instead, she ended up wearing her own bra, carefully layering tissue over it to smooth out the bra straps. Hughes's creation, she said, was "absolutely ridiculous-looking." "[B]elieve me," she wrote in her autobiography, "he could design planes, but a Mister Playtex he wasn't."[54]

By 1950 most bras had modern features: cups, an adjustable torso band, and stretchable, adjustable straps (Warner claimed that it spent $1 million in R&D to achieve these, for which it received U.S. patent 298,067), and an optional feature of underwires. But why didn't the bra turn out to be just a transient fad, a passing amusement of the young? How is it that the corset become permanently bifurcated?

Breasts as a Matter of
National Security

We can look, in part, to war for an explanation. Two wars, actually. By World War I, 2 million women in America worked in business offices. By 1930, more than 10 million women held jobs—flying airplanes, driving taxis, collecting streetcar fares, and directing traffic.

As they became increasingly physically active, women had all the more reason to seek undergarments that gave their bodies both support and flexibility.

"The predominance of the brassiere is an outgrowth of a dress habit in South-ern California," proclaimed the *Corset and Underwear Review* in its November 1943 issue. "Everybody from 13 to 90 wears brassieres, except perhaps a very few flat-busted women. Even many of those are using a corrective type to help the develop-ment of their breasts."[55]

Some manufacturers, like Lockheed, required bras to be worn on the job ei-ther for reasons of "good taste" or because they thought bras were a structural ne-cessity for women working a forty-eight-hour week. Other companies even outfitted their wartime assembly-line women with plastic protective mammary gear. East of the Mississippi, the Strauss Company of Pittsburgh issued its female employees "a set of flesh-colored, moulded, vulcanized fibre breast protectors" that came in three sizes.[56]

Respondents to a survey taken by *Corset and Underwear Review* in 1943 and 1944 were not completely satisfied with wartime bras, but they liked them more than corsets. In large part this preference was a consequence of wartime shortages of rub-ber and its substitutes as well as shortages of metals. Before the war, nine tenths of the U.S. rubber supply had been imported from East Asia, but after Japan's attack on Pearl Harbor those imports ceased.

The War Production Board had a strong national security motivation to take control of national rubber supplies. Given that 1,750 pounds of rubber went into a medium-size tank while a battleship required 150,000 pounds, it was hard to argue that women's underwear was a national priority. But that's exactly what Maiden Form did.

Dr. Louis Landaw, a physician in Paterson, New Jersey, wrote a letter in support of Maiden Form's case that bras were essential to national security. "Breast supports are generally more essential than abdominal supports," he wrote. "The back and abdominal muscles can and should be easily developed to give necessary support. This is not the case with breasts since no control can be exercised over their size or the strength of their supporting muscles."

Unsupported breasts caused fatigue, Dr. Landaw argued, and they also served as "distraction to male associates." He closed his letter with what he apparently considered his most compelling claim: that "the breasts are an erogenous area and the friction of the outer clothing can prove disturbing to the woman herself."[57]

Clearly these lobbying efforts worked, as the bra was declared an essential item. Not that Maiden Form was not doing its patriotic share. It provided the U.S. military with undergarments but also mattress covers, bush shirts, and even parachute vests for carrier pigeons (basically a one-cup bra with straps and corset lacing); this pigeon straitjacket kept the bird still so that it could safely jump to earth with a paratrooper.

By May 1942 the quantity of elastic permitted in foundations was reduced to fifty percent of what had been used before the war, and corsets were largely made of nonstretch materials. War Production Board regulations specified that brassiere straps could contain only two and a half inches of elastic, and elastic insertions in the body of the bra could be no more than six to eight square inches, depending on the style.

Before the war, the bra had been worn primarily by the young and adventurous. World War II made the bra the support garment of choice for even the middle aged and conservative. By the time the war ended in 1945 and rubber and metal supplies for consumers were once more abundant, most American women had grown more comfortable in a bra than a corset. Which is not to say that the corset became extinct. It abbreviated itself to the girdle and transmuted into an elastic mold made sequentially of a parade of new wonder synthetics: neoprene, nylon, and spandex.

Dangerous Curves Ahead

In April of 1932, *Vogue* was already declaring that "Spring styles say CURVES!"[58] A year later, the amply endowed Mae West was wowing moviegoers with her performance in *She Done Him Wrong*. Lily of France was advertising a bra that "beautifully emphasizes the uplift bust," and Formfit assured that its bras would give breasts "youthful, pointed, uplifted lines."[59]

The bra itself was not up to providing curves where none existed. So falsie innovators filled the void. In 1932, Gabrielle M. Poix, a bra innovator, introduced Cuties, round bust pads made of layered net fabric that could be worn "without anyone, even the wearer, being conscious of them."[60]

So popular were Los Angeles–based designer Madelon Louden's NueDé forms—"Perfect As Nature Itself"—that she expanded distribution to East Coast stores in 1935. Louden claimed that they "originated in a motion picture studio in Hollywood." The forms were constructed of "flesh-colored chiffon that is shaded slightly darker over the natural looking tip" and came in five graduated sizes, ranging from "rosebuds" to "surgicals."[61]

In 1935, Hollywood-Maxwell produced bust forms made of crocheted angora, which the company boasted came "in larger sizes than last season's bust tips."[62] That same year the Maiden Form Company, an early pioneer of the brassiere, was urging its salesmen to push its new Masquerade line, a bra into which foam-rubber falsies could be inserted. While these falsies were perhaps closer to human flesh than any that had come before, they had a major drawback. After a few launderings they turned hard as rock.

By 1940 the Sears catalog offered two styles of Flatterettes. These bras featured little pockets into which pads of whipped Latex or shirred net could be inserted. Falsie production came to a screeching halt in 1941, however, when the U.S. government banned their manufacture so that rubber could be diverted to the war effort. It is doubtful that they would have been a popular item during World War II anyway, since they would have gotten in the way on the assembly line as women took over men's jobs in factories. Besides which, most of the men who would have been interested in their curvature, enhanced or otherwise, were off at war.

At the same time that the falsie industry was expanding to meet the market demands of the poorly endowed, breast reduction surgery, pioneered in the 1920s, was becoming increasingly performed by surgeons who considered extremely large breasts to be a debilitating condition (termed *gigantomastia*). Many breast reductions, wrote Lois Mattox Miller in the *Independent Woman* in 1939, "are motivated by vanity and the desire for a more fashionable figure; but most physicians and psychiatrists now admit that there are innumerable cases in which it is not only advisable but essential to a woman's mental and emotional well-being."[63]

But once the war was over, falsies achieved their greatest popularity ever. Christian Dior introduced his voluptuous New Look in 1947, proclaiming that without foundation there is no fashion. In 1948 the medical author of *The Hygiene of the Breasts* observed a collective impulse to "comply with the present Hollywood rule which requires that the bust measurement be one inch greater than that of the hips."[64] The job descriptions for female acting jobs in Hollywood during that era might as well have read "Only big busts need apply."[65]

This meant that ordinary women were trying to emulate the ample figures of screen stars like Marilyn Monroe, Gina Lollobrigida, Jayne Mansfield, and Anita Ekberg. Since most breasts are not naturally shaped like pointy-tipped projectiles, women filled out their bras with a new type of cone-shaped falsie referred to by some as an amplifier. Sales for these amplifiers appear to have rocketed skyward through the end of the forties and early fifties. In 1951 the Sears, Roebuck catalog offered a veritable cornucopia of falsies: twenty-two different types!

But by the mid-1950s falsie sales had plummeted. Why the rapid descent in

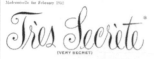
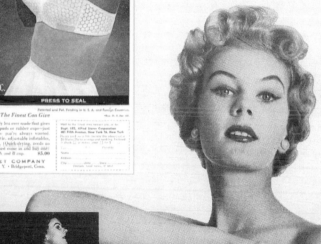
The Très Secrète was inflated through a little plastic straw.

The Bra-o-matic, a nylon taffeta strapless bra, could be adjusted by pressing a button that rotated the underwire and thus changed the degree to which the breasts were pushed up.

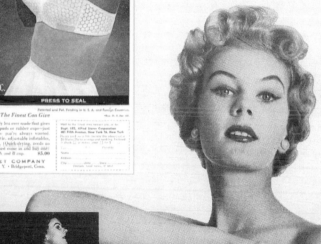
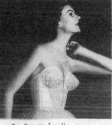

Water powered the Lady Bountiful's vacuum pump.

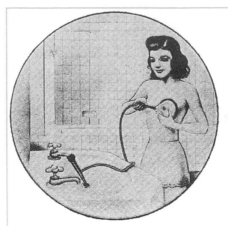

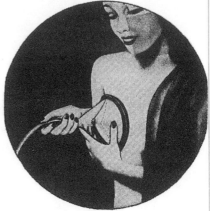

Easy To Use

(a) Attach vacuum unit to the COLD water faucet.

(b) Turn on the water — full force.

(c) Place plastic cup snugly over breast.

(d) Place thumb over the small opening on the tube near the cup, and hold the thumb there until the vacuum (created by the flowing water) pulls the breast out fully into the cup.

(e) After breast has been pulled into the cup, release thumb suddenly and allow the breast to return to original position.

(f) Continue this process — thumb alternately on and off.

How To Fit the Lady Bountiful

The above illustration shows the proper position of the plastic cup on the breast. Note that when the right thumb is pressed firmly over the small opening in tube, the vacuum created pulls the breast out to the proper position. When the thumb is removed from the opening (note dotted line) the vacuum is released and the breast reverts to its former position.

The LADY BOUNTIFUL operates on the natural principle of a vacuum and uses the perfectly natural processes of exercise to develop tissue which has remained dormant and inactive.

The women who are most highly satisfied with the results they have received are those who have exercised with the LADY BOUNTIFUL faithfully over sufficient lengths of time. To these satisfied users there is no question but that LADY BOUNTIFUL has helped them attain a more symmetrical development.

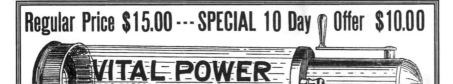
Vacuum power was a favorite entrepreneurial approach for pumping up the manly organs as well.

the popularity of falsies, given that the chesty look remained popular for certain women throughout the decade? In part it may have been the result of Dior's short-lived "flat look," introduced in 1954. (Marilyn Monroe quipped that there were not enough Diors in Paris to flatten her.)[66]

Dior's proclamation that the bra was passé notwithstanding, new advances in underwear technology—that is, the padded bra—brought a quick revival of the sweater-girl profile. Bra makers figured out how to incorporate the falsie into the bra, stiffening it by stitching foam rubber directly onto it; thus, the padded bra rendered obsolete time-honored falsies (although it must be noted that during the nineteenth century some women had sewn pads directly into their dresses, so the padded bra was never an altogether original idea).

Not that women had given up hope of increasing the size of their actual breasts. The $29.95 Abunda, with its two pink plastic breast-shaped cones, attached by a hose to the kitchen faucet, was advertised in the late 1950s as the means to achieve a perfect bust by hydromassage. As with its competitor, The Lady Bountiful, no water actually touched the breast; rather, a mild vacuum occurred when water ran past a tube connected to the breast-cup hose.

"Gentle, dancing waters . . . soothing, yet invigorating . . . massage and awaken the body to the call of increased circulation," read the Abunda advertising. "Hydro-massage truly works a magic only Nature can perform . . . a phenomenon impossible to be copied by Man."[67] On October 17, 1960, the U.S. Food & Drug Administration confiscated 380 of the devices plus 89 display units in Albuquerque, New Mexico, after an FDA investigation showed that the machine could not deliver the promises made in the company's promotional material.

Writer Nora Ephron humorously recalled that, in her days as a flat-chested preteen in the 1950s, she bought a Mark Eden Bust Developer, which was supposed to build up breasts through exercise. More impressive in effect, however, were the three padded bras she purchased in three different sizes. They allowed her to go from "nice perky but not too obtrusive breasts" in one week to "medium-sized slightly pointy" breasts in the next week. By the third week she was sporting "knockers, true knockers."

Indecent Exposure

During the 1950s and 1960s, Maidenform (having altered its name from Maiden Form) advertised its bras in its famous "I Dreamed" campaign. Models were portrayed bare chested save for their bra but otherwise impeccably dressed doing all manner of things—shopping, boxing, even running for public office.

"The Dream ads spoke for an American culture on the verge of a sexual revolution," writes Marilyn Yalom in A History of the Breast. "Breasts themselves were still carefully covered and packaged, but the very fact that women were shown in their brassieres in a number of unlikely public settings inched the fantasy of sexual freedom closer to reality."[68]

The Harvard Lampoon in 1961 ran a parody of the Maidenform Dream ads featuring a bra-clad I Dreamed model being arrested by two cops. "I dreamed I was arrested for indecent exposure in my Maidenform bra," the caption reads.[69]

Maidenform anticipated the braless trend with its Half-Way bra, which it introduced to the market a decade too early. "Literally half a brassiere," according to a company history, "it supported the bust beneath and left the top of the bust fabric-free, this for the benefit of extroverts who liked to boast they wore no bra at all."[70]

Others tried to invent the braless bra. The Bleumette, for example, was advertised in every major fashion magazine in 1957, a backless, strapless stick-on half-cup bra that ostensibly could be reworn. When making Vertigo that same year, Alfred Hitchcock playfully has Jimmy Stewart's platonic friend Midge, an advertising artist, sketching one of these feats of aerodynamics.

What ultimately threatened to dethrone the bra from its new perch was not a rival upstart foundation garment but rather the trend toward bralessness itself. Small breasts had never gone out of style. Even in the busty 1950s, Audrey Hepburn, with her trademark, highly tailored Givenchy look, was so small breasted that a bra was incidental. But increasingly during the 1960s bone-thin models like Twiggy dominated magazine spreads.

"Lingerie is finished," declared the French fashion icon Yves Saint Laurent.[71] It was a self-serving remark, given that he had just introduced a line of see-through clothes. Even so he captured the zeitgeist of the era. That same year, 1968, feminists staged a mock bra-burning at the Miss America contest. For bralessness was not just an aesthetic, it was a symbol of sexual freedom. The Pill, first imagined in the 1950s, was now on the market, and while women had been exerting increasing reproductive control for more than a century, it provided at least the illusion of unprecedented sexual autonomy.

Bralessness went mainstream when Marlo Thomas cast hers off on *That Girl*, her popular TV series about a single New York career woman. "God created women to bounce," Thomas declared. "So be it."[72] Thomas and hippie chicks notwithstanding, gravity—and the figure-shaping properties of the bra—prevailed. In 1968, American women bought more bras than they ever had before.

A Surgical Arms Race

Given the long innovative drive to create lifelike breast enhancements, it is perhaps inevitable that women ultimately resorted to surgery. Breast augmentation had been experimented with by legitimate physicians since Dr. Robert Gersuny of Vienna attempted the first paraffin injection in the 1890s. Paraffin was abandoned by the time of World War I (it had an unfortunate tendency to migrate to other parts of the body). Instead, doctors of the 1920s and 1930s transplanted fatty tissue from buttocks and belly into the breasts. Alas, this often was reabsorbed by the body—in lumpy and unflattering ways.

"Surgeons began the postwar years with a distinct lack of sympathy for the problems of small-breasted women, but this attitude changed quickly as women—encouraged by fashion magazines and inspired by movie stars such as Jane Russell and Marilyn Monroe to fill out Dior's 'New look'—clamored for new solutions," according to Elizabeth Haiken in her masterful history of plastic surgery.[73]

Not surprisingly, surgeons in Los Angeles led the way. In 1950 an article published in *Plastic and Reconstructive Surgery* for the first time proclaimed small breasts a deformity and even gave this newly recognized "disability" a name: hypomastia. This followed by some four decades the medical profession's identification of a similar "malady"—small-penis disease.

Small-breast disease was the focus of the August 1953 issue of *Pageant*, a popular Sunday supplement. The magazine reported that Robert Alan Franklyn had invented a novel way to help the more than four million women in the United States suffering from the ailment of "micromastia." Franklyn professed the humanitarian goal of wanting to help "girls and women whose neuroses had been traced definitely to the fact that they were flat-chested."[74]

Franklyn, whose medical credentials were legitimate if less than sterling (he did graduate from New York University Medical School, but there is no proof that he served residencies or was ever board certified), surgically inserted a mystery substance that he called Surgifoam but which is believed to have been regular old polyurethane.

During the ensuing decade, other surgeons in pursuit of the perfect augmentation would insert a number of other foreign materials into the breast: glass balls, terylene, wood, cartilage, polyvinyl sponges, and even Teflon. According to Joan Kron, plastic surgeon John Pangman, a breast-implant pioneer, implanted Ivalon sponges in Marilyn Monroe's breasts in the 1950s.

In 1956, *Cosmopolitan* magazine ran an article entitled "Monroes on the Increase." Indeed, many women first learned of breast enhancement through popular magazines, including about half of the women in a 1958 study at Johns Hopkins University, conducted by a plastic surgeon and a psychiatrist. The point was to discover the motivations of the women, a third of whom, like Marilyn Monroe, had Ivalon sponge implants.

All of the women in the study felt that "wearing padded bras or falsies was "phony" and like "cheating."[75] As one woman put it: "One might be in an accident and be found out and feel ashamed that one couldn't face people again." All but two of the thirty-two women were "extremely pleased" with their implants, with some saying that they "changed my entire life." This transformation of self-image held up over time, according to the study. Still, Ivalon was far from perfect. Breast tissue tended to invade the sponge, which then hardened, and it was found to cause cancer in rats. So the quest for a better implant material continued.

Silicone Summits

Silicone came of age just before World War II, in an era that celebrated all things synthetic. Made up of oxygen and silicon molecules strung together like beads on a necklace, it was a miracle industrial lubricant that would not break down at high temperatures. Soon, many health-care applications were found. Silicone rubber, for example, was used to replace damaged urethras.

Silicone did not initially make its way into women's breasts through the normal channels of medical research. Because of their underground nature, the origins of liquid silicone breast injections are nebulous. But according to a 1992 report in *The New York Times*, they were first performed on Japanese prostitutes who, catering to occupying American troops, felt that larger, Western-style breasts might garner more clients.

Industrial-grade silicone—not the purer, medical-grade stuff—started disappearing mysteriously off the docks of the Yokohama Harbor in the postwar years. Cosmetologists injected it straight into the breasts, along with some cottonseed or croton oil, so that immediate scarring would ensue and thus contain the silicone at the sight of injection.

Silicone breast injection did not really catch on in the United States until the 1960s—ironically, during the same era that Twiggy and her gamine look-alikes reigned on the pages of fashion magazines. One San Francisco topless dancer in particular, Carol Doda, is credited with spurring a bustward expansion in Nevada and California. After inflating from a thirty-six-inch to a forty-four-inch bustline, the blond, Watusi-dancing Doda proclaimed that "every girl should be as large as her dreams." She received weekly half-ounce injections of silicone for twenty weeks. This totaled nearly a pint per breast by the time she was finished.

Doda generously gave advice to customers. "Why lots of times a man will come in here with his wife or date; she'll be kind of flat and I can see her looking at me all through my act," said a colleague of Doda's who also got silicone injections. "Then she'll write me a letter—she's ashamed of her looks and wants to know who my doctor was. I always tell them."[76]

"These women, desperate for larger breasts, believed that a perfect method for breast enlargement existed and that the only reason hospitals did not offer it was

Woman's Home Companion *ad,* *1950.*

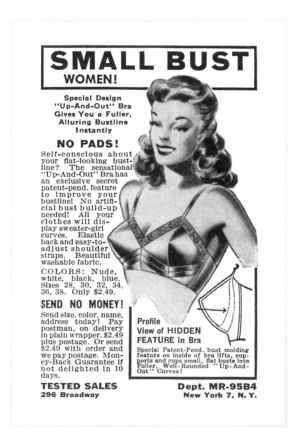

that physicians did not take women's concerns seriously," according to Elizabeth Haiken. "By going 'outside' regular channels, these women believed, they were criticizing organized medicine for not responding to their needs at the same time they were getting those needs met."[77]

But women were not the only ones getting silicone injected into their bodies. So were men who wanted bigger penises. Cases of a horrible new disease called "silicone rot," in which gangrene set in around the injected silicone and resulted in amputations, were reported by the medical profession in men as well as in women.[78]

So, too, were men pioneers in receiving silicone implants, silicone encased in a rubber envelope so that it would expressly not migrate. Harvey Lash developed the silicone penile implant in 1961 to treat impotence. That is the same year that Baylor University surgical resident Frank Gerow squeezed a plastic blood bag and, remarking how much it felt like a woman's breast, in an "aha" moment first conceived of the silicone breast implant.

"Patients were told that the implants were safe, that they would last forever, because that was what the doctors believed," writes journalist Mimi Swartz. "They're as harmless," Gerow used to say, "as water."[79]

The first silicone-implant recipient was Timmie Jean Lindsey, who showed up at a charity hospital one day in 1962 to see about removing her tattoos—red roses, "one over each breast, climbing like twin vines from her cleavage."

Gerow and his partner, Thomas Cronin, inserted the implants into Lindsey and six weeks later she was bar-hopping, wearing a crop-top blouse that hung on her breasts in a whole new way. "The men just—well, that was a boost to my morale," she told Swartz. "I thought I would never meet anyone. I thought I would never marry again. But, boy things began to look up after that."

Cosmopolitan magazine could not have agreed more. Breasts plumped with silicone implants were firm and round and would not sag or droop. "The fact of the matter is," *Cosmo* enthused, "that surgically augmented breasts have a *better* contour than the real thing."[80]

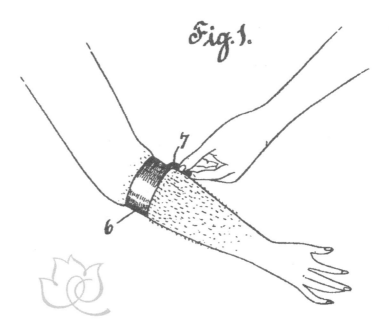

Fig. 1.

Hair

And I have known the arms already, known them all—
Arms that are braceleted and white and bare
(But in the lamplight, downed with light brown hair!)

— T. S. Eliot, 1917

In regard to the general hairiness of the body, the women in all
races are less hairy than the men. . . .

— Charles Darwin, 1871

When it comes to hair, women have devoted large portions of their lifetimes to curling it, straightening it, and coloring it. But perhaps the most basic beauty question hair-wise is not how to make it look more alluring but rather how to get rid of it. Whether a fuzzy forearm, a shadow on the upper lip, or some straggling hairs on the chin, hair removal has been a fundamental, though largely unchronicled, pulchritudinal preoccupation of women.

Hair removal, at least in American society, is in a different class from virtually any other womanly enhancement. For the goal is often not, as with most beauty inventions, to exaggerate femaleness but rather to minimize maleness.

When compared to some of their counterparts in other species, male and female humans look an awful lot alike. Consider the bright blue face of the male mandrill baboon, the lofty antlers of a male moose, and the gargantuan size of a male elephant seal, which can be as much as eight times as big as any given mate.

What does the male human have in terms of what evolutionists call sexual display? A modest amount of muscle mass, of course. A little size advantage. But beyond that, it's mainly body hair. So, perhaps, it is self evident why women have been scraping hair off various parts of their bodies for millennia: to prove they are not men.

The impulse to depilate stretches way back in time. The Koran, for example, tells of the Queen of Sheba's visit to King Solomon. When she was ushered into the great hall for an audience with the king, she saw her reflection in the floor of gleaming glass and, thinking that it was a pool of water, raised her robes high to wade

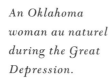

An Oklahoma woman au naturel during the Great Depression.

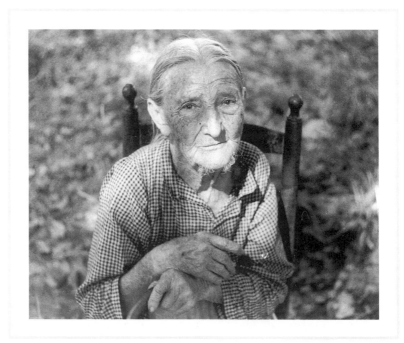

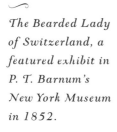

The Bearded Lady of Switzerland, a featured exhibit in P. T. Barnum's New York Museum in 1852.

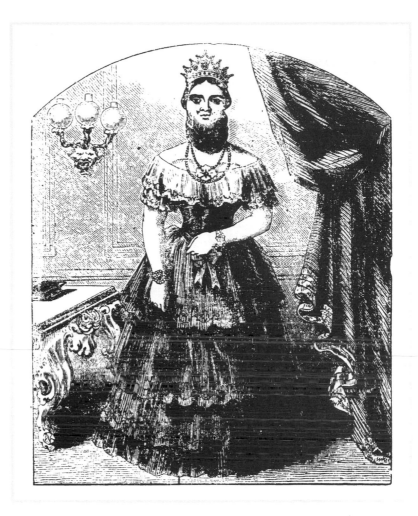

through it. The king was reportedly "amazed and disgusted" at the sight of her hairy legs.[1]

Certainly, throughout the ages, different cultures around the world have prized hairlessness on the body. But in the West a huge cultural shift occurred somewhere around the middle of the nineteenth century that made body hair on the American woman, particularly facial hair, especially repulsive.

Until then, women "in the change of life" could raise a crop of chin fuzz without great disgrace. And downy upper lips, while not revered as the symbol of femininity as they were in Asian cultures, were at least tolerated.

By contrast, from the time of the American Revolution to the Civil War, most men were clean-shaven. Indeed, "it had been so long since men wore beards that those who first tried to revive them were looked upon as freaks," according to Bill Severn.[2]

Consider the example of Joseph Palmer, a utopian schemer and friend of Emerson and Thoreau. When Mr. Palmer moved to Fitchburg, Massachusetts, in the 1830s, he was denounced as a "fiend incarnate" for wearing a beard. Even in more cosmopolitan Boston, his beard "attracted such a threatening street crowd that he finally had to be rescued by police."[3]

Around the mid-nineteenth century the fashion began to change for Western men. In London, an 1847 book was published by the title of *Beard Shaving and the Common Use of the Razor; an Unnatural, Irrational, Unmanly, Ungodly and Fatal Fashion among Christians.*"[4]

Napoleon III, who proclaimed himself emperor of France in 1852, sported a tuft of a goatee and a wide twirled waxed mustache, and his followers soon imitated his trademark look. Horace Greeley, the New York newspaper editor who admonished a generation to "Go West, young man," popularized the chin-saucer type of beard, while those who really did go west—gold-hungry prospectors on their way to California, for example—left their razors completely behind.

By the time the first shots of the Civil War were fired at Fort Sumter, sundering a nation in two politically, "there was a national unity in whiskers," Severn writes. "North and South, East and West, and for no clear reason, nearly all American men, middle-aged and older as well as young started to grow facial hair and went on growing it for a generation."[5]

But these male beards hardly appeared for "no clear reason." For the Victorian mind had become obsessed with body hair and its role in distinguishing not just between the sexes but also between races.

This was because the new science of anthropology, which was busy classifying humans by physiological traits such as skin color, physique type, and head shape, ostensibly gave credibility to the theories of racial determinism and white supremacy then percolating in the white consciousness.

Charles Darwin's theory of natural selection, published in 1859, was invoked to bolster this dubious anthropology, "emphasizing as it did the preservation of some species at the expense of others in the great struggle for life," according to historian Cynthia Eagle Russett writing in *Darwin in America*.[6]

Twelve years later, Darwin published his follow-up theory of sexual selection. Darwin argued that there was very little difference between the races of man. But he did note racial differences and these were trumpeted by certain members of the white ruling classes, who seized upon this as evidence of their own race's inherent superiority.

One of the purveyors of this "cult of the Anglo-Saxon" was Knight Dunlap, a professor of experimental psychology at Johns Hopkins University who wrote a book called *Personal Beauty and Racial Betterment*. Male body hair, he argued, indicated procreative fitness. Likewise, a lack of hair (except on the head and in the pubic area) indicated a woman's worthiness as a reproductive specimen. "The hairlessness of the female face and body, and the hairiness of the male face (or the evidence that the hair grows, although shaved off) are important elements of beauty," he wrote.[7]

The beard became an exalted symbol of virility by the late 1850s. "Deprive the lion of his mane, the cock of his comb, the peacock of the emerald plumage of his tail, the ram and deer of their horns, and they not only become displeasing to the eye, but lose much of their power and vigor," wrote Alexander Rowland. "The caprice of fashion alone forces the Englishman to shave off those appendages which give the male countenance that true masculine character indicative of energy, bold daring, and decision."[8]

Unlike Professor Dunlap, however, Mr. Rowland was no theorist; his arguments for the return of the beard were intended to drum up business for his hair products company. As whiskers were being associated ever more with masculinity, a bearded lady became an uncomfortable sight. Small wonder, then, that Western women became preoccupied with "excess" body hair during the last quarter of the nineteenth century. For a lack of body hair ostensibly indicated an advanced state of evolution and vice versa.

Not that this was a terribly logical argument. It made sense if Anglo-Saxons were trying to prove the evolutionary inadequacies of Jewish and Irish women, who did tend to sport more facial hair than the average Caucasian. But it made no sense at all—that is, if one assumed that such impulses to stereotype could ever make "sense"—when it came to women of African descent and Native American women. Those women, both targets of Anglo-Saxon condescension, were reputed to have much less facial hair than the average Caucasian.

Removing Roots

Members of the American Dermatological Association, a newly minted society in 1877, recognized an entrepreneurial gold mine when they saw one. They gave the age-old phenomenon of female body hair an ominous new name: hypertri-chosis.

Soon they had no lack of clients—women who complained of hair growing on their breasts, their abdomens, their necks, and even their tongues. George Henry Fox, an early practitioner of electrolysis whose office was at 18 East 31st in New York City, laid out the scenario in his 1886 tome, *The Use of Electricity in the Removal of Facial Hair and the Treatment of Various Facial Blemishes.*

"The growth of hair upon the female face is a deformity which is very fre-quently observed," he wrote. "Perhaps few physicians have an adequate idea of its prevalence. In nearly every 'museum of living curiosities' a bearded woman figures as one of the chief attractions, and it is quite probable that but a small proportion of bearded women are willing to advertise their misfortune for pecuniary gain."[9]

He then went on to itemize a half-dozen professional bearded ladies:

1. Mrs. Viola Meyers has a full beard, the hairs being soft, dark
and somewhat curly. The abnormal growth was noticed
during childhood. A full report of this case was published by

[Louis Adolphus] Duhring in the *Archives of Dermatology*, April, 1877.

2. Susie Conrad has a reddish-brown beard and weighs 300 pounds.

3. Annie Jones has a long dark-brown beard which began to grow in infancy.

4. Millie Rose, a French-Canadian woman, has a heavy mustache and beard.

5. Mrs. Krebs has not only a heavy beard but a considerable growth of hair upon the arms.

6. Mrs. Squires has a full beard upon chin and neck but the upper lip is comparatively free.[10]

Dr. Fox said he could not estimate the percentage of women thus afflicted. Hundreds of women, he said, could no doubt "raise a thick and long growth of hair which would deserve the name of a beard" but the number of women with moderate facial hair was "beyond computation."

"We note instances of this hypertrichosis on every hand, in the drawing-room, upon the street, or wherever ladies congregate, and could we but know the secrets of the boudoir we would be surprised to find how large a percentage of our female acquaintances resort occasionally, if not habitually, to the use of the depilatory, the razor, or the tweezers."[11]

Dr. Henrietta P. Johnson, a contemporary of Dr. Fox, eschewed the term *hypertrichosis* in favor of the daintier diminutive "facial hirsuties." But she offered similar observations.[12]

"I know of one beautiful and attractive woman who would not marry, lest the hairy tendency which had made her own life a wretched one, and which she had tried by every known artifice to conceal, might be transmitted to her female offspring," Dr. Johnson wrote.

"The number of women who do not in one way or another attempt to remove the conspicuous hairs from some part of the face by the use of tweezers, scissors, razors, or epilatory nostrums is decidedly in the minority."[13]

Dr. Johnson and Dr. Fox said they had yet to determine any pattern to those afflicted with "hirsuties." Some were athletic, others weak; some nervous, others phlegmatic; some fat, some thin; some blond, some brunette; some mothers, others childless.

Although women began to pursue hairlessness with vigor, the tools at their disposal in the second half of the nineteenth century were quite primitive.

Depilatory creams, not much improved from ancient formulations, often consisted of quicklime and a form of arsenic and as such were dangerous. "I have known several unfortunate ladies to produce ulcers and dangerous sores" with such compounds, warned Lola Montez, a notorious courtesan and actress who apparently knew a thing or two about facial hair.[14]

Since this was long before an efficacious slant-edged tweezers was mass produced, Montez also warned against tweezing ("a fruitless task, for they almost invariably break off the hair at the neck, instead of pulling it out at the roots"). Nor was she a fan of shaving ("even though the shaving were done every day, the blue or black roots of the hair show further than the hair itself").[15]

Montez also spoke dismissively about "the cauterizing remedy," and rightly so. Some in the medical profession attempted to arrest hair growth by inserting an unsterile needle into the hair follicle, the idea being that an inflammation would ensue and seal up the follicular canal, thus blocking the passage of any new hair growth to the surface of the skin.

But that was just one of several hair-removal horror shows. Other techniques involved injecting carbolic acid with a hypodermic needle or jabbing a barbed needle into the hair follicle and rapidly twisting it.[16] Perhaps the most potentially disfiguring approach was known as "punching," in which a slender cylindrical knife was pushed into the skin and the entire hair shaft, including the skin around it, extracted, like the core of an apple.[17] This method, not surprisingly, never really caught on.

Montez advocated what today might be called waxing. "Spread on a piece of leather equal parts of galbanum and pitch plaster, and lay it on the culprit hairs as smoothly as possible," she advised, "and then, after letting it remain about three minutes, pull it off suddenly, and it will be quite sure to bring out the hairs by the roots, and they will not grow again."[18] This type of waxing was likely effective in removing those fine downy hairs known as lanugo, but probably not terribly effective at pulling out the coarse darker hair that, for many women, was the real beauty challenge.

So when Dr. Charles Michel, a St. Louis ophthalmologist, reported in 1875 that he had successfully been extracting in-grown eyelashes with a battery-powered needle epilator since 1869, his colleagues lost no time figuring out how to employ the same technique to remove stray chin hairs and mustachios from ladies. For the first time, it seemed, women now had a way to remove unwanted hair permanently and safely.

Powered by direct current, the method was called electrolysis because it was thought to "electrocute" the hair. In fact, the electrical current caused a chemical reaction in the hair follicle that produced sodium hydroxide—essentially lye, the active ingredient found in caustic drain openers—thereby deadening the hair root. The standard office was outfitted with a large chair, a galvanic battery, a rheostat, a galvanometer, two insulated wires or conductors, one sponge-electrode, one needle holder, a case of jewelers' broaches (needles), and one pair of forceps for pulling out the hairs.

Dr. Johnson, the nineteenth-century electrolysis expert, provided step-by-step instructions in her book. "The patient being placed in position, near a northern window if possible, to secure the best light, is directed to hold the insulated handle of the sponge-electrode (wetted with warm water) in her right hand. The needle is then placed at the side of a hair and allowed to glide into the follicle. If the needle meet with any resistance, it should be withdrawn and re-introduced."

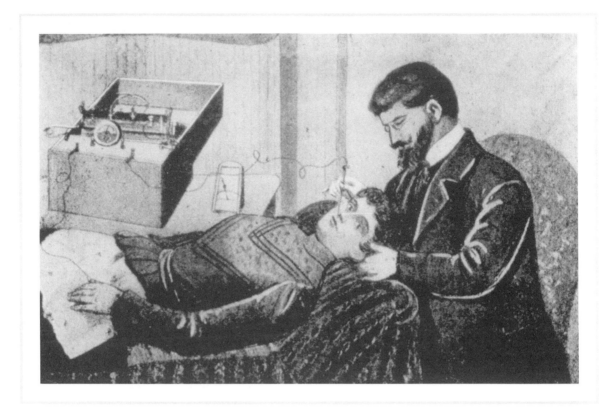

Early electrolysis: one hair at a time.

The circuit was completed by the patient herself, who was instructed to transfer the sponge-electrode to her left hand and press it into her palm. "When loosened by the electrolytic action, [the hair] seems almost to jump out of the follicle," Dr. Johnson continued. "It is well to have a small piece of black velvet in a convenient spot, on which the hairs can be laid. They sometimes stick to the forceps, and are troublesome; moreover, you can see the number removed."[19]

Dr. Fox advised his colleagues how to tell when hair was almost ready to be pulled: Look, he said, for "a blanching of the skin, and a little froth will appear at the mouth of the follicle."[20] Before the needle was withdrawn, "the patient should remove her hand from the sponge, in order to avoid the slight shock which would otherwise be felt."[21]

Dr. Johnson said that she removed no more than thirty hairs at a time, while Dr. Fox said that he usually destroyed from thirty to fifty hairs in a typical forty-five-minute session.

"I have removed over two hundred hairs at one sitting, when patients from a distance were anxious to leave the city," Dr. Fox advised. "But I deem it far better to spare one's eyes and to be more thorough, even if it involves a greater number of sittings."[22] This also guaranteed repeat business. Surely his most profitable patient was one particularly prodigiously hairy woman from whom, he noted, he had removed upwards of five thousand hairs.

Electrolysis practitioners contended that the experience was no more disagreeable than a trip to the dentist. Which, given the state of dentistry at the time, likely meant that it was not terribly agreeable. *Profitable Office Specialties*, a book published in 1912 advising doctors how to increase their profits, suggested numbing the skin first by slathering it with "a four to ten percent cocaine solution."[23]

Electrolysis had other drawbacks aside from discomfort. It was exceedingly slow (a one- to three-minute wait to treat each follicle), expensive, and required re-

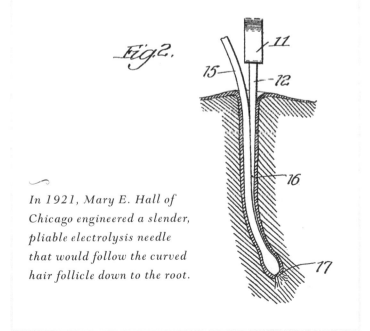

Fig. 2.

In 1921, Mary E. Hall of Chicago engineered a slender, pliable electrolysis needle that would follow the curved hair follicle down to the root.

11
15
12
16
17

peated visits. Although practitioners did not recognize it at the time, a hair could be permanently removed only when it was in a certain growth stage.

Electrolysis was relatively safe, but error was still possible. An inexperienced or inept practitioner could leave pitted scars and, if he or she accidentally reversed the electrical charge, would permanently tattoo his client with small black dots.

With the invention of multiple needles, brought to market by Paul M. Kree in 1916, electrolysis became somewhat less plodding. An operator could attach as many as ten needles at once. Alas, the multiple-needle machine, with its "octopus-like wiring" had the disadvantage of looking to the patron "like something specifically designed to produce pain."[24] And it was still incapable of clear-cutting large swaths of hair.

Hair Today, Gone Tomorrow

Given the rage for hairlessness, and the still imperfect methods of hair removal, it seems understandable that Kora M. Lublin's interest was piqued when in the late 1920s she came across a paper written by Raymond Sabouraud, a renowned French dermatologist, proposing a new hair removal approach. For forty years, Lublin, a beauty salon owner in New York City, had herself been searching for a satisfactory way to remove unwanted hair.

Though great improvements had been made in depilatories—improvements arising from innovations in the leather-curing business—they still smelled insufferably bad. One critic compared the scent to rotten eggs and stink bombs. By decreasing the concentration of hydrogen sulfide, one could decrease the smell, but the formulation would be proportionally more caustic to the skin.

"The deceptive thing about hydrogen sulfide," according to the 1930s exposé *Truth About Cosmetics*, "is that the odoriferous glands are quickly desensitized by the gas so that the user has the feeling that as she uses the product the odor disappears. Any one arriving even two or three hours later can inform her differently."[25]

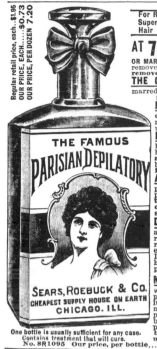
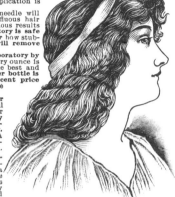
Sears, Roebuck catalog, 1902.

Dr. Sabouraud, the French dermatologist, appeared to have hit upon a new type of depilatory: a mixture containing a minute amount of thallium acetate. It did not smell bad but that, alas, turned out to be its only virtue. Previously used as a key ingredient in Rough On Rats, a rodent poison, thallium acetate had been taken off the market out of concern that it was so powerful that if accidentally consumed it could poison pets and children.

Apparently undaunted by possible dangerous side effects, Lublin began experimenting enthusiastically. By 1930 she had a product, whose name she proudly concocted from bits of her own name: Koremlu.

"Now, we have KOREMLU CREAM, 'Nature's rival,' that creates baldness only where it is applied and just where you want it," read the advertising material.[26] In its first year on the market, 120,000 jars of Koremlu were sold through department stores for the queenly sum of five dollars an ounce (ten dollars for three ounces).

The user was supposed to slather it on at night, as she would a cold cream. The problem was not that the product did not cause hair to fall out. It did cause baldness—but in all the wrong places. Lublin used a much higher concentration, 3.75 percent, than that recommended by Sabouraud. Moreover, the formulation was so haphazardly mixed that some jars contained as much as a 7 percent concentration of thallium acetate.

Hospitals reported patients "suffering from a strange new malady that paralyzed their lower limbs, doubled up their bodies with intense abdominal pain and constant nausea, made breathing difficult, blinded their eyes and loosened their hair," according to one account.[27] One twenty-six-year-old woman wrote Eleanor Roosevelt about her troubles, complaining that since using the cream her teeth were falling out, her feet were paralyzed, and she was losing her sight:

"In March of 1930 I started useing [sic] Koremlu Cream and a few weeks later I became very ill from then until now which is almost four years I have never been well all as the result of useing [sic] this cream.

"I could go on and on writing what this has meant and will mean in all of the years to come but I will sum it all in a few words by saying it took from me all I had that made life worth while[—]My eyes."[28] Complaints hurtled in from across the country, from Baltimore, Boston, El Paso. The health commissioner of San Francisco banned Koremlu. The Colorado state food and drug commissioner tried to do the same, but Lublin launched a saucy counteroffensive, protesting in a letter that it would be an impossibility for anyone using the product correctly to be harmed.

In the wild and woolly days of commerce before federal regulation of health and beauty products, Koremlu was by no means the only spurious product on the market. Nor was it only women who were the targets of unscrupulous entrepreneurs. Baldness remedies and impotence cures, for example, proliferated. Xervac, a baldness remedy invented by André A. Cueto in 1936, featured a helmet that resembled a big metal mixing bowl. The helmet was tethered, by way of a rubber hose, to a motor housed in a cabinet that "used a small vacuum force to massage the scalp and allegedly make hair grow."[29]

Ultimately, Koremlu was forced off the market, according to author Ruth de-Forest Lamb, "not by the action of a watchful government, not through the indignation of magazines refusing to carry its advertising, not through public-spirited dealers and jobbers refusing to handle this product, but only through the piling up of an immense amount of damage suits by people whose lives had been ruined by its use."[30]

With assets of only $2.93 to cover nearly $2.5 million in liabilities, Kora Lublin closed shop in 1932. The next mass-market depilatory, Nair, would not arrive on the scene for eight more years. It was safe but, not surprisingly, stinky.

And what about Monsieur Sabouraud? He abandoned the idea of thallium acetate early on— in favor of another hair removal technique that offered incredible results in a few easy treatments with no smell or mess. That technique? Radiation.

A 1910 advertisement for a hair-growing machine.

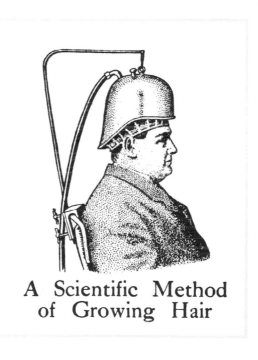

A Scientific Method of Growing Hair

The Wonders of X-Rays

Radiation promised a dignified, painless, and fast way to get rid of hair. "The rays were alluringly imperceptible," writes historian Rebecca Herzig. "Gone were the noxious smells of depilatories, the root-ripping pain of hot waxes, and the frightful appearance of multiple electrolysis needles."[31]

In late December of 1895, William Roentgen, a distinguished German physicist, announced his discovery of X-rays, a new kind of light that was imperceptible to the human eye. Before the end of 1896, John Daniel and William L. Dudley, two researchers at Vanderbilt University, were asked to use X-rays to locate a bullet in the head of a wounded child. To make sure the procedure was safe, Dudley first "tied a photographic plate to one side of his own head and sandwiched a coin between his head and the plate, then placed the X-ray tube a half inch away from his head on the other side and exposed the plate for an hour," according to Bettyann Holtzmann Kevles's revealing history of medical imaging.[32] Three weeks later, he had developed a bald spot exactly where his head had been exposed most directly to the X-ray tube.

This discovery inspired much "editorial merriment," with some newspaper wags suggesting that "X-rays might render daily shaving obsolete."[33] Though made in jest, this prediction would come true in a couple of decades. But it would be women rather than men who used it.

Initially, an X-ray machine was still a "novelty, a curiosity and a status symbol."[34] Photographers began offering X-rays in addition to studio portraits. "Celebrities set the pace," Kevles reports. "The czarina of Russia rushed to have her hand X-rayed. Kaiser Wilhelm II of Germany opted for an image of his arm. The British prime minister and his wife had their hands done, together, and Queen Emilia of Portugal sent her ladies-in-waiting to get their rib cages X-rayed to illustrate the evils of tight laces."[35] One inventor, hoping to market this marvel to the masses, patented a coin-operated X-ray machine.

While X-ray damage was reported, the public was less than concerned, as most of the victims were technicians or doctors who worked with radiation every day. Moreover, there was usually a long time lapse between the radiation exposure and the gruesome consequences that followed years or even decades later. But emerge they did. At a meeting of radiologists in 1920, "the menu featured chicken—a major faux pas because almost every one at the table was missing at least one hand and could not cut the meat."[36]

Despite the risks, a cadre of hard-core X-ray enthusiasts continually refined the technology. By World War I, Marie Curie, with the help of her daughter Irene, was transforming ordinary automobiles into mobile X-ray vehicles. To help better diagnose the injuries of those wounded in battle, Curie trained 150 female X-ray technicians and helped place 200 radiological installations near the French and Belgian army.

In the United States, draftees were routinely X-rayed off the battlefield to determine if they had tuberculosis. By the time the war was over, ordinary American citizens "now expected an X-ray as routine medical care."[37] Indeed, they also began to expect to be X-rayed at their local shoe store. At the end of World War I, according to Kevles, a large surplus of army portable X-ray units were transformed into gadgets marketed as the scientific way to measure feet. Foot-O-Scopes was the brand made by the United Shoe Machinery Corporation, but scads of fly-by-night companies manufactured knockoffs.

"All over the world, people who grew up between World War I and the 1960s recall the joy of standing inside the machine, pressing the appropriate button (usually labeled "Man," "Woman," and "Child" although the X-ray dosage was identical) and staring at their wriggling toe bones."[38]

Like the Foot-O-Scope, the hair-removal X-ray machine must have seemed a modern technological wonder. All a woman had to do was peer into a sleek mahogany-veneered cabinet for a minute or two every couple of weeks. At worst she might perceive a slight smell of ozone. And the unwanted facial hair shed easily within a few weeks after treatment.

X-ray hair removal salons grew faster than dark roots on a platinum blonde.

Marveau Laboratories appeared in Chicago, the Dunsworth Laboratories in Indianapolis (which promised that "Freedom from Unwanted Hair Opens the Gates to Social Enjoyments that are Forever Closed to Those so Afflicted"),[39] and the Tricho System in cities all across North America.

The mastermind of the Tricho empire was Albert C. Geyser, whose base of operations was in New York City at 270 Madison Avenue. By 1925 more than seventy-five machines were installed in beauty shops nationwide: Trenton, New Jersey; Wheeling, West Virginia; Tampa, Florida; St. Louis, Missouri; Minneapolis, Minnesota; Portland, Oregon; Seattle, Washington; and Montreal, Canada.

The Tricho was marketed as an award-winning innovation. And in fact in 1925 the company did win an award—the Grand Prize at the Paris Exposition Generale Commercial. Of course, so did every other firm in the "exposition," all of whom paid $400 for the privilege.

"The epilation laboratory is a vision of sanitary loveliness," purred a purveyor of an X-ray technique called the Martin Method. "The place is done in pure white enamel, not an atom of dust can enter here."[40] It was not cheap—three dollars a treatment, for ten to twenty treatments. But it worked beautifully. After a half-dozen treatments, the hair fell out, roots and all.

By the mid-1930s, X-ray hair removal seemed firmly entrenched as a feminine technology. But that does not mean that entrepreneurs had not attempted to market it to men. Indeed, a Tricho brochure from 1926 opens up noting that "When a man's arms, chest and back are covered with an unusually heavy growth of hair, it is unsightly, to say the least, and since such a growth serves no utilitarian purpose, it is superfluous."[41]

Arthur Nelson of Blairstown, New Jersey, must have been hoping to market the device to men when he wrote to the American Medical Association in 1934. "If this system is all they claim it to be it will save men many hundreds of hours wasted in shaving and money spent for razor blades, etc.," he said. But, he wondered, "if a man has the hair on his face removed by this system it will not cause him to become effeminate, will it?"[42]

In 1928, Dr. Oscar Levin, writing in *Good Housekeeping,* outlined the possible horrors resulting from X-ray hair removal. Immediately after treatment, the skin may become "inflamed, scaly, wrinkled, streaked with prominent blood vessels," he said. Months or years later, "growths may appear, which finally break down and ulcerate, and may even become cancerous."[43]

Also in 1928, the American Medical Association (AMA) received a letter from H. L. J. Marshall, president of the Beauty Sanitarium and Training School in New Orleans. The letter expressed concern about "one Mrs. Beatrice Lee" who was removing hair with an X-ray machine that had been disguised and presented as a harmless "Vibratory wave" apparatus. "This machine has been in operation in this City for over a year and I have seen several disfigured patrons bearing all the earmarks of X-ray telangiectasis," Marshall wrote.[44]

Marie Fink of Glendale, California, wrote the AMA in 1931. Proclaiming herself "a victim of that hated mar superfluous hair," she said she was inclined to try Roentgen treatments but she had "always heard of the dangers attached to the use of this measure" and was seeking assurance that it was safe before she tried it.[45]

Ignorance Is Bliss

Unlike Fink, many other women appear to have been either ignorant of the dangers or simply willing to ignore them, given the ease and effectiveness of the treatment. Mrs. B. Tellef, who lived at 4007 N. Lowell Avenue in Chicago, wrote the AMA about her younger sister who "has superfluous hair growing all over her face, and is worrying herself into the state of almost losing her mind." The sister had signed up for expensive treatments at the Tricho salon and Mrs. Tellef was worried not about safety but rather whether this was a cost-effective investment.[46]

Advertisements subtly acknowledged that X-rays could be dangerous but implied that X-ray hair-removal systems were now perfectly safe thanks to the ineluctable march of scientific progress. A pamphlet from a Tricho salon in Detroit soothingly equated X-ray hair removal with other common radiation procedures, which were indeed ubiquitous by 1940 in dental offices and emergency rooms.

The Tricho pamphlet also dazzled the prospective client with pseudoscientific prose: "In the Tricho System, we have the first biologic attempt to take advantage of an exceeding short blow or flash of $\frac{1}{40}$ part of a second, with a rest period eight times as long as the blow. We require less than one-half of a skin dose and since the hair papillae are located in the cutis vera, the penetration of our .4 angstrom wave length is limited to five millimeters as a maximum penetration."[47]

Though hair-removal entrepreneurs successfully maintained for decades that X-rays were a safe way to remove hair, this die-hard illusion vanished nearly overnight when, on August 6, 1945, a lone B-29 sailed over the industrial city of Hiroshima and dropped an atomic bomb. Although hair-removal radiation had little in common with the radiation released in the bomb attacks on Japan, the effects of enormous quantities of radiation were rendered vivid in the full-color photographs of *Life* magazine. Suddenly, all radiation was appreciated as dangerous.

Timing Is Everything

Nine days before the United States dropped the atomic bomb on Japan, one Dr. Henri E. St. Pierre sent off a patent application for a new invention.

Five years earlier, Dr. St. Pierre's "rather suspicious business" had drawn the unfavorable attention of two inspectors from the homicide squad of the San Francisco police department, who began observing him closely.[48]

The inspectors observed a steady stream of well-dressed ladies entering through the front door of an old three-story rooming house at 126 Jackson Street and then leaving through the alley exit a short time later. They all seemed to have appointments with St. Pierre, who was seen entering the building carrying what looked like a doctor's case.

The police inspectors thought St. Pierre was operating a fly-by-night abortion parlor. In fact, St. Pierre was extracting not fetuses but rather hair. He used a technique, known as thermolysis or diathermy, that he was in the process of refining. A Dr. Bordier in France was likely the first to use this technique to remove hair—in 1923. This technique used not the direct current of electricity but, instead, a newly discovered type of high-frequency radio waves. These were the same short waves that would be used in another invention, a new type of oven that would not reach the average American consumer until the early 1980s: the microwave oven.

Early on, the diathermy technique had some big drawbacks. For one, it relied on a "spark-gap"—a device that generated microwaves by passing sparks across a short gap in an electrical circuit. The only way to judge the intensity of the current, alas, was to listen and watch as the spark-gap fumed and hissed. But the advent of vacuum tubes, which could spit out microwaves with much greater precision and which could be easily calibrated with the twist of a dial, eliminated this disadvantage.

A second drawback was less easily overcome. While diathermy was much better than electrolysis at bulk hair removal, its long-term track record was poor. Indeed, hair removed with diathermy often grew back—luxuriantly. "The reappearance of a large percentage of previously treated hair was disillusioning," wrote Arthur Ralph Hinkel and Richard W. Lind, in their 1968 hair-removal textbook. "Alibis and excuses for such results ran the gamut from 'distorted follicles' to the 'hairy father' routine."

Hair follicles, it turns out, vary vastly in shape. Some are plumb straight. Others spiral like corkscrews. At the base of the follicle is a bulb and just as spring tulips sprout from bulbs, so, too, does hair. Diathermy was no good at uprooting the bulb.

St. Pierre's insight was to "blend" diathermy with electrolysis, to combine brawn with brains. Both methods are powered by the movement of electrons. But with diathermy, the electrons bounce back and forth as in a Ping-Pong game; with electrolysis the electrons are rushing forward like a train on a track. So how is it possible to blend the two?

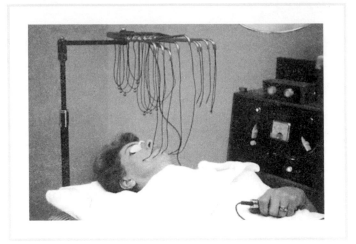

The multiple-needle electrolysis machine. What woman lost in dignity she made up for in hair-zapping speed.

"Envision a ping pong game going on in the club car of a speeding express train," wrote Hinkel and Lind. "Although the train may be traveling at more than eighty miles per hour in a straight line, carrying a ball along with it, the ball is still able to travel back and forth at its rapid pace across the table."[49] The result is that the root of the follicle is bathed in heated lye.

St. Pierre's combined system, as well as electrolysis alone, would continue to be widely used through the twentieth century.

A Close Shave

And now a few words about the razor. Why is it that women never adopted the razor as a way to remove facial hair? In part, perhaps, because it had been masculinized the way X-ray hair removal had been feminized. Nineteenth-century beauty manuals, for example, consistently warned that shaving would result in a heavier growth ultimately (though this was actually not true).

Around 1915 women did begin using razors—not on their faces but rather under their arms.

Before World War I, underarm hair was not a cosmetic consideration. Fashions until that point, while often form-revealing, covered up most of a woman's skin.

The only place one might glimpse a furry pit was in the boudoir, where apparently it was not considered offensive. But as bathing costumes and fashions became more revealing, some upper-class women started the trend of shaving their underarms.

To accomplish this, they turned to a relatively new invention: the safety razor with disposable blades. Shrewd marketers picked up on this trend with a vengeance. In the May issue of *Harper's Bazaar*, Gillette offered its new Milady Décolletée razor. The ad did not specifically mention underarm hair, but it featured a model donning a fashionable togalike evening gown with her arms arched over her head, flashing her smooth, hairless armpits. "Summer Dress and Modern Dancing combine to make necessary the removal of objectionable hair," read the copy.[50]

This ad marked the beginning of what historian Christine Hope has dubbed "The Great Underarm Campaign." "The advertisers in *Harper's Bazaar* initiated an assault on underarm hair which was to last for approximately four years," according to Hope. "Seventy-two percent of the hair remover ads during this period specifically mention underarms and most deal with underarms exclusively."[51]

The Gillette sales force was told to emphasize that the Milady razor had been "brought out after frequent requests from Palm Beach, [the] Virginia Hot Springs and other pleasure resorts."[52] This was apparently a "somewhat ticklish subject in those barely post-Victorian times," according to King Gillette's biographer, Russell Adams.[53] Gillette salesmen were instructed not to use the word *shaving* in their pitches. Men shaved, the company informed them; women "smoothed."

Gillette asserted that the Milady model was the first razor designed specifically for women, and billed it as the "safest and most sanitary method of acquiring a smooth underarm."[54] In fact, although it was smaller than the male razor, it was virtually the same product that King Gillette had introduced for men a decade earlier.

The safety razor had been around for some time before Gillette appeared on the scene, but its blade still required regular, skillful stropping and honing. What Gillette offered was a cheap steel blade that required no care at all because it was meant to be tossed out after a couple dozen uses. "Up to the time that the Gillette razor went on the market there were hundreds of thousands of men who did not shave

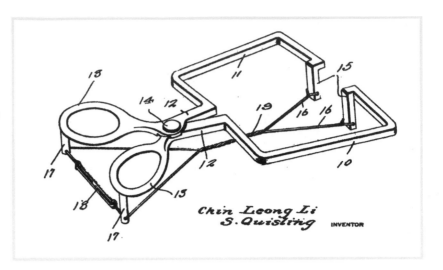

A hair-removal tool invented by Chin Leong Li and Sverre Quisling of Philadelphia in 1926. The idea was to grab the hairs and twist them out.

themselves, for the reason that they could not keep a razor in condition," Gillette himself claimed.[55]

Whether Gillette's company hatched the new market of women on its own or whether it was merely responding to a strong consumer demand is one of many vexing chicken-or-egg riddles in the history of advertising. Soon the disposable-blade razor was being aggressively marketed not just to the soignée subscribers of *Harper's Bazaar* but also to the middle-class readership of *McCall's*.

As a business strategy, it was a stroke of genius. While some women are genetically predisposed to sport facial hair, not all do. Other women develop facial hair only as they age or following an illness. But underarm hair is common to all women and it grows perpetually from adolescence well on through menopause. Moreover, since a razor does not permanently eliminate hair, a teenager who habituates herself to shaving her armpits acquires a habit that requires a steady investment in new razor blades over the course of a lifetime.

The Milady model helped bring an immediate spike in Gillette's business. In 1916 the company sold 782,028 razors—more than twice what it had sold two years before. In 1917 it sold more than a million.

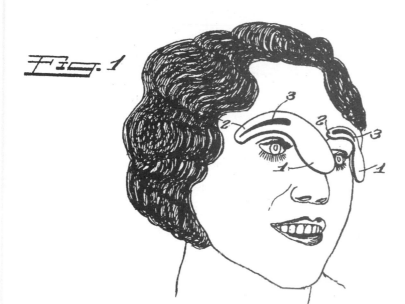

Fig. 1

A stencil for drawing in new, perfect eyebrows after the unruly natural ones have been plucked out.

Inventor: Gerd Wosse.

An elaborate eyebrow plucker, 1938.

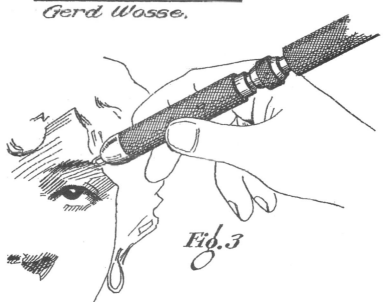

Fig. 3

It took another five years or so for the custom of underarm shaving to be fully embraced by the masses. In 1922 the Sears, Roebuck catalog for the first time offered dresses with sheer sleeves as well as products designated to remove hair from places other than the face, neck, and arms. Ads for both a depilatory and a woman's safety razor perch next to an illustration of a young woman admiring her smooth underarms before a mirror.

Underarm shaving was just one new habit that advertisers were urging consumers to adopt in the early twentieth century. Women were exhorted to rid themselves of socially fatal bad breath by gargling, to avoid embarrassing public accidents by using paper menstrual pads instead of rags, to make their homes more sanitary by purchasing rolls of toilet paper, and to eliminate the horrors of body odor with deodorant.

Meanwhile, Hollywood stars were raising the bar on facial hairlessness. The thin, arched, alienlike eyebrows sported by Marlene Dietrich and Jean Harlow, for example, could best be achieved by getting rid of real eyebrows altogether and simply drawing idealized brows in their stead. Celluloid beauties and their imitators—secretaries and telephone operators and store clerks—often found it was easiest to achieve a blank, stencil-ready brow with the simple swipe of a razor.

A Leg Up

By the time Sears catalog shoppers were being persuaded to shave their underarms, upper-class women were already wielding their razors elsewhere—on their legs. By the middle of the century, the male gaze was directed downward toward a "tanned, shapely, hairless leg."[56]

How this new habit became inculcated in American women is not clear. Although hemlines rose between World War I and World War II, razor advertisers rarely mentioned leg hair specifically. Rather, they featured illustrations of beauties

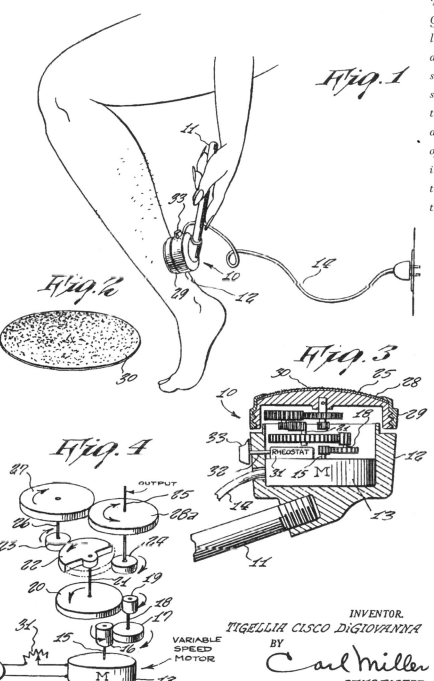

Tigellia Cisco Di Giovanna of Brooklyn patented a device that was supposed to lightly sand the hairs off the leg. Essentially a motorized update of Velvet Mittens, it doesn't appear to have made it to store shelves.

Fig.1

Fig.2

Fig.3

Fig.4

OUTPUT

RHEOSTAT

M

VARIABLE
SPEED
MOTOR

INVENTOR.
TIGELLIA CISCO DiGIOVANNA
BY
Carl Miller
ATTORNEY

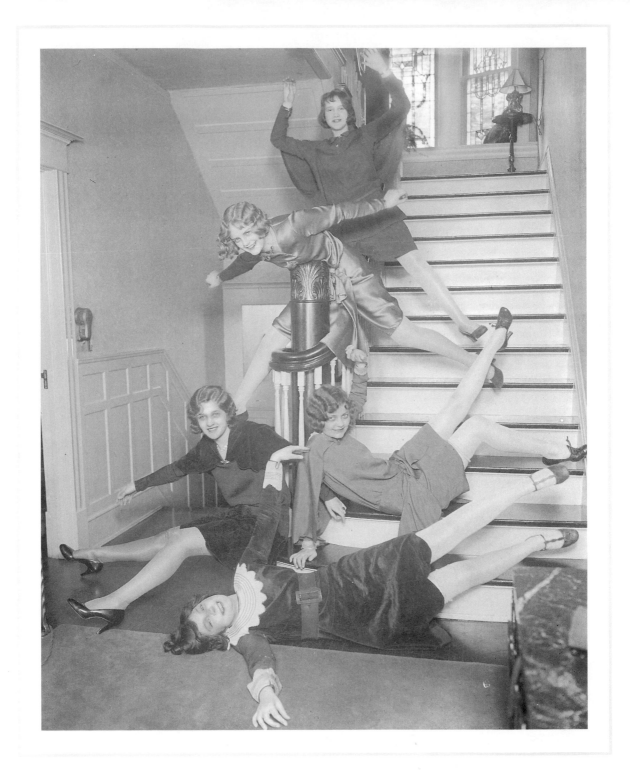

Colorado flappers show some leg.

with glorious gams under headlines like "Man's eye view" and "Let's Look at Your Legs—Everyone Else Does."

Virginia Kirkus was one of the earliest proponents in her 1922 beauty book. "Some people who consider themselves very particular look down upon the girl who shaves her legs and underarm hair, but as a matter of fact they have no more right to scorn her than scorn the man who shaves the hair from his face," she said. "Because the practice of underarm depilatory or shaving started with chorus girls is no reason for considering it beneath the dignity of the social leader. Lucky the woman who has no superfluous hair; let the rest of her sex get rid of it as best they can."[57]

Elinor Guthrie Neff, the beauty editor of *Harper's Bazaar,* advocated the shaving of leg hair with such missionary zeal that one suspects she must have held substantial stock in razor and depilatory companies.

"Ankle socks on the campus are a fine, old institution and all very well, but not on furry legs," she wrote in 1939. "If you must wear socks you owe it to your associates to get into the habit of using some safe, dependable depilatory. And we mean regularly—not just once in a blue moon as a kind of isolated experiment."[58]

Two years later, Mrs. Neff sniffed, women who do not shave should be forced to wear heavy hose. "If they are modern enough to demand silk stockings then they should certainly prepare their legs so that no thick 'forest' of hair is visible through the sheer fabric."[59]

Before World War I, virtually no American woman shaved her legs. But by 1964, ninety-eight percent of all American women under the age of forty-four did. While Mrs. Neff's opinions were undoubtedly influential, this great cultural shift was likely due to the convergence of other, more powerful forces during the late 1930s and the 1940s—Betty Grable's legs, for example. Grable scissor-kicked skyward in a pin-up pose, thereby raising the leg-beauty bar for the average woman, whose own legs were getting increased exposure as she danced the wildly popular, skirt-swishing jitterbug. At the same time, Wallace Carothers, a brilliant but troubled researcher at DuPont, was concocting the latest in synthetic wonder materials—nylon—which would showcase female legs in an entirely novel way.

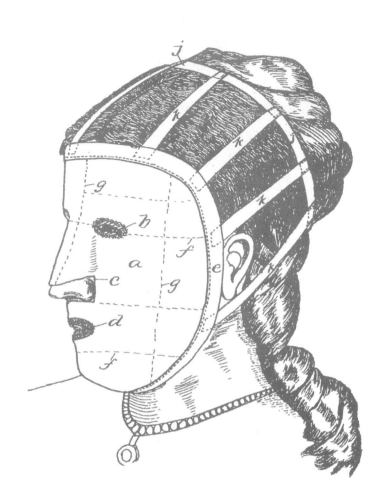

CHAPTER 5

Skin

Today there is no excuse for a woman to grow old, unless she is ill. . . . If you want to keep up with this modern, wonderful world, you must be young in thought, feeling and appearance . . . and all you have to do is stretch out your hand to receive the magic bounty of glamour that modern science has prepared for you.

— Lily Daché, *Glamour Book*, 1956

MARY: *But it's such a scary feeling when you see those little wrinkles creeping in.*

NANCY: *Time's little mice.*

MARY: *And that first gleam of white in your hair. It's the way you'd feel about autumn if you knew there'd never be another spring—*

NANCY: *(Abruptly) There's only one tragedy for a woman.*

MARY: *Growing old?*

NANCY: *Losing her man.*

MARY: *That's why we're all so afraid of growing old.*

— Clare Booth Luce, *The Women*, 1937

*S*mooth, radiant skin is a sign of health and vigor, and a key cue in the nonverbal courtship between man and woman. Firm, unwrinkled skin tells a man that a woman is in her reproductive prime.

Indeed, as the British novelist Fay Weldon has observed, youth *is* beauty. Virtually any young woman—regardless of the symmetry of her face, size of her nose, length of her chin, or width of her jaw—radiates beauty from the mere fact of her dewy skin.

Thus, it is no surprise that, although cosmetics have waxed and waned in acceptance and popularity, wrinkle eradicators catering to the less-than-young have always been a reliable feature of the American empire.

Newspapers from the early 1800s recommended a homemade skin tightener that could be made by boiling the white of eggs and alum in rosewater until it turned to a paste (a recipe that, perhaps, could trace its lineage to Queen Elizabeth, who sought to smooth out her high, well-plucked forehead with a similar concoction of egg white, powdered eggshells, alum, borax, and white poppy seeds).

Another recipe in an early American newspaper for a beauty cream was called Eau de Veau, which translates rather less euphonically from the French to "Calf Water": "Take a calf's foot and boil it in four quarts of river water until it is reduced to one half the quantity. Add half a pound of rice and boil it with the crumbs of white bread, steeped in milk, a pound of fresh butter and the whites of five fresh eggs, with their shells and membranes. Mix with them a small quantity of camphor and alum and distill the whole."[1]

Later in the century, Sarah Josepha Hale, editor of *Godey's Lady's Book* and high priestess of feminine propriety, proscribed the use of cosmetics for her readers. Nonetheless, she had her beauty secrets. She softened her hands with a lotion made of lard, rosewater, and coconut milk. And she warded off crow's feet with her nightly

Roll your wrinkles out

ELECTRIC WRINKLE ROLLERS

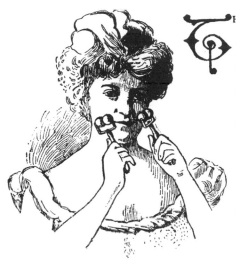

THESE developers are scientific instruments for a rapid and healthy development of the face and neck, and take the place of hand massage. Thin cheeks, soft muscles and flesh are rapidly built up by their use. Five to ten minutes' treatment will give the cheeks the glow of youth. The flesh becomes firm and hard and new life and action is excited in the pores and wasted tissues of the skin, giving it a delicate and refined appearance. The ELECTRIC WRINKLE ROLLERS used in connection with the Juvenis or Wrinkle Treatment does away with the fear that most ladies have in regard to not being able to treat themselves at home.

You can treat yourself, for these Electric Wrinkle Rollers do all the work for you. The results from their use are truly marvelous.

The Electric Wrinkle Rollers are turned from beautifully grained Central America wood, highly polished in natural color, and are an ornament to any lady's toilet table. To treat the face and neck, wash in tepid water, using my Virgin Soap, then dry the face. Hold a roller in each hand, contract the muscles of the cheeks by drawing the corners of the mouth backwards by muscular effort. Now vigorously and rapidly roll the cheeks up and down, back and forth, finishing with strokes from ear to mouth. Then treat the forehead from side to side so as to roll out the wrinkles in the brow and between the eyes. The neck may be treated in the same manner. You should not continue this treatment longer than from five to ten minutes.

Always roll firmly up and gently back, and firmly out and gently in.

As is well known, massage is the most active agent of the century for treatment of the entire body as well as for the face and neck. It brings into circulation the sluggish blood, drawing it to the surface, feeding with rich, warm blood the hollow, sunken cheeks; encourages perspiration the greatest bleach of nature, and frees the pores from all dirty accumulations that have been collecting for—I will not say how long.

My Electric Rollers are the only rollers on the market that can be used while creme is on the face without injury to the rollers. A pair of these rollers will last a lifetime.

Sent, prepaid by mail, on receipt of price, $2.50 per pair.

Wrinkle Emollient, to be used in connection with the Rollers, $1.00 per large jar.

MRS. NETTIE HARRISON DRUG CO,

**Manufacturers of High Grade
Toilet Preparations and Perfumes**

Nineteenth-century ad.

beauty ritual, which was to soak heavy brown butcher's paper in fresh apple vinegar, wrap her forehead, and then sleep through the night thusly mummified.

Fairy Tales
for Grown-up Girls

Most early skin-care preparations were homemade or bought from the local pharmacist until the second half of the nineteenth century, when the railroad made possible regional distribution and printing press improvements led to widespread dissemination of popular magazines and trade cards.

The first beauty cream entrepreneur to make the leap from homebrew to mass distribution was probably Harriet Hubbard Ayer. Born in 1849 into a Chicago family "better endowed socially than emotionally,"[2] as Mary Lisa Gavenas has wittily observed, the pretty Harriet married at the age of sixteen, the year the Civil War started. After she lost a child and her home in the Great Chicago Fire, she steamed across the Atlantic to France in an effort to forget her tribulations.

In Paris she made the acquaintance of a perfumer, one Monsieur Mirault, whose shop was located on the Boulevard Malsherbes. M. Mirault purported to have the recipes for the beauty creams used by the legendary French beauty Juliette Récamier—recipes he claimed his father and grandfather had mixed up especially for her.

Upon her return to Chicago, Hubbard became a society hostess who, clad in Parisian Worth gowns, entertained celebrities passing through the city; opera diva Adelina Patti and writer Oscar Wilde were among her guests. By 1886, however, Harriet's marriage had dissolved. She moved to New York City and, as a woman of reduced means, found it necessary to support herself and her children.

Hubbard found a backer with deep pockets, a financier named Jim Seymour, who put up a robust $50,000 (the equivalent of several million dollars in today's currency) for her to start her own beauty line. She licensed the Récamier formula and repackaged it in jewel-like glass jars under her own name.

Hubbard's chief contribution to the world of beauty was not innovation but marketing. "Harriet wrote ads that were fairy stories for grown-up girls," writes Gavenas. She dropped names, waxed poetic about Madame Récamier, and told "tales of miraculous makeovers that begot marriage proposals from rich and handsome men."[3]

Sales were brisk from the beginning. But in three years' time the business relationship went sour between Hubbard and Seymour. Hubbard went to court, alleging that Seymour, whose son had married her daughter, was trying to have her put away in an insane asylum as a ploy to take over the company.

Seymour did manage to get Hubbard, sane or not, carried off in a straitjacket. According to Hubbard's murky account in her autobiography, she escaped the asylum with "the aid of a mysterious Freemason to whom she communicated her plight in coded French."[4]

When she reentered the real world, the forty-five-year-old Harriet, renounced by her family and without financial resources, recovered with remarkable aplomb. She approached Joseph Pulitzer about a job on his newspaper and became America's first beauty editor. Meanwhile, her daughter and Seymour retained control of the Hubbard line.

From Catarrh Cure to Wrinkle Cream

Perhaps the first nationally distributed commercial beauty cream in America was Pond's cold cream. Cold cream, of course, is ancient. The Roman physician Galen is credited with the invention, though he may have actually gotten the idea for it from Hippocrates. But Americans, characteristically, have continually sought to improve it.

Theron T. Pond, who began his career as a chemist in Utica, New York, extracted from the bark of a witch hazel shrub in 1846 a "pain destroying and healing" potion that became known as Pond's Extract. Pond set up a small distillery in the rear of his apothecary and began producing his elixir.

From 1882 through 1907 the T. T. Pond Company advertised Pond's Extract as one versatile concoction. Supposedly useful as an aftershave lotion, a dentrifice, and (like the original formula for Lysol) a contraceptive douche, Pond's Extract was also hawked as a treatment for sore throats, catarrh, diphtheria, neuralgia, earaches, and insomnia.[5]

In 1907 the company introduced a "vanishing cream," a forerunner of what would become Pond's Cold Cream. The Pond's Girl ad campaign in 1910 offered this advice: "Avoid Sunburn, Freckles and Chaps. The Out-of-Doors Girl can easily avoid the unpleasant effects of sun and wind on her delicate skin by always using Pond's Extract Company's Vanishing Cream."[6]

Did it actually make freckles go away or keep them from forming? Not likely. This was long before the discovery that PABA (para-aminobenzoic acid) could block melanoma-stimulating ultraviolet rays. At least, however, it did no harm, unlike many skin "whiteners" on the market that contained such dangerous ingredients as lead or mercury.

The company's main innovation—and this must be credited to an anonymous company inventor or inventors rather than Theron Pond, who had died back in the mid-nineteenth century—was that it did not go rancid. Other cold creams, which had as a base animal fat, had to be kept chilled in the early twentieth century so they did not spoil. The Pond's cream, since it had a mineral-oil base, lasted a long time.

Perhaps just as important to the Pond Company as its mineral-oil formula, however, was its precocious understanding of the value of celebrity endorsements. Until 1907 its advertisements look as if they were meant to appeal to dottering old men who scuffled around all day in slippers. After 1907 the company beckoned to pampered upper-class females—or rather those who strove to emulate them.

Various American heiresses, European royals, and other high-profile women gave Pond's their imprimatur. Among them: Mrs. William Borah, wife of the senator from Idaho; Mrs. Nicholas Longworth, the notoriously catty Alice Roosevelt, daughter of Teddy Roosevelt; Queen Marie of Romania; Mrs. Marshall Field, the Chicago department store doyenne; and Mrs. Alva Belmont, a socialite suffragist and president of the National Women's Party.

"Personal contacts" who provided the advertising firm J. Walter Thompson leads on potential society endorsers got $1,000 for each high-profile endorsement that panned out. The endorsers of course earned a stipend, but they generally gave it away to their favorite charity.

In 1924 a Pond's advertisement featured Mrs. Reginald Vanderbilt (the mother of Gloria Vanderbilt, whose signature would be embossed in the 1970s upon the rumps of women clad in designer jeans) in a full-length photograph wearing a sequined evening gown and enough lipstick and eyebrow pencil to look like Theda Bara, the notorious screen vamp of the era. Later, Mrs. Nicholas R. du Pont (of *the* du Ponts) would enthuse over Pond's in a *Good Housekeeping* advertisement. "I can't imagine using a finer face cream," she declared. Under her stately gaze, the ad copy urged readers to "Get yourself a big jar of snowy Pond's Cold Cream—today!"[7]

Fashion historians have explained the abrupt shift in the feminine ideal from the full-bosomed, bustle-bottomed Edwardian lady to the slim-hipped and flat-chested flapper of the 1920s by pointing to heavy casualties during World War I. "Young women of the twenties with their youthful faces and boyish figures thus replaced the men who had been killed in battle," wrote historian Fenja Gunn. This new quest for youthful looks "encouraged cosmetic manufacturers and beauty salons to produce a range of preparations and treatments designed to erase wrinkles, discourage double chins, and generally preserve a youthful complexion."[8]

Cosmetics historian Gilbert Vail is less philosophical, attributing the trend not to postwar angst but native feminine vanity. "American women have always been in the vanguard of novices willing to try any sort of innovation which might help them to become more ravishing, and beauty operators had little difficulty in inducing them to accept whatever new treatment they recommended," he writes.[9]

The Grandes Dames of Beauty

Whatever the cause for the spike in demand for wrinkle cream, the beauty industry—which just as much as law, medicine, and architecture was becoming increasingly professionalized during this era—mushroomed. From sales of $100,000 in 1906, cosmetics sales grew over the next thirty-two years into an industry worth more than $180 million.

The story of beauty cream innovation in America culminates, perhaps, in the fifty-year-long catfight between those two grande dames of glamour, Elizabeth Arden and Helena Rubinstein. Arden and Rubinstein actually had a lot in common. They were both brilliant entrepreneurs who built blockbuster businesses out of beauty. Despite their common ground, they hated each other. Helena Rubinstein, informed by journalists that a horse had bitten off the tip of Elizabeth Arden's finger, reportedly quipped: "Is the horse all right?"[10]

Arden, whose Jet Pilot won the 1947 Kentucky Derby, was crazy about horses but could not stand the smell of the liniment they were rubbed down with. So she ordered that trainers rub the horses down with her scented Ardena skin tonic. One trainer, who had the temerity to suggest that what was good for a human was not necessarily good for a horse, was summarily dismissed. Indeed, Arden was characterized in her *New York Times* obituary as a "woman who treated horses like women and women like horses." She left behind two bitter ex-husbands and a trail of disloyal workers.

Those inclined toward armchair psychoanalysis might trace both the entrepreneurial chutzpah and the dyspeptic temperament of this cosmetics tycoon to insecurities deeply rooted in her inauspicious beginnings. On the other hand, maybe she was just naturally ambitious. In any case, Florence Nightingale Graham was born in Ontario, Canada, on New Year's Eve in 1878, the daughter of an immigrant truck driver. When she came of age she held a series of decidedly unglamorous jobs, the last one as an office assistant to a dentist.

But in 1908 she took a bold step. Nearly thirty years old, she moved to New York, first taking a job as a treatment girl with Eleanor Adair, a respected doyenne of the beautification business. Graham, who was paid only in tips, soon moved on to the new salon on Fifth Avenue just opened by Mrs. Elizabeth Hubbard (no relation to Harriet Hubbard). But the two had a falling out over money. They split up, and Florence, with a $6,000 loan from a cousin, set up her own establishment on the premises, forcing Mrs. Hubbard to set up her rival establishment two doors down.

The first thing Florence had to do as the proprietess of her own business was come up with a name. "Florence Nightingale," her namesake, was more likely to evoke battlefield hospitals than glamor. Instead she took the first name of Elizabeth (it had a regal ring to it but, more practically, Mrs. Hubbard's first name was still printed on the windows of the salon). "Graham" was too plebeian by Florence's sights as well. No one is certain of the origins of "Arden," some conjecture that it came from a Victorian novel, but overnight Florence Graham was reborn as Elizabeth Arden.

Arden was by all accounts an excellent facial masseuse. But was she a true innovator in the beauty cream department? Margaret Allen, in *Selling Dreams*, suggests Arden borrowed heavily, first from Mrs. Hubbard's recipes and later from Paris salons.

Indeed, during a 1914 visit to Paris, Arden had no time to linger before masterpieces at the Louvre or climb the Eiffel Tower. Instead she went on "an orgy of salon visiting," hitting four different ones every day. Although Arden denied it, Margaret Allen contends it is likely that one of these salon's was Madame Rubinstein's Maison de Beauté Valaze. When she returned home she was laden down with pots and tubes from virtually every salon in Paris.[11]

Arden immediately got started reverse engineering, hiring A. Fabian Swanson, a chemist, to analyze the composition of her Parisian booty. But Arden was not content merely to reproduce the creams. All of the creams of the day were hard and greasy, so Arden set about trying to create one that was light and fluffy.

One afternoon an excited Swanson showed up at the salon. "I've done it!" he exclaimed.[12] When Arden peered into the jar that Swanson proffered she saw a substance with the fluffy texture and white-on-white color of stiffened egg whites—exactly what she had sought.

She promptly dubbed it Venetian Cream Amoretta and advertised it as a "famous French formula" despite its Italianate name and the fact that it had been brewed in a New York chemical laboratory by Fabian Swanson.

Thrilled with his face cream, Arden ordered Swanson to go off and invent a new skin tonic. He returned shortly with what would become her Ardena Skin Tonic, which was composed quite simply, a later chemical analysis would reveal, of water, grain alcohol, boric acid, and perfume.

As for Helena Rubinstein, the historic record reveals little about the composition of her famous creams, except that the early ones likely contained lanolin and pine-bark extract. She was by all accounts a larger-than-life character. Perhaps the most evocative description of Rubinstein is offered by Patrick O'Higgins, her associate and biographer. O'Higgins recalled his first meeting with the portly purveyor of pulchritude thusly:

"The Princess, Madame Rubinstein, appeared. She wore her usual bowler hat and a matching yellow chemise dress with balloon sleeves and a drawstring neck from which multiple strings of carved emeralds hung to the uncertain level of her waist. One small hand, decorated with a diamond the size of a bottle cap, held a piece of sausage . . . 'Polish sausage!' she said, chewing away. Large gypsy circles of ruby and emerald cabochons swung from her earlobes and brushed each of her well-rounded shoulders. . . . She led me at a trot into a room some forty feet long whose walls, confirming my first hasty glance, were papered with row upon row of paintings. . . . Was selling paintings one of her side lines? I wondered. "Vodka?" the Princess broke my reverie. She offered me two hunks of sausage, pointed her little finger to a bottle in a crested silver bucket and repeated: "Vodka? Good! Serve yourself!

Drink! Eat!'' She rolled her 'r's like a Broadway actress impersonating a Russian grand duchess.''

Despite her notorious rivalry with Arden, the only time Rubinstein felt truly threatened was the day Charles Revson introduced his beauty cream innovation, Eterna 27, in 1962. That same day Madame Rubinstein, according to a company executive who happened to walk into her office at the time, was leaning out the window and shaking her fist at the Revson offices across the street on Fifth Avenue. "What are you doing? You're killing me, you rat! What's the matter with you?" the diminutive nonagenarian screeched in her heavy Polish accent.[13] It looked, the executive recalled, as if she might fall out the window. It would not be the last time that Charles Revson drove a rival to apoplectic rage.

Plug Me In . . .

In the late nineteenth century, historian David Nye tells us, electricity was invoked as "the panacea for every social ill and the key to a whole range of social and personal transformations." It promised to "lighten the toil of workers and housewives, to provide faster and cleaner forms of transport, and to revolutionize the farm." It promised more than that, however. It also promised to eradicate wrinkles and to bring women to orgasm.

Perhaps a little background is in order. Rachel Maines, in her highly original book *The Technology of Orgasm*, posits that during the late nineteenth century the electric vibrator brought relief to doctors who theretofore did a brisk business earnestly using their hands to bring women to sexual climax ("hysterical paroxysm," to use the technical medical term of the era). Indeed, this was the prescribed treatment for hysteria. Even Freud practiced it before he decided that the root of hysteria was above the neck rather than below the belly button. And it is quite possible that

Alice James, the neurasthenic sister of famous brothers William and Henry James, underwent "vulvular massage" treatments.

"For physicians in this line of work, the vibrator was a godsend," Maines asserts.[14] In 1906, Samuel Spencer Wallian, sang the praises of "rhythmotherapy," noting that with manual massage the physician "consumes a painstaking hour to accomplish much less profound results than are easily effected by the other [the vibrator] in a short five or ten minutes."[15] The mechanization of massage "significantly increased the number of patients a doctor could treat in a working day."[16]

By 1918, Sears, Roebuck included a page titled "Aids that Every Woman Appreciates," which depicted, among other appliances, electric radiators and egg beaters as well as vibrators. Because of consumer demand, the vibrator (at this stage meant to be externally rather than internally applied) was only the fifth electrical device introduced into the household, arriving just after the electric sewing machine, fan, teakettle, and toaster and long before the electric vacuum cleaner and iron, which would not come to market for another decade.

But, according to promotional material, household versions of the vibrator had myriad applications, including the treatment of wrinkles. Electrical stimulation of the facial muscles probably made them more taut, at least temporarily. The beautifying effect, however, was likely as fleeting as an orgasm.

The vibrator's greatest appeal in the salon business was perhaps not for the client but for the beauty operator. For what it offered was relief from manual labor—the same manual labor that exhausted those poor physicians treating hysterical patients.

Facial massage is a hallmark of beauty routines across cultures, but it is a tiring enterprise. *Profitable Office Specialties*, a book written in 1912 for doctors and other entrepreneurs, described the optimal manual technique in its inimitable rococo prose: "The digits of both hands, with the exception of the thumbs, are applied to the cheeks, between the malar eminences, and the ascending ramus of the mandible, and execute shaking movements, whilst the tips of the fingers approach, and move away from each other in the quickest possible time. After a number of vibrations on one

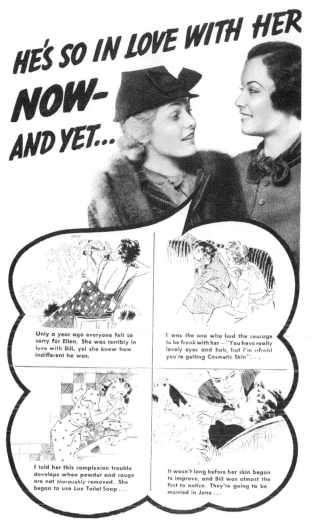

Women's magazine ad, 1936.

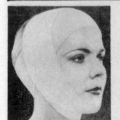

YOUTH-MOLDE

The NEW Head Band and Chin Strap that is ELASTIC without rubber and WASHABLE

Keep your chin and neck firm and young with Youth-Molde (double style). Wear this light, comfortable, active chin support for a half hour a day or longer. See how it supports sagging muscles, reducing flabbiness, or double chin, and re-molding normal contour. A practical beauty aid...$1.00.

Youth-Molde Head Band (single style) protects hair when using cosmetics—also for all outdoor sports...50c. Sold at drug and department stores. If your dealer cannot supply you, write us.

Becton, Dickinson & Co., Rutherford, N.J.

An ad from the 1930s.

A European version of the Elizabeth Arden ionization mask.

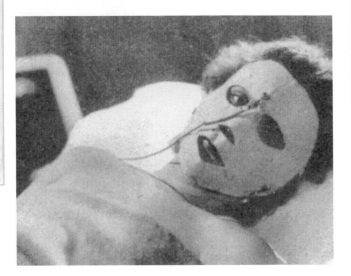

part of the face, the vibrating fingers are transferred to another part. The thumbs hang free in the air."[17]

Phew. No wonder the book recommended that the shrewd practitioner purchase a "vibro-hand apparatus." "You can execute the delicate touch with the finger tips, and vibratory movements from this instrument, with little or no exertion from the operator," it advised.[18]

Violet Ray machines offered a variation on the vibrator theme. They were supposed to "increase secretions" and have a "soothing effect on the nervous system" by "spraying thousands of volts of High-Frequency electricity into any weak, sluggish, or painful organ or muscle, purifying and causing the flow of warm, rich blood to surge through the treated part."[19]

Like vibrators, they were supposed to treat a medical dictionary's worth of ailments: abscesses, alopecia, anaemia, asthma, ataxia, "barber's itch," boils, "brain fag," bunions, carbuncles, constipation, gray hair, lumbago, piles, pyorrhea, sciatica, ringworm, writer's cramp, and, of course, wrinkles.

The standard machine came equipped with numerous electrodes. The Marvel Violet Ray electrode number SI, for example, was shaped like a smoking pipe with a flat head. Ostensibly it not only made skin look young again but also eliminated freckles, cured whooping cough, and firmed up flabby breasts.

After four decades of respectable use, the vibrator and its ilk were relegated to the attic, however. Erotic films appearing on the scene in the 1920s ripped the mantle of medical respectability off the vibrator and revealed it to be what it indeed was: a sex toy.

Electrons Battle Dandruff, Psoriasis, and Wrinkles

That by no means heralded the end of the beauty industry's long love affair with the electron. During a 1920s excursion to Vienna, Elizabeth Arden chanced to hear a lecture given by one Professor Steinachon on the subject of "diathermy treatments," which consisted of mild microwave heat being applied to the skin for treatment of arthritis, rheumatism, and injured muscles.

If it works for those ailments, Arden mused, why not for chin wattles and crow's feet? Thus was born the one invention that can be directly attributed to Miss Arden: her Youth Mask.

These papier-mâché face masks were shaped directly from a plaster cast of the patron's face and made conductive with tinfoil. Then they were fitted over the face and hooked up to conducting cords springing from a "diathermy machine," essentially a box that supplied a low level of microwave energy. Arden claimed that this treatment beautified the skin by reviving dead cells and increasing circulation. The medical profession never corroborated these claims, but the Arden salon clientele voted with their faces. It was a very popular treatment of the twenties. Hordes of hopeful beauties paid two hundred dollars for a course of thirty-two treatments.

Medical induction coils had been used since 1835 to tone muscles. By the 1930s, electrical products were pervasive in beauty parlors. The Marinello company, which trained black as well as white beauticians, was one of many companies to supply beauty parlors with something called a Wall Plate. It hooked up either to a direct or alternating current or, if the shop was not yet on the power grid, could be powered by a dry-cell battery. It was a huge advance, apparently, over previous electrical

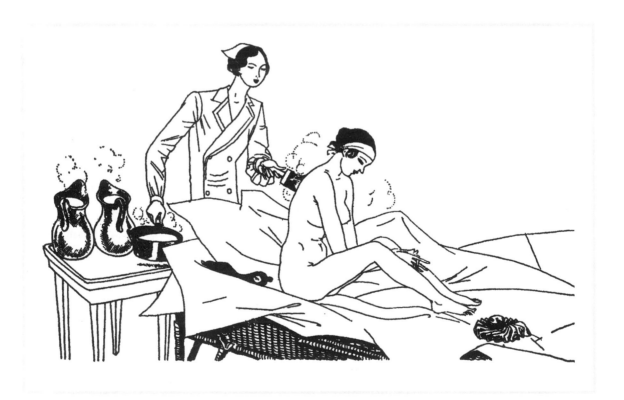

The hot-wax bath. The best part of the ordeal was leaving the beauty salon.

beauty machines, which were large, unwieldy friction machines that worked only when enough static electricity had been stored up in the condenser.

The Marinello machine was a tall, shallow box with cords that attached to different "electrodes" designed to treat dandruff, eczema, psoriasis, and "eczematous scabs" as well as wrinkles. "The nerves are stimulated; dormant or sluggish muscles are revitalized and made firm," according to a Marinello trade book.[20]

Adjusting the electrical current was an art, however. If just right, "the patron feels properly refreshed by the treatment." If too strong, however, "its overstimulating effects often produce a violent headache, and an extreme nervous irritation which negatizes all the intended benefit of the treatment, and may be actually harmful."[21]

A rival method was the Derma-Vac Facial System, which ostensibly worked miracles not just on wrinkles but also blackheads and whiteheads. The beauty operator was supposed to mix two teaspoonfuls of something called Melto Pack with water to make a paste that was to be spackled on the patron's face. After three to five minutes, the Melto Pack was removed. "Cover the eyes with moistened witch-hazel pads while lamp is being used. . . . Lightly but firmly 'roll' the Melto Pack off the face; 'Do not "wipe off" the melto pack;' 'roll' off as directed."[22]

After something called Vita Lotion was patted over the face, the operator selected from four different glass applicators that, through suction, were supposed to deliver miraculous results not only by making skin youthful again but also by slimming double chins, filling out acne pits, and even smoothing dowager humps.

Another skin-rejuvenating innovation, the hot-wax bath, Arden claimed to have brought back to America from her time at a Bavarian spa. The point of the bath was weight loss, as well as a general purging of "bodily poisons." Despite its Germanic heritage, Arden rechristened it the Ardena Bath.

As a salon treatment, according to the 1933 *Vogue Book of Beauty*, the Ardena Bath and similar treatments at other salons offered unparalleled luxury. This, however, probably had more to do with the hour-long massage following the wax wrap than the actual treatment, which was described thusly: "You are put into a large

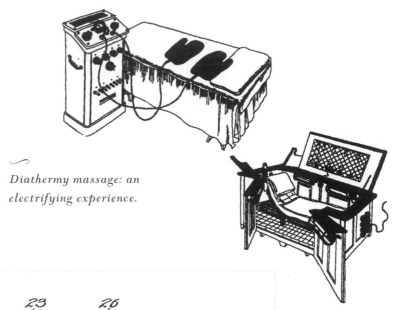

*Diathermy massage: an
electrifying experience.*

Fig. 1.

*The fat-roller,
patented by
Chicagoan Louis
W. G. Flynt in
1916.*

*Inventor:
Louis W. G. Flynt.*

white wicker crib lined with vast sheets of spotless paraffin paper. Then you are painted all over with a hot wax-like substance. . . . Once you are coated like a mummy, with an ice-bag over your heart, you are wrapped in layers of crackling white paper, then in blankets, with an ice-bag around your neck. There you lie, glorying in the fact that everything that should not be in your system is rapidly being drawn out of it."[23]

Vogue offered this highly evocative, though not terribly scientific, explanation of how the treatment worked: "The theory is that Nature abhors a vacuum. So a temporary vacuum is created between your body and the wax. Nature will then do something about it—she will try to fill the vacuum with the secretions which are forced from your body."[24] In any case, the dammed-up sweat would rush out of the pores as soon as the wax was peeled off.

Those in need of more serious artillery in the war against fat could opt for a whirl though the giant roller, a contraption of wooden cylinders designed to "smooth" the pounds away. Although it's not clear whether Arden herself patented such a device or licensed the use of it from someone who had, the U.S. Patent Office issued patent 1,175,513 for what appears to be an awfully similar invention.

Sloughing Off Age

It was inevitable, of course, that the antiwrinkle brigade would turn to chemicals for help. One popular skin treatment that originated in the nineteenth century still prevails today: the phenol peel.

Who invented the phenol peel? One theory, proffered by Joan Kron in her thoughtful meditation on the face-lift, is that during the 1870s a nurse in a European hospital accidentally spilled some carbolic acid on her face as she was reaching for a bottle of it. Carbolic acid, which is also known as phenol and is a derivative of coal tar, was introduced into hospitals earlier in the century as a disinfectant after Joseph Lister postulated that germs transferred from unclean hands and instruments were the cause of many infections. In any case, the nurse quickly cleaned her skin with a germicidal powder to prevent infection and bandaged the wound tightly. Once healed, the nurse's skin was amazingly smooth and youthful-looking—so she repeated the experiment on the other side of her face and voilà, got the same result.

This story is perhaps apocryphal, but by the 1880s "skinning" (or "écorchement," the French term for phenol peeling) was "a thriving, unregulated business, carried out in beauty institutes, shady salons, and private homes."[25]

Popular though it was, it was far from safe. A 1908 *Ladies' Home Journal* article, for example, offered the grotesque example of one skinning that had left a woman's face looking "like a piece of raw beef."[26] On the other hand, the author noted, a successful peel resulted in a complexion that was as soft as a fuzz-free peach.

According to *Profitable Office Specialties*, a phenol peel required that the face be painted with three coats of carbolic acid. After the acid dried, the entire surface was to be covered with rubber adhesive strips, which remained on for three or four days. "The skin is allowed to remain, however, until nature desquamates the integument," the book cryptically advised. In other words, apparently, until patient's face, in snakelike fashion, sloughed off the old skin as fresh skin grew underneath.

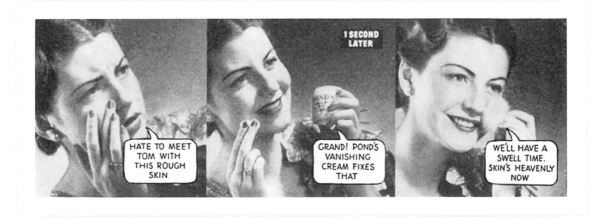

Miracles, miracles.

This method was allegedly so effective it worked not just on wrinkles but also on deep-seated smallpox pittings.[27]

One of the first reputable salons to offer phenol peels, according to Kron, was the John H. Woodbury Dermatological Institute in New York. Woodbury and his brother William would go on to establish a soap empire. But in the meantime one of their cosmetologists, Ella Harris, absconded with the skin-peel formula and opened a salon in San Francisco.

When Harris died suddenly, one of her clients, an actress named Irehne Hobson, seized opportunity. "Dear, sweet aunt Irehne broke into Harris's salon, found the formula, and had it analyzed by a chemist," remembers Arthur Gradé, her nephew, who also went on to a long career as face-peeler to the stars.[28]

"Before long, there were as many peelers as manicurists in Hollywood, most with invented European lineage," Kron writes. "And they were all plotting to get one another's formulas and clients."[29] Gradé claimed the phenol peel was a boon for Mae West, who did not start making films until she was forty. Not so for silent screen star Mae Murray, who had so many peels "she smiled to one side."[30]

Pinned Up, Not Peeled Off

While phenol peels carried a much bigger risk than conventional creams or electrical treatments, they also offered potential for greater improvement. So, too, did face-lifts—only to a greater degree in both departments.

The first modern face-lift is thought to have taken place in 1901, performed on a Polish aristocrat whose name has been lost to history. "She dreamed up the operation and convinced Berlin surgeon Eugen Hollander to perform it on her," according to Joan Kron, the author of *Lift*. The face-lift, argues Kron, is an operation that has been "consumer-driven since day one."[31]

Sarah Bernhardt, the world-famous French stage actress, was quite possibly the first celebrity to get a face-lift. She did so at the age of sixty-three—just before she filmed her first movie, *Queen Elizabeth*, in 1908.

Bernhardt was not so vain that she lied about her age, according to one biographer. However, she did cling "stubbornly to the self-delusion that in appearance she was younger than most of her associates."[32] After the face-lift, apparently, she did look younger than her age. When she returned to France, French cosmetic surgeon Suzanne Noël recalls in her memoirs, "all the newspapers remarked that, by means of a practical operation performed on the scalp, [the actress] had regained a surprising degree of youthfulness."[33]

Mrs. Martha Petelle, a sixty-year-old character actress, was far less well known than the celebrated Bernhardt but she was the chief attraction at the 1931 International Beauty Shop Owners' Convention. During the convention, plastic surgery pioneer J. Howard Crum performed a face-lift on her in public in the Grand Ballroom of New York City's Pennsylvania Hotel. For her part, Mrs. Petelle submitted to the operation "voluntarily and with much apparent joy," motivated by the hope that more work would come her way if she looked younger.

Dr. Crum, a graduate of the Bennett Medical College in 1909, proclaimed the procedure a success. Fifteen hundred people showed up to gawk at the spectacle. According to Thyra Samter Winslow, a reporter from *The New Republic*, "the operation, as publicly performed, appeared amazingly simple—about as easy as peeling a banana."

"Areas in front of the ear and on the back of the neck . . . were marked off with iodine. A solution of Novocain was injected. . . . The surgeon drew up the sagging face. Snipped it. Sewed it together into a semblance of youth. He bandaged the two long, narrow wounds. And the old lady, much younger looking, certainly, had her hair waved and her photograph taken!"

Even though a face-lift operation might be painful and potentially leave one's face "more than a bit lopsided," Winslow sarcastically suggested, desperate souls might find it worthwhile.

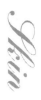

"If you're getting on, and are beginning to be psychopathic about your appearance, regaining a semblance of youth may mean more to you than anything else in the world. And an operation including many injections of Novocain, cutting, fifty stitches or so, five hundred to a thousand dollars, very real danger of infection and the chance of being disfigured for life, may seem a small price to pay for the possibility of looking younger again."[34]

In his book *The Making of a Beautiful Face; or, Face Lifting Unveiled*, Crum admitted that plastic surgery could be seen as "an encroachment upon the province of Mother Nature." But the benefits outweighed the risks, he contended. "An aging and unattractive face will often have as disastrous an effect on a woman's life as would some physical deformity." Plastic surgery was "the one reliable method whereby time and age may be pushed back and the happiness of woman advanced."[35]

Clearly, at this stage plastic surgery was largely the province of hucksters and charlatans. The author of *Profitable Office Specialties* acknowledged that such procedures might seem ridiculous to traditional physicians: "Yet it is these operations which fatten the purse of many unethical and ethical physicians," he advised.[36]

In 1922, Ethel Lloyd Patterson, a "woman standing with reluctant feet where thirty-nine and forty meet," was researching a magazine article about face-lifts. Upon approaching a conservative surgeon for an interview, she was rebuked. "I would not touch any woman at any price who came to me and asked me to remove the legitimate trace of her years," the surgeon said. Fifteen years later, the *New York Herald Tribune* was giving its readers the same advice. "No reputable surgeon attempts" to lift faces.[37]

Indeed, until the 1950s, even aging cinema stars prolonged getting a face-lift as long as possible, preferring less-risky options such as skin peels, electrical facials, or the "Hollywood Lift"—a "special contraption made of glue, silk thread, and rubber bands" that makeup artists deployed to pull sagging faces taut (which was not without its own disadvantages—it tugged painfully on the ears and its rubber bands tended to snap inconveniently during the middle of a scene).[38]

The Hollywood Lift appears to have been perfected by Adolph M. Brown, of

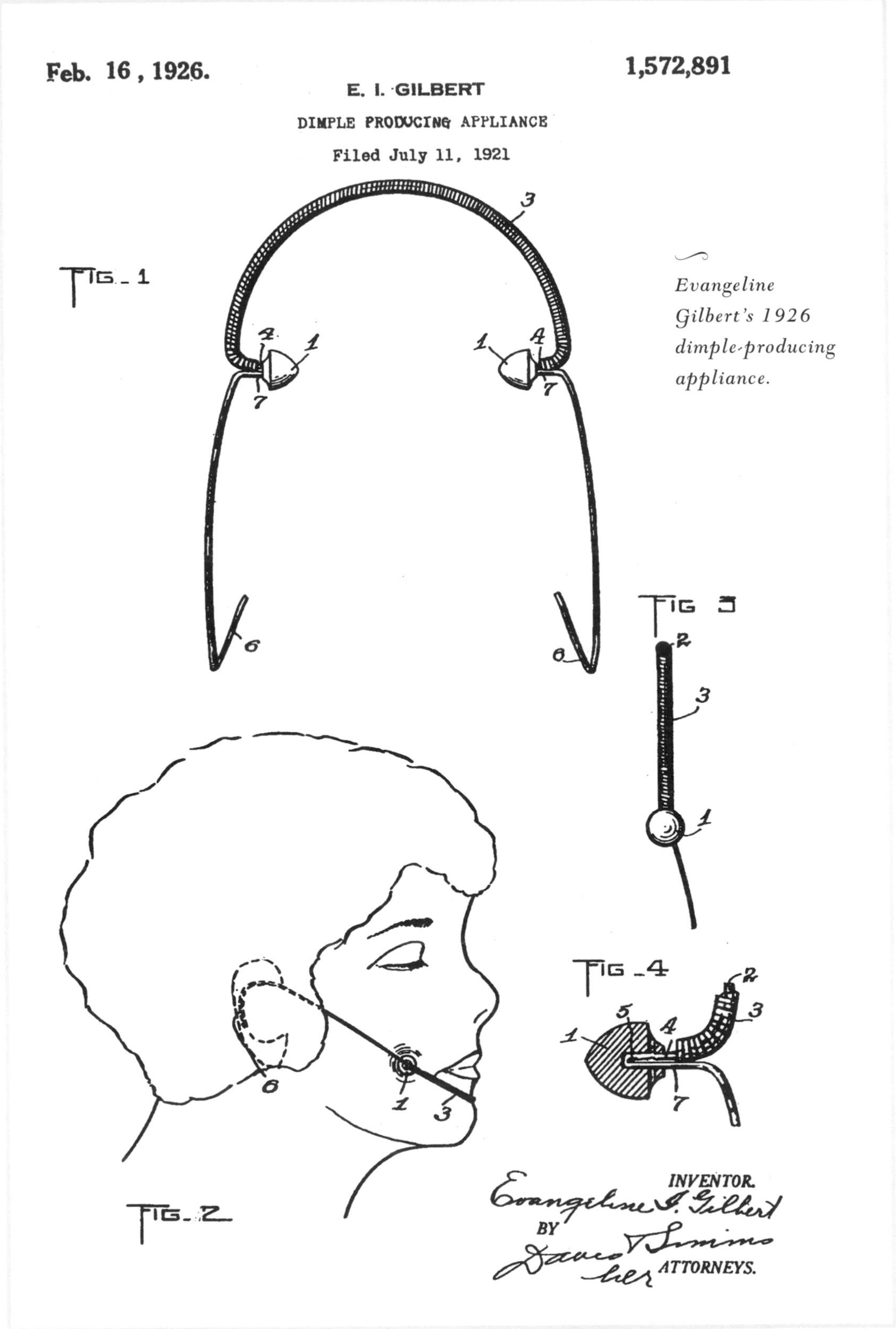

Feb. 16, 1926.

E. I. GILBERT

DIMPLE PRODUCING APPLIANCE

Filed July 11, 1921

1,572,891

FIG. 1

Evangeline Gilbert's 1926 dimple-producing appliance.

FIG. 3

FIG. 4

FIG. 2

INVENTOR.

Evangeline I. Gilbert

BY

David Simms

her ATTORNEYS.

Beverly Hills, California, who received at least four patents covering his method of minimizing "facial senescence," as he put it. Smooth facial skin tissue is an "especially important desideratum as women increasingly occupy professional and business positions," he noted in 1959.[39]

Precedent for Brown's instant face-lifter went far back. For more than sixty years previously, inventors—most of them women—were tinkering with the same idea. In 1895, Elizabeth Ent of Philadelphia patented a "Device for Removing Wrinkles and Hanging Cheeks and Chins of the Human Face," which gripped the tops of the cheeks and was tightened with pinions.[40] Abbie M. Hess and Alfred Lee Tibbals of Kansas City, Kansas, patented a face-lifter in 1913 that gripped the ears, pulling them upward. The device not only eliminated double chins and wrinkles, the inventors claimed, but it also relieved "partial deafness."[41] In 1937, Elma Knauth of New

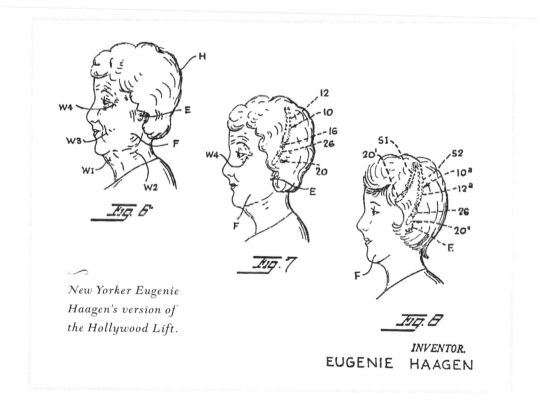

New Yorker Eugenie Haagen's version of the Hollywood Lift.

York City claimed that her beauty appliance "may be compared in its performance with the work of a sculptor engaged in portraying a face as it was at a more youthful period."

Mechanical face-lifters appear to have reached their baroque era in 1966, when Edna Jurgovan patented a type of butterfly bandage that, camouflaged by a preposterously large earring, was supposed to pull up the slack from cheek wattles.

Surgical Fountain of Youth

A face-lift, like any surgical procedure, was fairly risky before antibiotics came into routine use. Anesthesia became more refined and antibiotics became widely available at about the same time as the invention of Cinemascope film and television, both of which provided such realistic close-ups that viewers in the back row of the movie house could discern nose hairs and blackheads. Postoperative healing became more of a sure thing just as screen actors were feeling even more pressure to look even more youthful. With the face-lift, a surgical wizard could perform exactly the sort of fountain-of-youth sorcery that wrinkle cream and beauty contraptions had promised for eons but were never able to truly deliver.

Just as they were first to experiment with many other beauty innovations, the rich and famous were first to make the pilgrimage to plastic surgeons. Plastic surgery became a respectable, even glamorous profession as word quietly spread of celebrities who had face-lifts: Lucille Ball, Joan Crawford, Gary Cooper, Bette Davis, Fred Astaire, John Wayne, Gloria Swanson as well as Woolworth heiress Barbara Hutton.

But plastic surgeons quickly aimed their scalpels at a less glamorous but equally profitable market: the middle class. In 1957 surgeon Walter C. Alvarez pitched the face-lift to the hausfrau. Writing in *Good Housekeeping,* he compared plastic surgery to sewing. "After the surgeon loosens the skin so that it can be moved," Alvarez said, "he pulls it up and outward to straighten out the wrinkles, and he shapes it to the face, just as a seamstress might fit a dress over the shoulders of a woman. . . . He puts a few "basting" stitches to guide him later and cuts off the excess. . . . Then with a fine and almost invisible suture (stitching), he brings the two edges of the cut together."[42]

In June of 1960, *Harper's Bazaar*, the women's magazine for the soignée upper crust, waved the wand of respectability over the face-lift procedure. "The Wish to Be Beautiful is part of every woman," wrote Geri Trotta, who proclaimed that cosmetic surgery had emerged from "the unwholesome hush of conspiracy, the aura of guilty secrecy."

Trotta matter-of-factly explained that a face-lift took from four to five hours and that the liftee needed to stay in the hospital for several days. While a woman should not feel compelled to advertise the fact that her fresh look had been accomplished with the aid of a scalpel rather than a new makeup foundation, "she might larkily admit it to her friends as she might mention dyeing her hair."[43]

The next year *McCall's* magazine told its middle-class readers that it was a myth that only "vain, rich, idle women" sought plastic surgery.[44] By 1963 the lift went truly mainstream when the *Ladies' Home Journal* published "The Diary of a Face Lift," which was ostensibly written by an anonymous housewife who had saved up for the operation by squirreling away part of her household allowance and taking on odd jobs. It was not a comfortable procedure, she acknowledged. Fluid had to be drained from her neck and as the stitches healed her scalp itched ferociously. But it was worth it. When she returned from a six-week recuperation away from home her best friend passed judgment. "Oh," she said, "I hate you."[45]

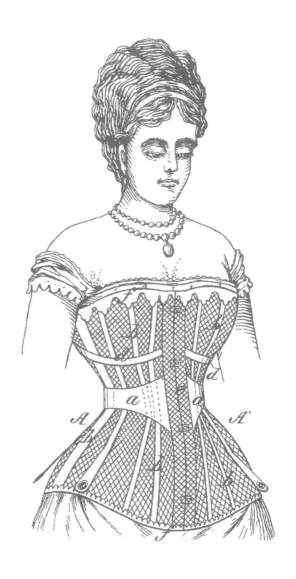

CHAPTER 6

Waist

"Nothing could be more amenable to reason—or unreason—as set forth by the creators of fashions than the human figure. With the greatest of amiability it lends itself to a corset which molds it like a lump of potter's clay into the lines of the latest styles. With every radical change in fashion there follows inevitably a change in the figure and the corset."

— *Delineator*, October 1914

A cross virtually all cultures, it turns out, men are particularly attracted to a certain waist-to-hip ratio in women. The ideal ratio is .7, meaning that the waist would be seventy percent as big as the hips. This is the ratio, believe it or not, of such disparate beauties as Marilyn Monroe, Twiggy, the *Venus de Milo,* and virtually every Miss America since Margaret Gorman first won the title in 1921. (For those with less than hourglass shapes, however, it is comforting to consider the measurements of the paleolithic sculpture *Venus of Willendorf.* If built to human scale, her proportions would be 96-89-96, meaning that her waist is almost ninety percent as big as her hips.)

Given this male predilection, it is no wonder that women have long sought assistance in minimizing the size of their waists. For several centuries the corset coyly provided a waist for the waistless without provoking controversy. The average corset, concludes cultural historian Valerie Steele, helped women achieve, on average, a waist-to-hip ratio of a nearly ideal .72.

Given that women deployed the corset effectively as an instrument of seduction for several centuries, how is it that the corset had gone virtually extinct by the early twentieth century? Basically, the corset was being engineered to become more effective (in the sense that it constrained the figure more effectively) at precisely the same time that new freedoms demanded a more flexible torso for women. So—and this may shock those who place great faith in the idea of an ineluctable march forward of technological progress—corset innovation for decades was heading in the opposite direction of social progress.

Body Armor in the Battle of Love

The corset was engineered and reengineered many different times over the course of the nineteenth century. The corset of 1900 evolved into a creature that was vastly different from its great-grandmother. Imagine the difference between a simple country chapel and a Gothic cathedral pushed skyward by flying buttresses. They are both buildings that house the sacred, true, but there the similarity ends.

So how did the corset become so transformed? As with the hoop skirt, ladies of the Spanish, and possibly Italian, court pioneered the cutting-edge Western versions of the corset. By the early fifteenth century, they were wearing a new invention called a "body," which was essentially the lady's counterpart to a knight's armor—though of course it was deployed not in war but rather in the battle of love.

The "body" was constructed of two hinged pieces of stiffened material that was further strengthened with slats of wood or whalebone known as "stays" (later to be called "boning"). Although some striking metallic corset specimens have survived, they were not, alas, some fantastical instrument of bondage dreamed up by a forefather of the Marquis de Sade. Rather, it seems they had the more prosaic goal of correcting misshapen spines.

The French and English appropriated the corset but lost no time introducing a new innovation, the busk: a long rigid stomach-flattening strip inserted down the middle of the front of the corset. By the sixteenth century, aristocratic women commissioned elaborate busks of ivory, boxwood, mother of pearl, and even silver to be inserted in their luxuriously hand-stitched corsets of silk or damask.

"Made by specialist craftsmen and often engraved with amorous verses, the busk itself became an erotic object, the subject of boudoir poems and public gestures," according to cultural historian Marilyn Yalom. "It was considered daring to pull the central busk out of the bodice and to gesture with it as a form of flirtation."[1] One such inscription, written in the voice of the busk itself, went like this:

> *I have from Madam this grace*
> *that I may rest long on her bosom,*
> *from where I heard a lover sigh*
> *that he would well take my place*[2]

Meanwhile, the merchant class had to reinforce its corsets with less poetic material—uninscribable turkey cartilage, for example. And working-class women wore something called a corselet, a looser-fitting, buskless garment that nonetheless gave shape to the waist and supported the breasts. Worn over a shirt and skirt, the corselet laced up the front rather than the back.

Waisting Away

The corset had been a controversial article of clothing at least since the philosopher Jean-Jacques Rousseau exhorted women to return to nature, cast off their corsets, and breast-feed (a noble idea, though it is curious that it came from someone who had earlier cast off his own wife and children). Many French women did make the revolutionary gesture of abandoning their corsets. The striking Madame Tallien, the ruling fashionista of Paris who claimed to preserve her beauty by bathing in crushed raspberries, showed up to a ball in the fall of 1795, naked save for the sleeveless, form-revealing silk sheath draped over her magnificent body.

Corsets then went out of fashion for the trim-figured during the first two decades of the nineteenth century as the empire waist (or rather lack of waist) became the rage so that breasts could take center stage. But by about 1825 the straight lines of the Greek-revival silhouette undulated into a Romantic passion for small waists and swelling skirts.

And that's when things get interesting, corset-wise. For in the ensuing decades the industrial revolution ushered in not just steamboats and railroads but also myriad new and improved ways to construct corsets that would transform the way women looked.

Early on, these inventions were of two sorts. One kind gave rise to corsets that could be more tightly laced, affording any given woman the opportunity to eye-catchingly exaggerate the difference between the size of her waist and the size of her hips.

The other category of inventions changed the collective profile of Western women by democratizing what had once been an article of status and privilege and turning the corset into something it had never been before: an affordable, highly finished product available to the great masses of common, laboring women.

Until the late 1820s, ladies attempting to cinch their waists to the extreme would have faced the prospect of ripping their laces right through the eyelets. That's because the eyelets were reinforced with stitches and nothing more. In 1823, however, a London inventor by the name of Rogers came up with the idea of metal eyelets. His idea did not make it to market but a Parisian inventor, Daude, came up with an early version of a two-piece metal eyelet, which he patented in 1828. This both obviated the need for intricate hand-stitching and made it possible to lace up a corset more tightly than before. Indeed, it is an innovation that has survived into the twenty-first century.

"My daughters are living instances of the baleful consequences of the dreadful fashion of squeezing the waist until the body resembles that of an ant," a tradesman wrote in 1928. "Their stays are bound with iron in the holes through which the laces are drawn so as to bear the tremendous tugging which is intended to reduce so important a part of the human frame to a third of its natural proportion."[3]

During the 1830s, corsets became stiffer still thanks to the use of cording, light boning, and intricate geometric or floral stitching. About a decade later, Madame Dumoulin, a French corset maker, introduced a corset without gussets—diamond-shaped or triangular inserts that provided for the breasts. She sculpted a form-fitting shape, according to the February 1844 issue of *Les Modes Parisiennes*, by sewing together seven to thirteen separate pieces that "decrease or increase gradually to follow the contours of the figure."[4] As we shall see, she started a trend that in the decades to come, when combined with other innovations, would profoundly augment the corset's ability to remold a woman's body.

While metal eyelets and fitted pieces were allowing women to squeeze their waists tighter, several other innovations put the corset on the path to mass production. A major obstacle, however, was figuring out how to make a corset that a woman could put on and take off by herself.

Before the nineteenth century, corsets had been the province of aristocratic and bourgeois women, who in the absence of a husband or lover could turn to a servant to do the unlacing in the back. A joke recycled frequently by satirists depicted a husband who, upon unlacing his wife in the evening, would remark with astonishment that the laces of her corset were knotted differently from how he had knotted them in the morning.

In 1829, Jean Julien Josselin patented the first two-piece steel busk that a woman could fasten and unfasten herself. Alas, it had the unfortunate tendency to unhook itself at inopportune moments. Moreover, steel at that time was of such poor quality that it was inclined to rust or simply break apart.

In Britain, one of the best-known corset makers was Madame Roxy Anne Caplin, proprietress of a stay-making business and "ladies anatomical gallery" at 58 Berners Street in London. She and her husband dreamed up many improvements. They patented their own version of a mechanical corset as early as 1838. It had pul-

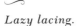

Lazy lacing.

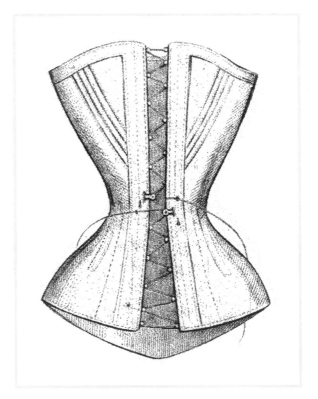

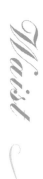

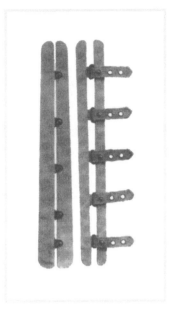

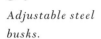

Adjustable steel busks.

leys and wheels behind and springs and grooves in front to allow a woman to get in and out of it herself. One can only imagine the fun fetishists might have had with this. Alas, it did not work very well, being only a minor improvement over the first pulley-equipped mechanical corset, which was unveiled at the Exposition Universelle of 1823 in France.[5]

It was not until 1840, with the invention of stretchy lacing, or "lazy lacing," that a woman could easily don body armor by herself. In the next decade, the two-part steel busk finally became a practical solution as quality steel became more abundant (for more on how this wonder material helped transform the appearance of women, see the history of hoop skirts in Chapter 8). A number of inventors, both in Europe and in America, came up with new versions. The most popular of these was a version that has remained to the twenty-first century: metal loops situated on one of the steel strips fasten onto metal studs situated on the other.

Conspicuous Invention

The Victorian era was an era of possessions, an age when clutter conferred class. Calling-card receivers, overstuffed parlor sets, hallstands, carpet sweepers, ice-boxes, antimacassars, lambrequins, pianos, sewing machines, and bric-a-brac and bibelots and gadgets that womankind had theretofore made do without now suddenly seemed necessities. Historian Vernon Parrington called the Gilded Age a "world of triumphant and unabashed vulgarity without its like in our history."[6]

It was also a time of unprecedented wealth. Before the Civil War the United States was home to only nineteen millionaires. By the 1890s there were more than four thousand. Robber barons like Andrew Carnegie and John D. Rockefeller and William K. Vanderbilt flaunted ostentatious wealth. Their domestic palaces rose along Fifth Avenue in the style of "French chateaux, Italian villas, Renaissance palazzos, and architectural concoctions that defied definition."[7]

But much of what had been the stuff of luxury in another era now became, with the advent of mass production, the province of everyman and everywoman. The promise of pulchritude beckoned from every quarter, especially from plate-glass windows in the grand department stores—Stewart's Marble Palace in New York City, Wanamaker's of Philadelphia, Marshall Field's in Chicago, Jordon Marsh in Boston.

Those who were not born to beauty could now purchase it.

This message was most compelling on the pages of the fashion magazines. Improvements in printing processes made images not just cheaper to duplicate but more real than ever. In the twenty years of ebullient economic expansion following the Civil War, the number of periodicals in America jumped nearly fivefold. Nationwide, in cities and on farms, in the East and the West, in the North and the South, American women were thumbing through the same pages of *Harper's Bazaar, Frank Leslie's Ladies' Journal,* the *Delineator, The Queen,* and *Demorest's Monthly Magazine.* Small newspapers may have featured hometown reports on the front page but

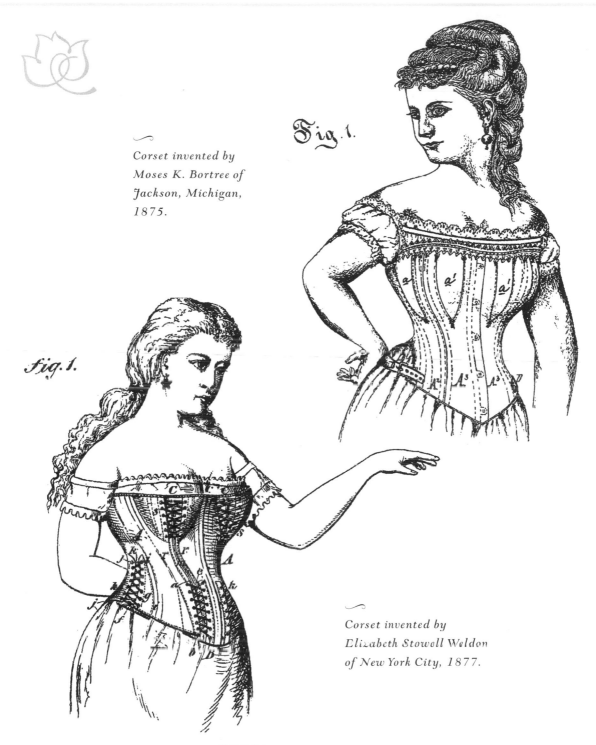

Fig. 1.

Corset invented by
Moses K. Bortree of
Jackson, Michigan,
1875.

fig. 1.

Corset invented by
Elizabeth Stowell Weldon
of New York City, 1877.

INVENTOR.
Elizabeth Stowell Weldon

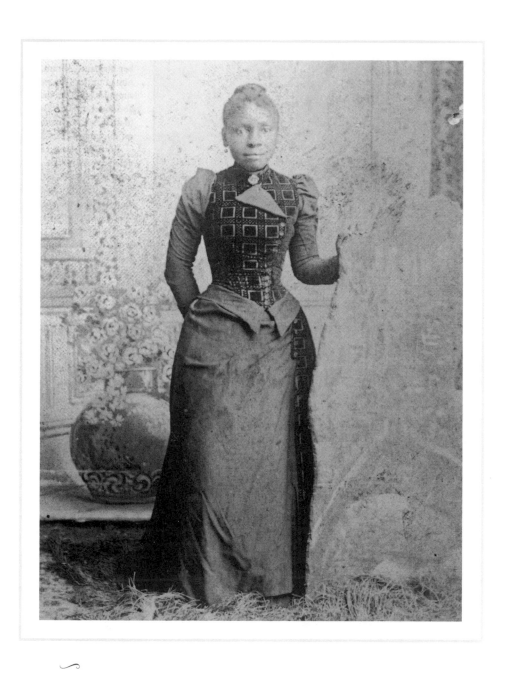

*A schoolteacher from Norfolk, Virginia, corseted into
a perfect hourglass figure.*

inside were preprinted syndicated "women's" and "farm" pages that offered news that was identical in hundreds of local papers across the country.

This point in time marks an important watershed in American history for consumer items. During the Gilded Age, abundance elbowed out necessity as the mother of invention. Just as abundance—a surplus of goods competing for dollars and attention of consumers—gave rise to the institution of advertising, so, too, it ushered an era during which much of "innovation" often would become indistinguishable from marketing.

During this era Thorstein Veblen coined the term *conspicuous consumption* to describe how people established their social status by buying material goods. But there is an important corollary to this theory that apparently did not occur to Veblen. This theory could easily be called "conspicuous invention"—and we have to look no further than the corset for ample evidence to support it.

When cosmetics were largely the province of hussies and actresses, a corset was the main instrument with which an ordinary woman could alter her form. And what an array of choices from which to choose! More than a thousand corset improvements were patented in the years between 1870 and 1900.[8] All these changes for a single consumer item that had first been "invented" centuries earlier. This is quite possibly more patents than were issued during the same period for the then-revolutionary form of communication known as the telephone system, covering everything from handsets and switchboards to electromagnets and vibrating diaphragms.[9]

Bodies Like Antique Sculptures

At the same time as all this furious innovation, both real and illusory, a quiet revolution was taking place that contributed greatly to the demise of the corset: exercise. Since the Civil War, calisthenics had become popular among both men and women. Then came the bicycle. At first, the only kind of lady for whom the bicycle was suitable was a stage acrobat. Although a side-saddle ladies high-wheeler bicycle

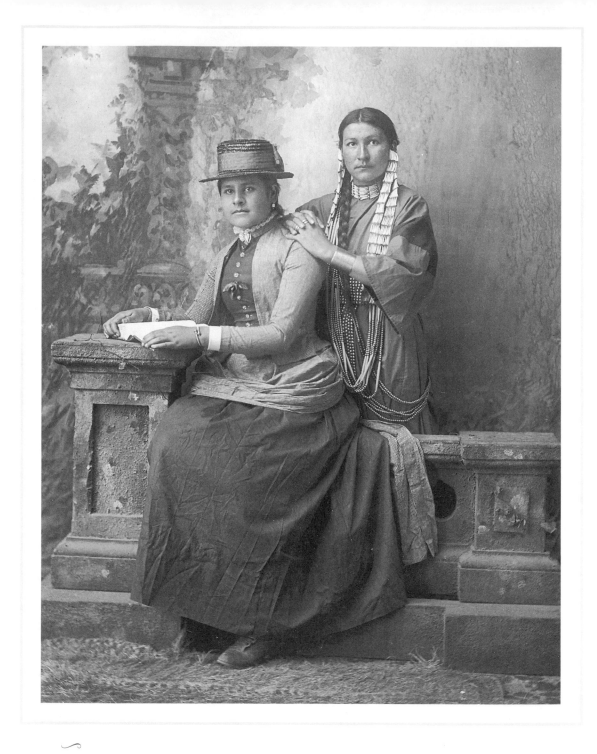

SHOOTING STAR, a Dakota woman, sits for her portrait corseted while her sister, Grass Woman, poses in native costume.

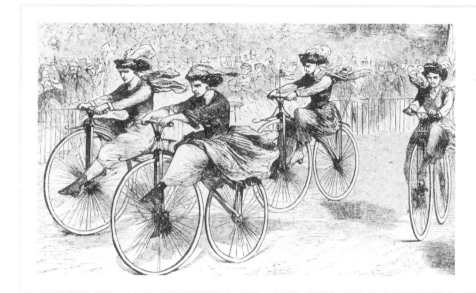

Daring athletic French female cyclists, before the invention of the safety bicycle. This illustration appeared in Harper's Illustrated Weekly *in 1868. It was copied from a European magazine, according to art historian Julie Wosk, but altered so that the ladies' legs were covered.*

was invented sometime in the 1880s, pedaling on only one side of the bicycle posed obvious balance challenges even for women who were masterful horseback riders.[10]

Later a much more reasonable vehicle appeared. The Victor was a dropped-frame version of the so-called safety bicycle, a machine with two wheels of equal size rather than the high-wheelers with a big wheel in front and a small one in back. It offered a new mode of exercise for women that required not so much mobility in the torso as deeper breathing, which the corset ostensibly restricted.

"They say that bicycling is all the rage now and that if I take the right time I shall see all the swell ladies on the wheel in bloomers," wrote Mrs. Alexander Graham Bell to her husband from Paris in 1895. "I believe no one attempts to ride a bicycle in any other garb."[11]

Teresa Dean commented in her 1889 book that while a few years earlier it had been unusual to see a woman riding a tricycle, the large, slow-moving adult-size ones that were fashionable at the time, "now our avenues are lined with ladies on the 'two-wheeler.' How gracefully they glide along, noiseless, untiring, at the rate of twelve or fifteen miles an hour, and how sensible they look."[12]

*Women dove out of
their corsets and
into the water.*

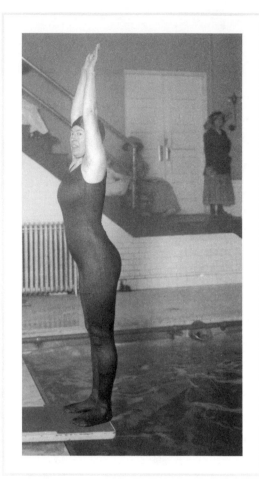

No doubt the bicycle, as many historians have already noted, was instrumental in getting ladies to get their bodies moving. But swimming may have had the most profound effect of all. As Maxine James Johns demonstrates in her fascinating, unpublished 1997 dissertation on women's swimwear, a public bath movement started in the mid-1800s in the United States, with the earliest bathhouse being built in New York City in 1852. By the turn of the century upwards of millions of people were swimming in public baths in other big cities such as Chicago and Boston. But outdoor swimming baths were also found in many less-cosmopolitan spots: Columbus, Ohio; Erie, Pennsylvania; Alhambra, Montana; Waco, Texas.

The main point of these baths was to wash the great unwashed—immigrants and rural folks who were streaming into cities at a rapid pace. But people did more than bathe in these large pools; they also learned to swim.

Ultimately, not just working women but also "ladies" from upscale New York neighborhoods swam in the baths. "In the all-female arena, they unselfconsciously learned to swim from competent instructors who were convinced, and convinced others, that women of all ages and physical ability could and should learn to swim," according to Johns.[13]

During 1877, one Chicago bath was reserved from five P.M. to six P.M. for "a dozen or two expert swimmers," according to the *Chicago Tribune*—women whose bodies were like "antique statues."[14] In New York, the Berkeley Ladies' Athletic Club offered not just a swimming pool but also three bowling alleys and gym equipment designed with ladies in mind by one Dr. Dudley A. Sargent, the "physical director" at Harvard. Women and girls gave exhibitions that featured dumbbell exercises, drills, fancy stepping, fencing, club swinging, apparatus work, and "heavy" gymnastics.[15]

Scribners Magazine published Sargent's article on the physical development of women in 1889, in which he reported a study of a dozen women running both with and without corsets. His findings? After running one-third mile in loose gym garments, the women averaged 152 heartbeats to the minute. After running the same distance while wearing a corset that reduced their waists by one inch, they averaged 168 heartbeats a minute.

By the time the Australian swimmer Annette Kellermann crossed the English Channel in 1905, ordinary women had been swimming for several decades. So they were likely receptive to the proclamation by Dr. Sargent that Kellermann's body approximated perfection (alas, we have no record of her waist-to-hip ratio) and constituted an ideal that young girls should emulate. Kellermann was no shrinking violet. In 1907 she was arrested for indecent exposure in Boston for appearing on a beach in a revealing one-piece jersey swimming suit.

Daring young flappers followed suit. Zelda Sayre, during the years she was being courted by an army lieutenant and aspiring writer named F. Scott Fitzgerald, scandalized Birmingham society girls by racing about in a flesh-colored stocking suit.

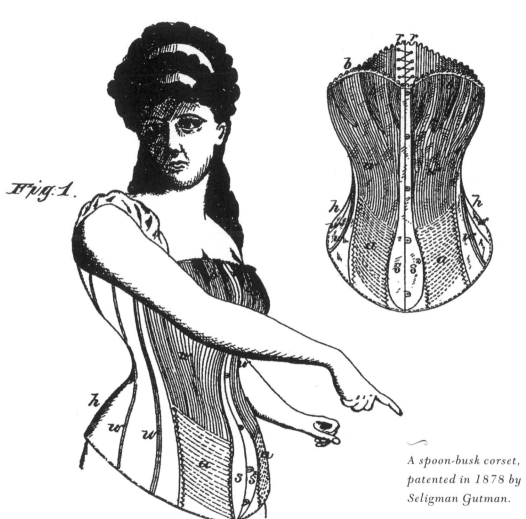

Fig. 1.

Fig. 2.

A *spoon-busk corset,*
patented in 1878 by
Seligman Gutman.

When the straps to that proved irritating, she peeled it off with panache and, completely nude, made a swan dive into the cool pool below.[16]

As women's bodies became more toned, their own muscles began taking over the function of the corset, whose purpose was to hold in the torso as well as uplift the bust. "It must not be forgotten," writes Norah Waugh in *Corsets and Crinolines*, "that twentieth-century education, with its accent on games and physical training, had by now produced a woman whose firm young body was adequately supported by her own muscles."[17]

Yet even as women were becoming increasingly athletic, the corset of the day was constructed in an increasingly restrictive way, whether one chose to tight-lace or not.

That's because the corset of the 1870s had evolved into quite a different beast than it had been even a decade earlier. To begin with, the process of steam molding came into practice in 1869. A corset that had been cut and reinforced with stays—the firm but flexible strips of material such as whalebone—now could be stretched around a copper mannequin with a pluperfect figure, starched to kingdom come, steamed, and then dried into a stiff mold into which real living women with less than ideal figures could pour themselves.

As the human body is less pliable than, say, hot wax, a variety of contrivances were invented to ease this process. The spoon busk, for example, was introduced in 1873. It was called a spoon busk because, yes, it was shaped like a big long spoon with a very flat bowl. That bowl rested right against the lower part of the tummy with the ladle extending up against the breast bone. (Rather than a spoon, the French likened the busk to a pear, calling it a *busc en poire.*)

Woman could not aspire to a couture figure with mere homemade foundation garments. The shapes proffered by ready-made articles were not achievable on a home sewing machine, even though Isaac Singer's credit plan made sewing machines as prevalent in parlors as cast-iron stoves had become in kitchens across America.

Ugly Children and Swollen Feet

Though it was simmering during much of the 1800s, anticorset sentiment did not reach a boil until the last part of the century. In 1874, Luke Limner wrote a widely reprinted screed against the corset, listing ninety-seven "diseases produced by Stays and Corsets according to the testimony of eminent medical men."

The litany of ills visited upon corset-wearing women, he alleged, included tuberculosis, cancer, chlorosis, dropsy, kidney disease, fainting, liver inflammation, hunched backs, hysteria, melancholy, epilepsy, miscarriage, ugly children, and swollen feet.[18] Meanwhile, a group calling itself the Ladies' Sanitary Association declared that "There ought to be the word Torture, or Murder, in large letters on every pair of stays."[19]

American feminists also tried to banish the corset. The New England Women's Club, founded by Julia Ward Howe, even set up a store in Boston to sell alternative, more humane undergarments that, while lighter and looser, still had the cut of a corset. In 1899, Thorstein Veblen, the cranky American economist, joined the anticorset chorus in his *Theory of the Leisure Class*. Veblen railed against high heels and corsets as devices by which rich men could render their wives unable to work, so that these women were no longer so much people as status objects.

"The corset is, in economic theory, substantially a mutilating undergarment for the purpose of lowering the subject's vitality and rendering her permanently and obviously unfit for work," Veblen grumbled.[20] Though he proffered an original analysis of the corset, he was hardly original in his criticism. From the late 1860s through the 1890s the British medical journal *The Lancet* frequently published articles lamenting the unhealthy repercussions of tight lacing.[21]

In 1904, Dr. Arabella Kenealy bolstered her argument against the corset by describing an experiment with monkeys. "A number of miniature corsets, exactly

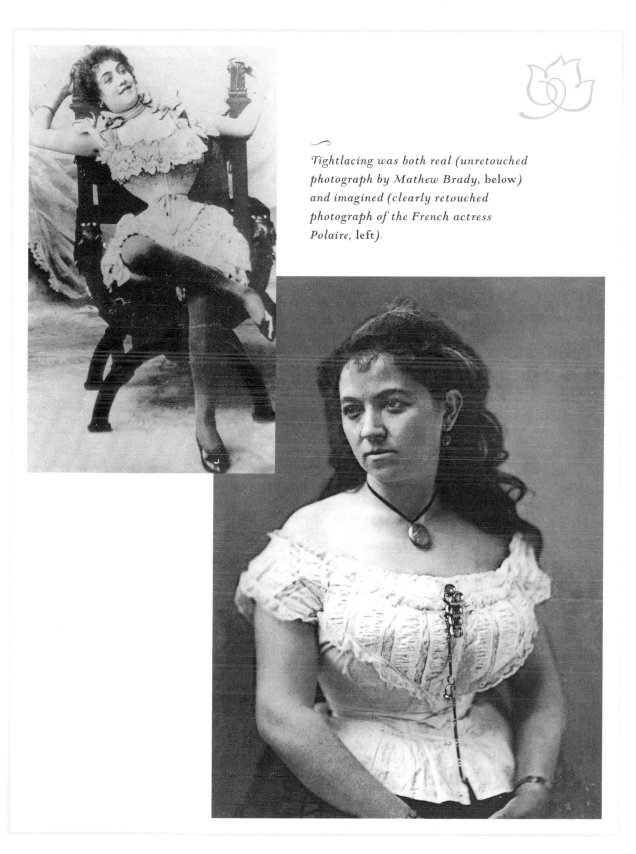

Tightlacing was both real (unretouched photograph by Mathew Brady, below) and imagined (clearly retouched photograph of the French actress Polaire, left).

similar to those worn by women, were fashioned to size, and a number of poor little creatures encased in them," Dr. Kenealy wrote. Those wearing the S-curve (as opposed to hourglass-shaped) corsets died "within days," she said. The others, with more conventional corsets, lived longer but poorly.

"These rudimental martyrs to a civilized vice fell off grievously in appetite and spirits," wrote Dr. Kenealy. "They . . . moped and lost flesh, alternating between extreme languor and marked nerve-irritability."[22] A fascinating experiment but, given that the "experiment" took place in an unnamed placed at an unspecified date, one suspects that Dr. Kenealy's colorful rhetoric sprang from emotion rather than scientific observation.

Yet the corset continued to have its ardent defenders. In the United States, the Women's National Medical Association declared itself in favor of corsetry. Popular writers championed it as well. Teresa Dean, in her 1889 book *How to Be Beautiful*, facetiously questioned whether the inventor of the corset should have supplied operating instructions on how to lace it appropriately, since she herself considered the corset to be the ultimate in "comfort, grace and beauty."

"This unending war against corsets that has been raging for about two score years and ten is certainly as good an advertisement as the most enterprising manufacturers can wish for," Dean wrote. If tightlacing has "wiped off from the face of the earth a few brainless women," so be it, she declared.

"If a woman's vanity, poor taste or ignorance leads her to 'draw the strings' until a serious injury is the result, she should by all means discard the corset, just as she would flee from any other temptation she has not the will power to resist."[23]

Some twenty years later, Havelock Ellis, the high-profile sexologist of the time and onetime paramour of birth-control evangelist Margaret Sanger, expressed a similar sentiment. In an article entitled "An Anatomical Vindication of the Straight Front Corset," Ellis claimed that female humans required corseting because the evolutionary shift from "horizontality to verticality" was fraught with structural challenges for women.

A woman might be "physiologically truer to herself if she went always on all fours," he wrote. The shift in gravitational pull on her feminine viscera caused such "profound physiological displacements" that the corset is "morphologically essential."[24] Curiously, however, Ellis did not make any parallel observations that gravitational pull might make jock straps also morphologically essential (after all, they had been invented in 1874).

In 1910, the same year that Ellis's article was published, the champion of U.S. women's amateur tennis addressed the hotly contested subject of whether women should wear corsets while playing golf or tennis. She wore one herself while playing, she said, and felt they were "desirable for many reasons." One of these reasons? That corsets simply made women athletes look better.[25]

As the debate over tightlacing raged, doctors and dressmakers alike responded to warnings of the dangers of tightlacing by inventing "improved," "hygienic," "rational," "sanitary," or "reform" versions of the corset.

One comfort corset was introduced by the eccentric Dr. Gustav Jaeger, promoter of the Sanitary Woolen System. He argued that his wool corsets had "all the advantages of girded loins without the disadvantages." They were not for the fashionably inclined, however, as they had all the sex appeal of an old sock.

Unlike the corsets designed by Jaeger, however, many, indeed most, of these "healthful" corsets ended up being far more restrictive than the ones they were meant to replace. Their makers boasted that they were designed by medical doctors and emphasized their salutary effect.

But in fact these new corsets were on a par, medically, with patent medicines popular during that era, like Lydia E. Pinkham's Vegetable Compound (one part herbs, three parts alcohol). Not that women could be faulted for turning to Lydia Pinkham's potions in an age when bloodletting was considered state-of-the-art medical care. But it should be noted that the medical "profession" during the nineteenth century was riddled with charlatans.

Perhaps the single biggest influence on corset design toward the end of the nineteenth century was Dr. Josephine Ines Gaches-Sarraute, a French woman who was both a physician and a corsetiere. In 1896 and 1897, Gaches-Sarraute published claims in French medical journals about the superior construction of her corsets. Convinced by her claims, physicians from Amsterdam to Tokyo exhorted their patients and peers to follow her advice. One of Gaches-Sarraute's many lay American proselytizers was Mrs. E. B. Duffey, who extolled their virtues in *What Women Should Know*, her 1898 book of beauty hints.[26]

In America, Lucien Warner and his brother, Ira De Ver, both trained as physicians, hawked their version of a healthful corset. The business had been started by Lucien, who unlike his brother was unable to establish a successful medical practice.

Initially, Lucien rode the circuit, selling vitamins from the back of a horse-drawn wagon and lecturing on liver ailments until a new entrepreneurial idea snapped into his head: Why not sell a new "healthful" corset? The first corset he produced actually had shoulder straps and a nonconstricting waistband. It resembled closely, in fact, a corset already produced by Mrs. Lavinia Foy, an inventor who started out in New Haven, Connecticut, and relocated to Boston; she successfully challenged him on her patent.

Soon Warner was selling instead a "straight front" corset similar to the type promoted by Gaches-Sarraute. "The altruistic principles upon which the business was founded (such as suspending weight from the shoulders and not compressing the waist) were sacrificed by the good doctors on the altar of fashion and financial exigency," according to a John W. Field and Bernard Smith, Warner biographers.[27] Ira De Ver soon joined the business and both brothers were millionaires within four years.

Dr. Gaches-Sarraute and her imitators, the Warner brothers, transformed the hourglass corset, which, when it was not tightly laced, restricted the waist only modestly, into rococo contraptions that cinched the waist to breathtaking degrees.[28] Featuring "straight front" busks and constructed of numerous longitudinal sections, these medically inspired corsets forced excess flesh up toward the bosom and down toward the derriere. They were increasingly reinforced not with whalebone, which was extremely expensive, but with steel, an unforgiving material that was billed as being unbreakable. It in fact did break when the pressure from flesh became too great, sometimes inflicting puncture wounds.

Corset anatomique et scientifique de l'Académie de Paris

Breveté S. G. D. G.

Exécuté par Mⁱˡᵉ E. AGIER, 22, Avenue de l'Opéra, PARIS

MEDAILLE D'OR à l'Exposition Franco-Anglaise de Londres 1908 (Première Exposition où ait figuré le " CORSET ANATOMIQUE ")

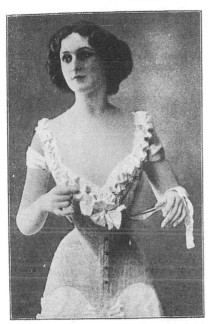

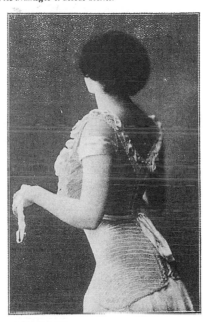

Le plus grand désir de Mⁱˡᵉ E. Agier est que chaque femme montre son corset à son docteur, à la disposition duquel elle se tiendra pour toutes explications et démonstrations qu'il pourrait désirer.

Mⁱˡᵉ E. Agier est heureuse de signaler à sa nombreuse et fidèle clientèle sa dernière innovation, le merveilleux " Corset Gant ", sans baleines ni coutures, ne se distendant jamais.

Mⁱˡᵉ E. Agier s'engage à annuler la commande de tout corset, essayé au magasin, qui ne réunirait pas les conditions et les avantages ci-dessus décrits.

Ce corset, non seulement transforme le corps de la femme par sa forme extra-esthétique et élégante, mais il lui donne une grâce incomparable en même temps qu'une souplesse et une légèreté du corps jointe au plus grand confort. Il est construit de telle façon qu'il ne presse sur aucun organe, mais bien au contraire, la femme peut se serrer indéfiniment, sans jamais se faire du mal. La compression s'opère sur les os du bassin, au bas de l'abdomen et au bas des reins qu'il maintient en bonne position, ainsi que tout l'organisme de la femme, qui fonctionne avec aisance.

Toutes les maladies occasionnées par le port de mauvais corsets peuvent être combattues avec succès par le Corset anatomique.

Démonstration des avantages du Corset anatomique

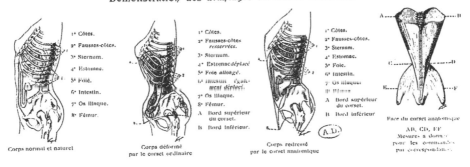

A Torso of Steel

Steel came more and more into favor not mainly because it was cheap. Other suitable materials were either scarce or deficient in some way. Cane and cork were flexible, but because of the tight construction of the corset they often broke. Braided horsehair was not stiff enough to brace the fashionable silhouette. Whalebone had long been a precious commodity and buffalo cartilage, which had proved a worthy substitute, also became rare.

At the turn of the century, the steel-boned S-curve corset became increasingly grotesque, with the waist becoming tinier and tinier and the tailbone arching farther and farther to the rear. Women, always in search of novel ways to remold themselves, initially loved it. The aim was to achieve an S-shaped figure—a posture more goose-like than human. The epitome of that new fashion figure was the Gibson girl, immortalized by Charles Dana Gibson but also favored by other artists, including Harrison Fisher, Howard Chandler Christy, and Edward Penfield.

"Edwardian underclothes developed a degree of eroticism never previously attempted," wrote C. Willett and Phillis Cunnington. Women had "invented a silhouette of fictitious curves, massive above, with rivulets of lacy embroidery trickling over the surface down to a whirlpool of froth at the foot."[29]

The curious paradox here is that, as it was reinvented and reinvented, the corset became more and more standardized. Instead of providing a vast array of choices that fit women's individual bodies and responding to their changing lifestyles, manufacturers produced fashion corsets that were more and more uniform structurally even though their superficial differences were increasingly varied.

Yellow Apricot and Peacock Blue

Earlier in the century, corsets were sedate, private affairs. "Dyed colors are occasionally attempted," notes costume historian Karen Brown-Larimore, "but are not 'acceptable' to a proper lady of the 1830s."[30] By the 1840s new dyeing technology made red and black corsets essential building blocks of the fashionable wardrobe. In the ensuing decades, as dyeing techniques improved further, well-off women could buy silk or satin corsets in every hue, from amber gold and cardinal red to yellow apricot and peacock blue. The masses could choose from cotton or linen corsets made from a more subtle palette: gray, putty, and tan. White remained a fashionable option for all classes.

During the 1880s the corset became more decorative still. To be "dainty" was the ultimate compliment of the era, and ladies' underwear was nothing if not dainty. Corsets were embroidered in colorful floral designs that complemented the shade of the corset itself. They were threaded with ribbons and beading and brimming with lace.

As advertising proliferated, firms gave the illusion of variety as they trumpeted the advantages of one design over another. There were some exceptions. Early on, in 1867, Joseph H. Beal, Edward J. Sawyer, and Granville S. Webster of Boston patented a paper corset they claimed was "light and sufficiently strong and elastic, at the same time being cheap of construction."[31]

Doing the Unthinkable

But corset innovation at this point was found chiefly in the finishing materials and in the marketing, not in the design itself. Take, for example, the "electric" corset, quite a popular item in an era that worshiped the new wonder of electricity. Dr. Scott claimed that his corset would cure "internal weakness, pains in the back, palpitation, nervousness, hysteria" as well as extreme obesity. The authority for these claims? A Dr. W. A. Hammond, who is variously described as "Late Surgeon-General of the United States" and "formerly Surgeon-General to the U.S. Army."[32]

This is how the corset worked, according to an advertisement for Scott's Electric Corset that ran in *Harper's Weekly* in the 1880s:

"In place of the ordinary steel busks in front, and a rib or two at the back, Dr. Scott inserts steel magnetods which are exactly the same size, shape, length, breadth and thickness as the usual steel busk or rib. By this means he is able to bring the magnetic power into constant contact with all the vital organs, and yet preserve that symmetry and lightness so desirable in a good corset. It is affirmed by professional men that there is hardly a disease which Electricity and Magnetism will not benefit or cure."[33]

Each corset (retail prices ranged from one to three dollars) arrived with a silver compass which the wearer could use to verify that the corset was indeed electric. "Do not be misled by the advertisements of peripatetic vendors of rubbishing appliances in which there is nothing Electric but the name" warned an advertisement in *The Graphic,* a London newspaper.[34] In fact, what the little compass "proved" was merely that the steel stays had been weakly magnetized. But this was enough for most customers, given the murky definitions of "magnetic" and "electric" that were ricocheting about the average nineteenth-century mind. His corsets created "no unpleasant shock whatsoever," Dr. Scott averred.[35] And no wonder.

By about 1910, women individually and then collectively began to reinvent themselves by slackening their waistbands and drawing attention to other parts of

In my action-free SPENCER
I feel rested ... and
fit for work or play!

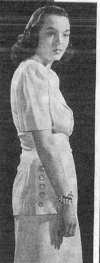

On the go all day long? Then enjoy the freedom-plus-support of an action-free Spencer! It will be light, flexible, easy to slip on and off—and, if you choose, can be made of an airy, easy-to-launder mesh!

Your Spencer Body and Breast Supports will be created just for you to solve your figure problems—and the health problems that come from imperfect posture. No more ugly bulges, tired back, weary feeling! You have trim new figure lines and radiant vitality. For keeps, too—because your Spencers will be *guaranteed* never to lose their shape.

Write or Phone for FREE Information

MAIL coupon below for fascinating booklet showing how a Spencer will help you! Or PHONE nearest dealer in Spencer Supports (look in yellow pages under "Corsets".—or in white pages under "Spencer Corsetiere" and "Spencer Support Shop".) No obligation!

CASUAL CLOTHES SHOW UP YOUR FIGURE! Ordinary supports do nothing for "spare tire", sagging abdomen, back bulge. No restful lift! *Right: see how tired and sloppy she used to look!*

CLOTHES LOOK SMARTER OVER YOUR SPENCER! Wear easy classics, dainty sheers, even slacks,—and *look* as well as you feel! *Far right: same woman, same dress, but wearing her Spencers!*

DOCTORS KNOW!
Doctors prescribe Spencer Supports to improve general health by improving posture; to aid treatment of back derangements—arthritis and other chronic diseases—displaced abdominal organs—breast problems—maternity—post-operative and other conditions.

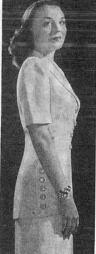

their bodies—the ankles and feet, for example. Paul Poiret, the Paris couturier du jour, grabbed credit for starting the fashion of hobble skirts—skirts whose hemline was so tight as to make walking nearly impossible save for in the tiniest and most mincing of steps.

"Like all great revolutions, this one had been in the name of Liberty—to give free play to the abdomen," he boasted in his memoir. "It was equally in the name of Liberty that I proclaimed the fall of the corset," he said. "Yes, I freed the bust but I shackled the legs."[36]

In 1911 the Illinois State Legislature considered a bill to prohibit both hobble skirts and bifurcated "harem" skirts. Defying pressure from social and governmental institutions, women who had refashioned themselves with the hobble skirt soon morphed their bodies into the flapper silhouette.

Corset makers were flummoxed by this trend. In 1921, G. B. Pulfer, the treasurer and general manager of the Kalamazoo Corset Company, issued a rallying cry to his fellow corsetieres in an article entitled "Fighting the Corsetless Evil."[37]

Why will women never abandon corsets? he asked rhetorically. "Fear!" Pulfer thundered. "Fear of ill health, fear of sagging bodies, fear of lost figure, fear of shiftless appliance in the nicest of clothing, fear of sallow complexion. Fear sends them to the corsetiere, trembling; the same corsetiere from whom they fled mockingly a couple of years back, at the beck of a mad style authority who decreed 'zat ze body must be free of ze restrictions, in order zat ze new styles shall hang so freely.' "[38]

Good Housekeeping, whose typical reader was a Midwestern matron wearing sensible shoes and price-shopping for a new icebox, tried to help out its loyal advertising base by publishing in 1921 a series of articles on how to choose a corset. One such tip: "If there is a surplus of flesh over the abdomen, place the hand inside the corset and smooth the flesh back toward the sides, not up in the front."[39]

All this effort was to no avail. The corsets responsible for that low-slung dowager silhouette so popular earlier were now simply god-awful uncomfortable to the many women who had been liberated from their strictures. Moreover, women had a new class of weapon in their beauty arsenal: cosmetics. The face would soon eclipse the waist as a focus of female allure.

Vogue magazine presciently analyzed the situation in an article entitled "Woman Decides to Support Herself." Women had grown used to loosely constructed waists because of recent trends in both fashion and sports, the magazine said. When couturiers—and corset makers—tried to reimpose a constricted waist, "the unexpected, the unprecedented, happened." And what was that? "Women refused to wear them; they actually did that unheard-of thing."[40]

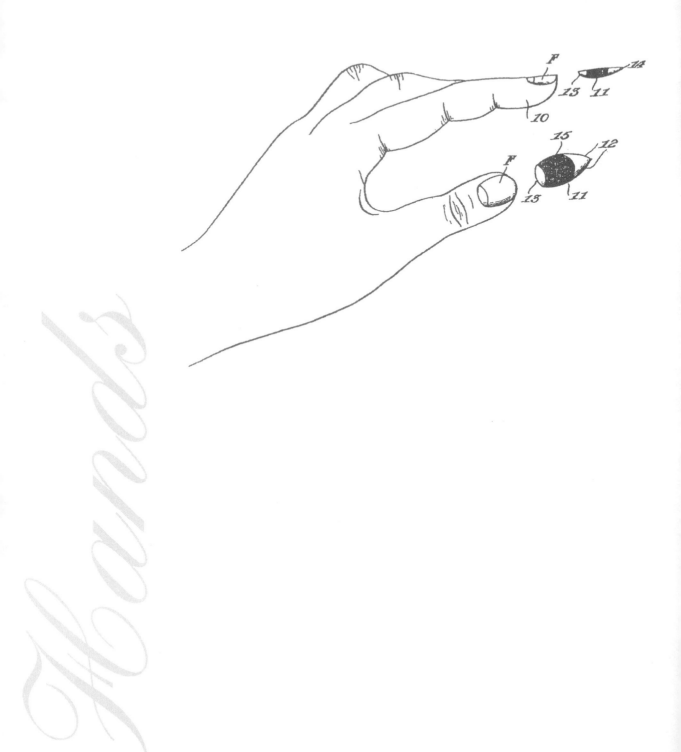

CHAPTER 7

Hands

The beauty of her whole figure, her head, her neck, her hands, struck Vronsky every time as something new and unexpected. He stood still, gazing at her in ecstasy.

— Leo Tolstoy, *Anna Karenina*[1]

I got home and told my wife and parents that I had a job. They said, "Great! Where?" I said, "With the Revlon Company. They make nail polish." My wife said, "Nail polish?" It was a dirty word. She never used nail polish or lipstick or anything else in those days.

— Charles Hastell, on being hired by Revlon in June 1933, quoted in *Fire and Ice*[2]

Given that hands are not intrinsically sexy, it is unlikely that they evolved as a way to attract a worthy mate. Hands are indispensable as tools for foraging, building shelter, starting fires, and holding babies, of course. But as sexual ornaments they pale in comparison to hips, lips, breasts, buttocks, or even those highly functional appendages, the legs.

This is what perhaps makes nail polish such an astounding invention. It transforms purely functional parts of a woman's body—the fingernails but also the toenails—into shiny little baubles that grab hold of the flitting eye of the male.

With hands, beauty equals idleness. We wear rubber gloves to do the dishes and slather our hands in lotion so we escape dishpan hands. Enormous jewels on our hands and long decorative fingernails make our hands look beautiful and give the impression that we are ladies of leisure.

Of course, the Western woman is by no means the first female to come up with the idea of ornamenting her hands. For centuries if not millennia, Indian and African women have dyed their fingertips with henna or other natural plant dyes. Rings made of precious metals and stones have called attention to hands throughout the ages.

But nail polish is perhaps the most revolutionary makeup innovation of the past century. Nail polish, a cheap product that is synthetic to its very core, reflects light and color with an intensity heretofore achieved only with expensive jewels. A woman time traveling from Elizabethan England or even ancient Greece or Egypt would likely not be terribly surprised at many of the cosmetics of the twenty-first century. Although the ingredients and packaging have changed, the effect of today's mascaras and lipsticks is not unlike kohl highlighting the eyes or ceruse brightening the lips.

Not so with fingernails.

The history of nail adornment might be best broken down into two periods, B.N. and A.N.—Before Nitrocellulose and After Nitrocellulose.

Before nitrocellulose lacquers came on the scene in the twentieth century, Western ladies seeking that manicured look turned to either powder or cream polish, which had as its base bee's wax or tin oxide or a form of silicon dioxide. Buffed onto the nails with a chamois cloth, these would produce a nice luster but would at best yield only a slight pink shade. As anyone who has had his or her nails buffed knows, the effect is far subtler than that imparted by the high-gloss, color-saturated nail polish of today.

Nitrocellulose had been around long before anyone thought about using it for nail polish. In the 1830s, European chemists discovered that dipping cellulose (otherwise known as wood pulp) into nitric acid made for a powerful explosive. Too powerful, alas, given that it tended to explode in the laboratory. Eventually, however, nitrocellulose became the basis for a smokeless gun powder. And later it formed the basis for celluloid, which revolutionized photographic film but also heralded the age of plastics as it was molded into false teeth, knife handles, combs, brushes, collars, and cuffs.

Before World War I, nitrocellulose lacquers were used in the woodworking industry on a limited basis—to varnish umbrella handles and wooden heels, for example. And in the early twentieth century, Germany held a strong technological lead in chemical industries and provided most of the world's lacquers and dyes. But during World War I blockades, the United States resourcefully appropriated German patents and licensed them out to American companies until hostilities ceased. Consequently the American chemical industry mushroomed and the United States, as a member of the victorious Allies, gained a postwar advantage that Germany did not recover until the 1970s.

During the 1920s the lacquer business grew symbiotically with the automobile industry. In 1921, seventeen factories were producing five million kilos of these lacquers. Just four short years later the United States had eighty-five such factories, churning out forty million kilos of the stuff. Indeed, without the creation of rapidly drying nitrocellulose automobile lacquers, Henry Ford's assembly-line production system might not have been possible.

Henry Ford famously said that his customers "can have any color they want so long as it's black." That was not just because he thought his customers needed nothing more than a no-frills utilitarian vehicle. At the time, black lacquer dried a lot faster than lacquer infused with other colors.

By 1923, however, DuPont came out with its Duco, a fast-drying pigmented

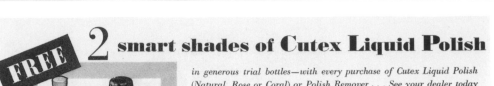

FREE

2 smart shades of Cutex Liquid Polish

in generous trial bottles—with every purchase of Cutex Liquid Polish (Natural, Rose or Coral) or Polish Remover . . . See your dealer today

The world's authority on the manicure makes this offer so that, without extra cost, you may try the new fashion of Variety in Nail Tints

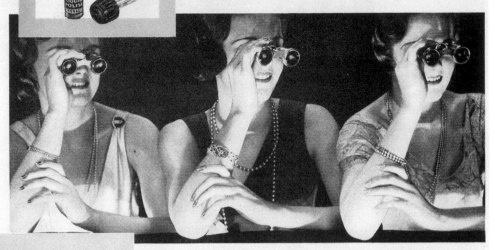

Tinted Nails or Natural? BOTH — say great Beauty Experts

Natural just slightly emphasizes the natural pink of your nails. It goes with every one of your costumes but is best with bright colors—bright red, bright blue, bright green, purple, orange and yellow. It is the most popular tint today.

Rose is a lovely feminine shade that you can wear with any color dress, pale or vivid. Blondes often prefer it to all other shades. It is subtle and charming with pastel pinks, blues, lavender . . . with dark green, black and brown.

Coral nails are bewilderingly lovely with white, pale pink, beige, gray, "the blues," black and dark brown—either daytime dresses or evening frocks. Smart also with deeper colors (except red) if not too intense.

Cardinal is deep and exotic. It contrasts excitingly with black, white, or any of the very pale shades. Good with gray or beige; very smart with the new blue. Wear Cardinal in your festive moods and be sure your lipstick matches!

Colorless is conservatively correct at any time. Choose it for bright or "difficult" colors.

TAKE ADVANTAGE *of this grand new Cutex offer. Be sure to get your complimentary package—containing 2 smart shades in generous trial bottles—FREE with every purchase of Cutex Liquid Polish in Natural, Rose or Coral, or Cutex Liquid Polish Remover.*

VARY your nail tint with your gown—the Beauty Experts say. It's time to stop wrinkling your lovely brows over whether to tint or not to tint your nails. And just put your best thought on *which tint* to wear with *what dress.*

If you find that color schemes tax your imagination, nobody cares if you refer to the panel on the left.

And once you get going you'll find this new nail fashion can do a lot for you.

Rose nails worn with any of the new aquarelles will take you to tea anywhere you say. And Coral nails with a white chiffon frock are guaranteed to bring you a positively confusing number of dance partners!

Anyway, you'll never again wear the same color nails with red, green, blue and pink dresses, will you? You might as well wear the same hat.

And right here is a good place to mention quality as well as color. Cutex has both! It comes in five perfect shades; absolutely won't crack, peel, streak or fade; and keeps its lustre one whole week!

And last, but not least, if you're a neat girl, it has a new bakelite cap with brush attached so that the tip never touches your table top.

Run around to your nearest dealer for the two lovely sample shades to start with. Free, with the special offer!

THE EASY CUTEX MANICURE... Scrub nails. Remove old cuticle and cleanse nail tips with Cuticle Remover & Nail Cleanser. Remove old polish with Polish Remover. Brush on the shade of Cutex Liquid Polish that best suits your costume. End with Cutex Nail White (Pencil or Cream) and the new Cutex Hand Cream. Before retiring, use Cutex Cuticle Oil or Cream.

NORTHAM WARREN · NEW YORK · LONDON · PARIS

Cutex *Liquid Polish* .. only 35¢

Look carefully in this 1930s ad and you can see the "moon manicure," which left the tips and the moons of fingernails white.

lacquer. General Motors' president Alfred P. Sloan Jr. began boldly painting his automobiles with DuPont's new colored synthetic lacquers to lure customers with novel styling. H. Ledyard Towle, a GM color consultant, boasted that he could "make a stubby car look longer and lower" through studied use of color.[3]

General Motors was not the only motor car company to wield a paint palette. In F. Scott Fitzgerald's 1925 masterpiece *The Great Gatsby*, Tom Buchanan drives a blue coupe and Gatsby's Rolls-Royce is a rich cream color. The car that Daisy Buchanan tragically crashes is a bright yellow. By 1927 an advertisement in the *Ladies' Home Journal* features a well-to-do woman reclining pensively on a sofa. "Paige-Jewett motor cars match milady's mood," the copy reads.[4] Tiny roadsters— blue, green, red, tan, white—swirl around her.

The hands of "milady" in the ad's illustration are not lacquered, but ultimately women decided that colored enamel could do for their nails what it had done for cars: make them glamorous. Nitrocellulose lacquers, made possible by the invention of new plasticizers and resins, were used to varnish automobiles, golf balls, pianos, and billiard balls. They also indelibly transformed the hands of women. Without them, cosmetics historian Gilbert Vail noted in 1947, "the manicuring art would not have been able to turn ordinary nails into the flawless colored and brilliant jewels that they are today."[5]

The first patent for a nail polish was granted in 1919. Its color was a very faint pink. Indeed, throughout the early 1920s, nail polish was available in any color so long as it was pink. Pale pink. Cutex in 1924 started offering a rose-colored enamel.[6] It's not clear how dark this rose was, but any girl whose nails were tipped in any pink darker than a baby's blush risked gossip about being "fast."

The vogue for painting fingernails more opaque colors likely originated in France, where it was adopted by Paris society and the elite who summered on the Riviera. *Vogue*'s beauty editor wrote in 1928 that "One of the first things that the knowing American woman does upon her arrival in Paris is to make an appointment for a manicure at Madame Mille's, that little place in the rue Saint Honoré which was formerly known as Carmichael's. The excellence of Madame Mille's liquid polish and the

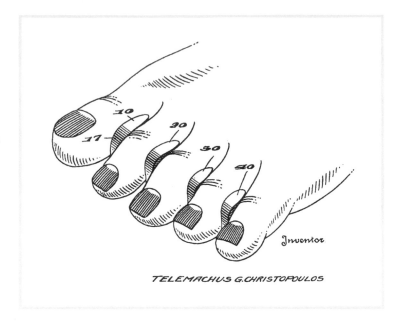

Toe-spacing device to keep polish from smearing on the feet.

exotic delicacy of the tint imparted to the nails have made her justly famous."[7] Generally, the polish was applied just on the middle of the nail; the half moons and tips were left white, leading Beatrice Kay, the manicurist at MGM movie studios, to dub this the "moon manicure."

From Pink to Black and Blue and Silver

In a bold move that would change the course of (fingernail) history, the exotic Princess de Faucigny-Lucinge grew her nails long and painted them a rich crimson. The effect was startling. It took a while to catch on but by the summer of 1930 "a handful of film stars and society beauties who were sunning themselves in the South of France suddenly realized that pale rose nails looked rather anaemic with sun-tanned fingers."[8]

They, too, discovered blood-red nail varnish, "which both pleased their artistic sense and gave them the satisfaction of knowing they were causing a sensation," according to Neville Williams in *Powder and Paint*. The ultra chic flashed their "platinum tips"—an opaque silver polish brushed on the ends of their already red nails.

Photographs of society queens basking in the sun with bright fingernails and toenails were published in newspapers. "The vogue spread like wildfire to other continental resorts, and holiday-makers returning to England via Paris, still wearing their sun tan, found that the smartest stores had stocked up with a wonderfully rich range of coloured nail varnishes."[9]

In 1932, American women introduced their own nail color trend by sporting black nail polish (shades of Henry Ford?), but this was short-lived. Before long nail polish was available in every color fathomable: blue, green, mother of pearl, wicked red, crimson red, blood red, bull's-eye red, and, since this was the era of art deco and all things shiny and sleek, gold and silver.

Publicity as "Honest Fiction"

Who brought these colors to the American woman?

The nail polish craze may have been ignited by French élan and fueled by Hollywood glamour, but it was Charles Revson, the founder of Revlon, who inspired the average female to burn with desire for bright shiny nails. No bold innovator he, Revson nonetheless contributed incremental improvements to the science of nail polish while, even more important, proving himself to be a marketing genius who could popularize a new product while ruthlessly elbowing aside the competition.

Robert Hoffman, inventor of the Hoffman professional hair dryer system, remembered Revson once telling him: "Copy everything and you can't go wrong." This was Revson's formula for forty-three years, according to a rollicking biography by Andrew Tobias: "You let the competitors do the groundwork and make the mistakes. And when they hit with something good, you make it better, package it better, advertise it better, and bury them."[10]

It seems ironic (or, conversely, inevitable, if one subscribes to the theory that all cosmetics are a male-imposed conspiracy to oppress women) that Charles Revson, who by some accounts was one of the great misogynists of twentieth-century America, would become so instrumental in the purveyance of such a distinctly feminine commodity. Few women employees, with the exception of the brilliant copywriter Kay Daly, stayed for long at Revlon. And wives (especially Revson's own wives) were outright banned from company trips.

If Charles Revson was a chauvinist in the workplace, he was a downright pig at home, according to Tobias's report. His extramarital exploits were to become the talk of the cosmetics industry, and the treatment of his wives verged on the sadistic. Revson claimed not to remember the name of his first wife. His long-suffering second wife eventually left him. And on the tenth anniversary of his marriage to his third wife, who was twenty-six years his junior, he presented her with a $30,000 check and five Van Cleef and Arpels bracelets—only to announce two days later that he had started divorce proceedings.

An old press release from Revlon, by contrast, gives a romanticized account of Revlon's beginnings:

"It was a bleak November morning back in the Depression year of 1931, and Charles Revson, then in his very early twenties [he was twenty-five], badly needed a job. Over a cup of coffee in the Automat, young Revson scanned the sparse Help Wanted ads in the paper—a perusal that similarly occupied thousands of other jobless men at the time.

"Two of the ads were for selling jobs; one for a man to sell household appliances—the other, a man to sell cosmetics. Each required applicants to appear in person, and at the same time the following morning. Charles knew there would be a long line at both places. He had never sold either household appliances or cosmetics. So, tossing a nickel in the air, he let chance decide where he would go; heads, cosmetics; tails, household appliances.

"The coin landed on the table, heads up, and at dawn the next morning, Charles Revson was waiting for the office to open. He got the job. A little more than a year later, Revlon was born.

"That was the last time anything concerning Revlon was left to chance."[11]

How much of this account is true? Hard to tell. "Publicity," Charles Revson would later say, "is honest fiction . . . there has to be a basis of fiction about it, otherwise it's not readable. Who the hell wants to read it?"[12]

Though it is difficult—nay, impossible—to ever completely separate corporate mythmaking from historical fact, we do know that Charles Revson at some point during 1931 went to work selling nail polish for Elka, a company in Newark, New Jersey, that did not offer much élan. The only other members of the company were the owner, who was an older man, and a hunchback woman who demonstrated the nail polish at beauty shows.

The company did have one thing going for it: a distinctively different product. While all other nail polishes on the American market in the nascent industry at that point were still pale and translucent, Elka's was opaque.

Elka appears to have been a spin-off company of Ellis-Foster of Montclair, New Jersey, which was co-founded by Carleton Ellis, a pioneer in the field of enamels and the author of a comprehensive 1923 treatise on synthetic resins and plastics. Ellis received 753 patents in his lifetime, and is probably best remembered as the inventor of modern margarine (an animal-fat version had been invented earlier by a Frenchman in the nineteenth century; Ellis figured out how to make it from vegetable oil so that it would sit around for eons before going rancid).

In 1932, Ellis received a patent for a nail enamel containing nitrocellulose, though he called it a "fingernail glossifier."[13] It was not the first nail polish patent that mentions nitrocellulose, but Ellis seems to have made a major improvement. The solvents used with nitrocellulose were commonly known as banana oil and reeked with the smell of rotten fruit. Ellis substituted odorless anhydrous methanol, which he claimed was more suitable "for boudoir use."[14]

Northern New Jersey would become a hotbed of nail polish manufacturing, but initially nail polish innovators were spread across the country. In 1936 the Egyptian Lacquer Manufacturing Company of Chicago patented its own nitrocellulose formulation. Four years later Henry C. Fuller, of Washington, D.C., who patented his proprietary nitrocellulose recipe, described the not-insignificant hurdles a nail-enamel innovator faced: "Satisfactory nail enamels must spread easily, not run at the edges, [and] dry within one and a half minutes leaving a smooth glossy surface that is not tacky," Fuller wrote. Not only that, but the enamel had to stay shiny and be durable enough to stick to the nails for up to a week.[15]

Revson Polishes His Own Nails

Revson, who never claimed to be an innovator himself, nonetheless recognized the potential of Elka's product. But he decided that he could do better away from Elka, and set up Revson Brothers in New York, from which he was authorized to sell Elka nail varnish regionally. When he asked the company to let him distribute the stuff nationwide, the company refused. So twenty-five-year-old Charles and his brother Joseph decided to start their own company. Soon they hooked up with Charles Lachman, a thirty-five-year-old man who had married into the family that owned Dresden, a small chemical company in New Rochelle, New York.

By Tobias's account Lachman contributed little but the "l" from his name to turn Revson Brothers into the Revlon Nail Enamel Company. The Revsons provided three hundred dollars in cash, while Lachman's connections allowed the company to get nail polish from Dresden on credit. The Revlon company, in its various promotional accounts, has described Lachman as a "brilliant young chemist." Martin Revson, Charles's youngest brother, saw things differently. When it came to chemistry, Martin rather indelicately put it, "he did not know his ass from a hole in the ground."[16]

In any case, Charles Revson soon persuaded Lachman to "retire," though for the rest of his life he would draw a salary and bonuses. Lachman may not have made any original contributions, but the chemist at Dresden, Taylor Sherwood, deserves a place in the nail polish pantheon, as it was he who brewed an opaque nail polish that mimicked Elka's.

Charles Revson was not a chemist, but he was a pioneer in what today would be called focus-group research. He relentlessly asked women, especially those who did not use Revlon products, what they thought of his nail polish. Morever, he used himself as a guinea pig.

"Charlie never went to bed without putting lipstick on his lips and nail polish on his nails," recalled Jack Price, a salesman who traveled with Charles in the early days of the company. "He would leave a call with the desk to wake him at two and at four and at six to see how it was wearing."[17]

As is the case with most fledgling companies, the early years of Revlon were lean. Charles lacquered each of his fingernails with a different shade of polish before going on sales calls to beauty salons; it saved him the cost of printing up a color chart. Robert Hoffman, the hair-dryer innovator, recalled that he gave Revson a corner of his hair-drying booth at a beauty show because Revson could not afford to rent his own. To get to another beauty show, down in Atlanta, he and Revson drove down in Hoffman's old Ford to Washington, where they stayed with Hoffman's cousins because they could not afford a hotel room.

The next day Hoffman's uncle gave them a huge tin of potato chips to bring on the train for the next leg of their trip to Atlanta. Though he had no cash, Revson checked the two into the best suite in the hotel and then wired his brother for money. His thrifty brother wired back that there would be no money coming. "We had to entertain," Hoffman said, "so we went out and bought the cheapest bottle of whiskey we could find, and all our entertaining was done in this big suite with a giant can of potato chips in the middle of the floor."[18]

Revson's big breakthrough order came from a small booth at the Midwest beauty show in Chicago's Sherman Hotel in the spring of 1934. "I started my sales talk by showing the prospect how to apply our cream nail polish, then a new type,"

Revson told a trade paper years later. "Before the week was out, I was teaching beauty shop operators and clerks how to demonstrate and use the polish. That group grew so big I had to rent the booth next to ours, and that additional space made my exhibit larger than our entire plant."[19] During that trip, Marshall Field's made a whopping order of four hundred dollars, which Charles assured the buyer Revlon could fulfill.

When he wired the news, his brother wired back asking whether there had been an error in transmission, because there was no way they could fill such a large order. Charles wired back to confirm the order just before catching the train back to New York. He and Joseph spent the rest of the week working around the clock to fulfill the order.

Revlon's first advertisement appeared in *The New Yorker* because that magazine's readership included the sort of "classy dame" Revson wanted as a client. The small ad (which cost the company $335.56—its entire annual budget for consumer advertising) boasted that Revlon's new summer shades in nail polish, Sun Rose and Chestnut, had been "originated by a New York socialite" and produced for her by the House of Revlon. "Never mind the fact that 'the House of Revlon' was a few bare rooms where people poured from big bottles into little ones and trimmed applicator brushes," Tobias observed, "or that Charles did not even know a New York socialite."[20]

The Depression years of the 1930s may have seen breadlines and record unemployment, but women were apparently saving enough to buy nail polish (the cheapest of which sold for ten cents a bottle).

The lean economic years of the 1930s notwithstanding, profits for Cutex nail polish climbed steadily year by year. And DuPont, which had produced the automobile paints, clearly had its eye on this burgeoning market. It received at least two nail polish patents in the early 1940s, though it never commercialized them (perhaps because it had other consumer ideas percolating, chiefly nylon).[21]

Revson weathered the Great Depression of the 1930s by selling nail polish, at premium prices, through hair and beauty salons.

A. C. Bailey of the Bailey Beauty Supply Company in Chicago claimed that he decided to distribute Revlon exclusively because of the superiority of the nail polish. "I went with him," Bailey recalled, "because I had checked with some of the finest beauty shops in the East, like Michael of the Waldorf, and found that this polish was incredible. It was chip-proof and had more stay-on power, had more gloss and luster, the colors were beautiful, and the formula was just terrific. We were carrying at that time about five brands of nail polish. Blue Bird, Chen-Yu, Glazo and a couple of others. We threw everything else out and carried only Revlon."[22]

Not all these innovations were for the good, however. Revlon introduced, and then soon withdrew, a base coat called "Ever-On" that so lived up to its name that it appears to have destroyed a good number of fingernails and led to at least one amputation. According to historian Gwen Kay, dermatologists suspected that this was due to the ingredient toluenesulfonamide formaldehyde. Ever-On was not the only product with a problematic formulation. Other long-staying polishes that caused severe allergic reactions were produced by different companies and included the trade names of Permannail, Adheron, Stazon, and Duragloss.[23]

Nail Polish Remover and Chicken Soup

Unlike lipstick, which served as the muse for dozens of packaging designers, nail polish did not initially inspire much novelty in the way of packaging. In part this is because the most obvious design for a nail polish container was a miniature version of a glue pot, which had been around at least since the nineteenth century.

Only a handful of patents issued in the 1930s were for nail polish bottles. One of the earliest, but by no means the first, was in 1937 to Joseph Revson, Charles's brother, for a glass bottle with a threaded cap for holding either nail polish or nail polish remover. For his part, Charles, ever the perfectionist, was very fussy about

*Revson's nail
polish patent.*

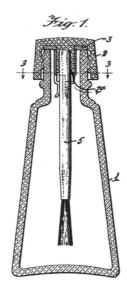

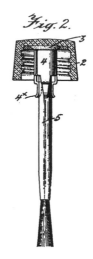

Fig. 1.

Fig. 2.

Fig. 3.

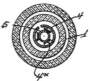

Fig. 4.

INVENTOR

Joseph Revson

BY   *H. Lee Helms*

ATTORNEY.

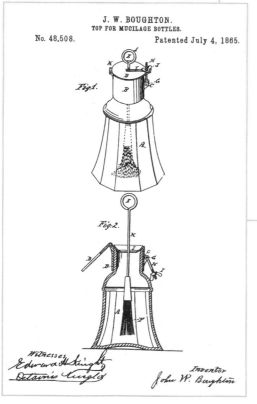

J. W. BOUGHTON.

TOP FOR MUCILAGE BOTTLES.

No. 48,508.   Patented July 4, 1865.

Fig. 1.

Fig. 2.

Witnesses:
Edward H. Knight
Octavius Knight

Inventor
John W. Boughton

Glue-pot patent.

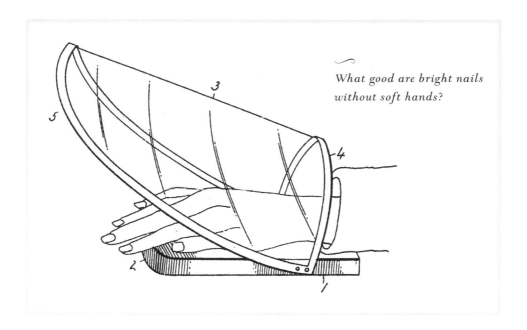

*What good are bright nails
without soft hands?*

trimming the applicator brushes—he wanted them perfectly even, with no straggly bristles.

But nail polish bottles did not have to look beautiful, at least in the beginning. For the most part women went to beauty shops to get their nails enameled. Nail polish enjoyed a symbiotic relationship with another two beauty inventions: the hair-straightening comb and the permanent wave machine.

In her 1937 play *The Women*, Clare Booth Luce evocatively describes the permanent wave machine as "an aluminum tree," a "hanging thicket" of wires and clamps.[24] The hot comb was a less monstrous affair but it, like the permanent wave, required a big investment from women in both money and time. Early wave machines required the patron to sit attached with the medusalike contraption tethered to their head for eight hours.

One of the characters in Luce's play flashes her Jungle Red nails and the plot twists as a gossipy manicurist unwittingly informs a patron that her husband has a mistress who happens to be the manicurist's friend Crystal ("Crystal's a terrible

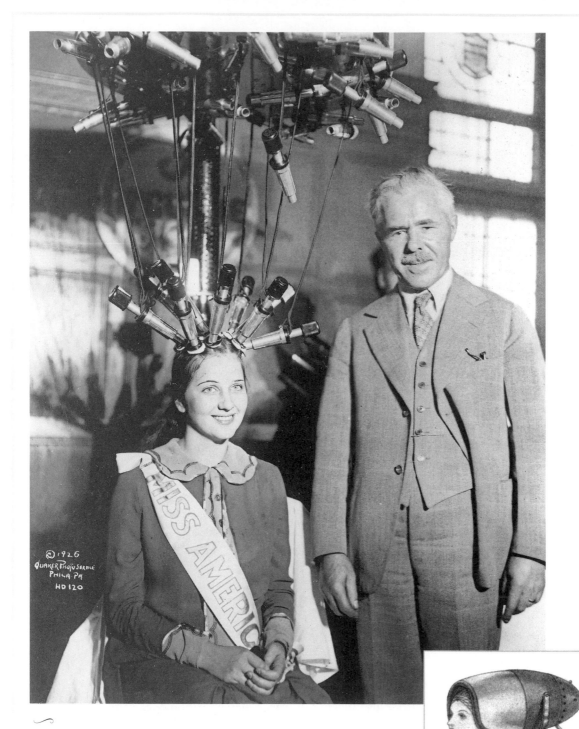

Permanent wave machines and other hair-dressing inventions were a boon to the nail polish business, making salon patrons captive audiences to manicurists.

girl—I mean, she's terribly clever. And she's terribly pretty, Mrs. Haines—I mean, if I was you I wouldn't waste no time getting Mr. Haines away from her.")[25]

By 1938, Revlon sales surpassed one million dollars, and the polish was carried in thousands of salons—some of them catering to more humble clientele than the classy dames Revlon wanted to cultivate as customers.

Annclore Harrell of Savannah, Georgia, remembered the beauty parlor her next-door neighbor ran out of her house. "Manicures featuring Revlon products were done at a little table that could be rolled around the room for convenience. Fingernail polish with names like Windsor Rose, Orchids to You, and Bravo shared space with soaking bowls and orange sticks and emery boards. At night, the heavy shampoo chair with the adjustable drain rack was pushed aside at the sink so dinner dishes could be

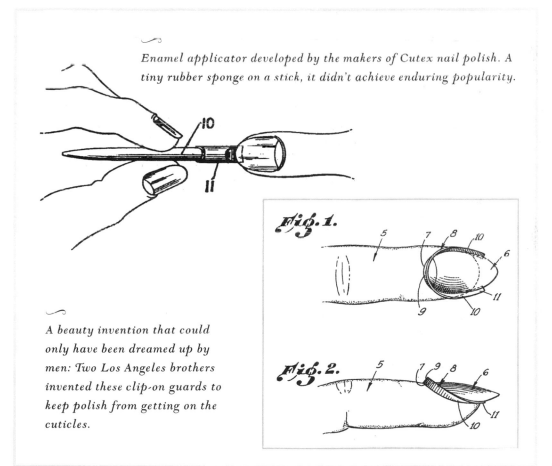

Enamel applicator developed by the makers of Cutex nail polish. A tiny rubber sponge on a stick, it didn't achieve enduring popularity.

A beauty invention that could only have been dreamed up by men: Two Los Angeles brothers invented these clip-on guards to keep polish from getting on the cuticles.

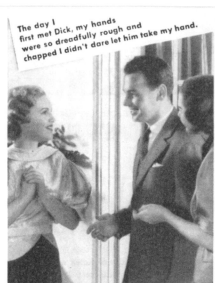

The day I first met Dick, my hands were so dreadfully rough and chapped I didn't dare let him take my hand.

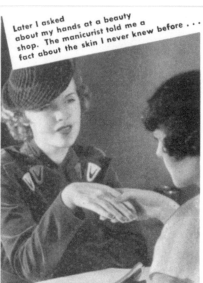

Later I asked about my hands at a beauty shop. The manicurist told me a fact about the skin I never knew before . . .

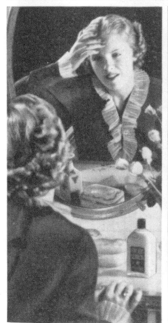

A FEW DAYS LATER while we were playing blind-man's buff at a party, Dick said . . .

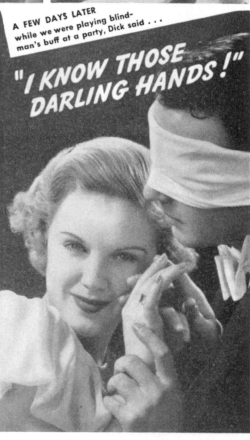

"I KNOW THOSE DARLING HANDS !"

HAND SKIN IS DIFFERENT . . .

instead of oil such as your face has, hands have a peculiar non-oily moisture that dries out easily. To make hands smooth, you have to put this moisture back. Jergens Lotion does this !

Easy to have hands men remember

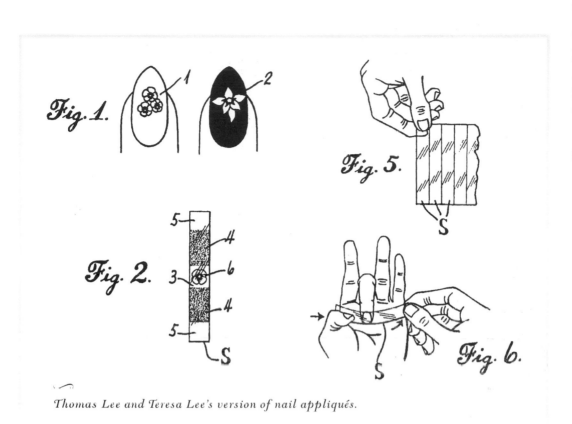

Thomas Lee and Teresa Lee's version of nail appliqués.

washed. The room smelled of shampoo and bacon, of nail polish remover and vegetable soup."[26]

    Critics charged that the fashion magazines were touting new products such as
nail polish merely to garner advertising dollars. "By persistent advertising and the
'cooperation' of fashion editors and authorities, some eight different shades are now
available to match each different costume for different times of day or different oc-
casions," M. C. Phillips wrote in her 1934 *Skin Deep: The Truth About Beauty Aids*,
a cynical look at the beauty industry. "Thus, the fashion editors, who so kindly co-
operated with the advertising department, would lead us to believe that it is quite im-
proper to appear on the tennis court without a certain shade of nail polish; that
another is needed for cocktails, still another for the theater."[27]

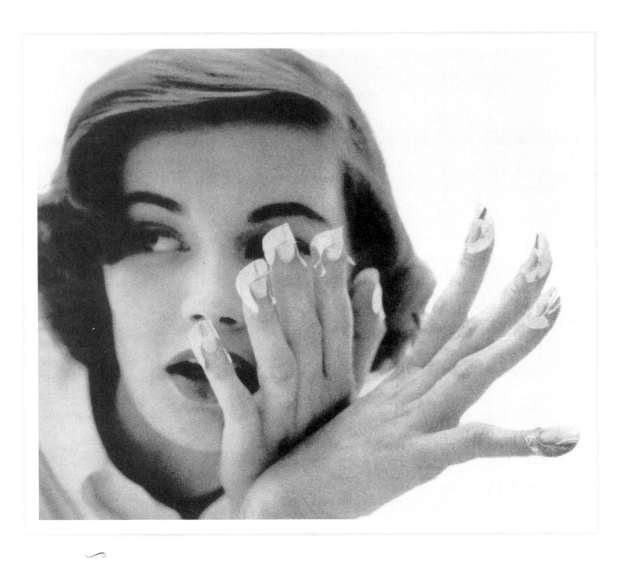

The dental profession's contribution to beauty: artificial fingernails.

Whether because of fashion-magazine manipulation or sheer free will, women embraced the endless novelty of nail polish. Girls would give their teams a hand, by lacquering their nails in school colors. In England, scenic vistas were popular. "It was not uncommon to see a gracious lady in London who had the beautiful Swiss mountains, the picturesque English countryside, the interesting Holland dykes literally at her fingertips," according to Gilbert Vail.[28] Actress Rita Hayworth started a rage for long, oval nails in bright red.

In Massachusetts, a Yankee inventor named Earl Tupper was toying with the idea of glue-on nail appliqués made of celluloid. He envisioned nail ornaments in the shape of shamrocks, hearts, and valentines in a rainbow of colors. But Tupper was distracted by other ideas as well: eyebrow dye shields, garter hooks, knitting needles, egg-peeling clamps, flour sifters, dish drying racks, an "instrument for starting menstruation in women who have delayed monthlies or are pregnant" as well as an "Egyptian Slave dancing girl Waist Ring."[29] These were all, apparently, ideas before their time. Tupper concentrated instead upon another of his inventions: a storage bowl made of extruded plastic featuring an airtight lid whose seal was verified with a "burp."

As with Tupperware, the next big ideas in fingernail technology did not arrive until the 1950s. Manicurists found a new use for the recent invention of aerosol hair spray: as a spray-on nail-polish dryer. "Nail wraps" came into vogue. Manicurists, instead of filing down split nails, repaired them by gluing on patches of tea bags, coffee filters, cigarette filters, or perm papers with Duco cement or airplane glue.[30]

But the most important advance in nail beauty came with nail elongators. The new wonder material that made these nail extensions possible arose not from the automobile industry but rather the dental profession. The latest in nail glamour? Dental fillings. Or rather nail extensions made of a new acrylic polymer originally invented to fill cavities in teeth.

Nail elongators would not become practical (if by practical we mean easy to apply) until the 1970s. Acrylic nails would render typing nearly impossible and make dishwashing out of the question, but they did bring unprecedented length and symmetry to women's nails. In this respect, nail elongators would bring to fingernails what surgical implants brought to breasts: a pluperfect perfection that in Nature simply does not exist.

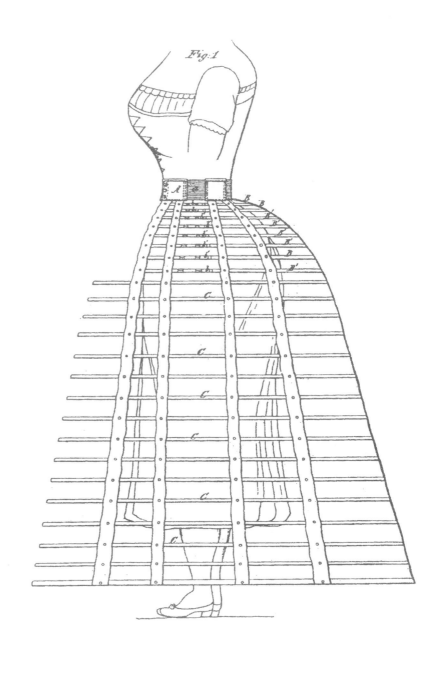

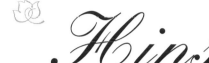

CHAPTER 8

Hips

It has been asserted by some that crinoline is to be abandoned, and we see some hoopless individuals perambulating our streets; and queer oddities they are.

—— *Godey's Ladies' Book, 1863*

Five years ago when hooped skirts were first introduced, every one predicted for them a speedy decline . . . but after encountering the shafts of ridicule and opposition in every conceivable form, they will not only remain a fixed fact, but have become a permanent institution, which no caprice of fashion will be likely wholly to destroy.

—— *The Mirror, 1862*

In 1855 the raven-haired bride of Napoleon III, Eugenie de Montijo, Comtesse de Teba, scandalized and delighted English society when, arriving for a Windsor ball, she swept into the Waterloo Gallery wearing an enormous hoop skirt. As the young arriviste empress glided by in her white-net confection, the matronly Queen Victoria pronounced her *"delicieuse."*[1]

It was a new type of hoop skirt that permitted the outrageous magnitude of Eugenie's gown. It was called a cage crinoline, and it was ostensibly the first fashion edifice ever erected from steel. Within the year, fashionable women in Western Europe and America and beyond would be mimicking the French empress and her ladies. And within the next several years, many more less-than-fashionable women—housewives, sweatshop seamstresses, and parlor maids—also would be swept away by crinolinomania.

Who invented this new type of hoop skirt? The true story of the hoop skirt is one that unravels a long-honored fashion myth. It is a story thick with intrigue and plot twists, riches and glory, secret alliances, and familial treachery. It is a story that cuts across class and gender and features players who range from seventeen-year-old skirtmakers and impecunious entrepreneurs to seafaring investors and millionaire merchants. It is a story that extends from the dank basement skunkworks of nineteenth-century inventors to the most fashionable stretch of Broadway in antebellum New York City.

But just as important as who invented the metallic hoop skirt is the question of why women so eagerly and rapidly embraced such a wildly inconvenient artifice at this particular point in time. The hoop skirt blocked street traffic, got caught in carriage wheels, and was even prone to catching on fire if it happened to graze the hearth.

Of course, Woman has continually used technology to transmogrify her single self into many women. Yet during this era women could have reinvented themselves by applying heavy eye makeup or turning their heads into towering edifices of hair. Instead they shifted attention to their hips, by armoring themselves with monstrous hoop skirts.

The hoop skirt craze reached its zenith as the first shot was fired in 1861 at Fort Sumter, sounding the beginning of the American Civil War. The fact that many

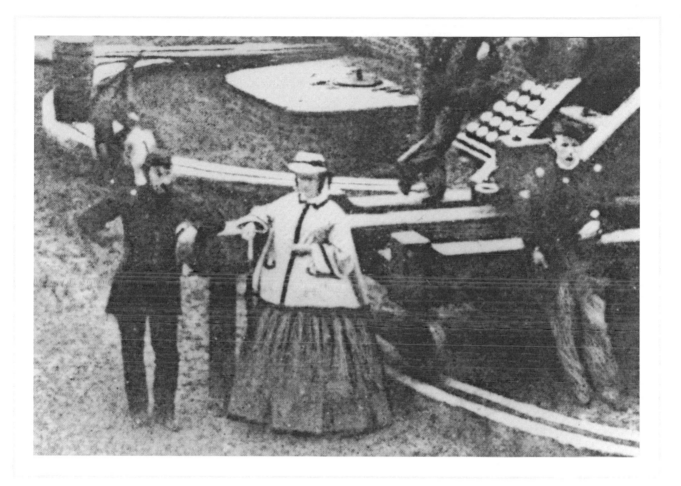

*During the Civil War Southern women smuggled
provisions hidden in their skirts across enemy lines.
One belle managed to smuggle a "roll of army cloth,
several pairs of cavalry boots, a roll of crimson
flannel, packages of gilt braid and sewing silk, cans
of preserved meat, and a bag of coffee!"*

Southern women used the ample skirts to smuggle goods for Confederate soldiers across enemy lines may have had something to do with its popularity in the South.

The ascendancy of the hoop skirt, however, has more to do with a confluence of many divergent circumstances than any single event. It can be attributed not just to the American Civil War but also the Seneca Falls Women's Rights Convention of 1848, the evolutionary theory of Charles Darwin, the building of the U.S. Capitol, the international bank panic of 1857, and the simultaneous appearance of myriad yet seemingly invisible technological developments.

A New Kind of Liberty

When she made her dramatic appearance at the Windsor ball in 1855, Empress Eugenie was only reviving a style that began in her native Spain. Indeed, the term *farthingale,* used to describe a hoop skirt, comes from the Spanish word *verdugos,* which means "saplings." The early hoop petticoats probably got their architectural support from saplings, at least until whalebone and cane came into popular use. (Although many fashion innovations have been adopted by men—corsets, for example—the historical record provides no pictorial or written evidence that this invention was ever a manly contrivance.)

Velásquez's portraits provide the most striking visual reference for the Spanish farthingale, which was flat in front and extended to the sides in an oval shape. But over the ensuing centuries the hoop would morph from an oval to a cone and back again.

From Velásquez forward, hoop skirts waxed and waned in size and popularity in Western aristocratic dress, but with little change in the structural engineering of the hoop itself. Around 1830, after a long reign of the Empire fashion of long straight skirts, women began to plump out their skirts not with hoops but with stiffened petticoats often made from crinoline, a fabric woven of horsehair and either cot-

THOMSON'S
CRINOLINA HAIR CLOTH
SKIRT.

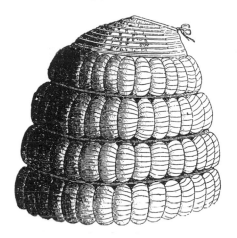

To ladies who still prefer the Hair Cloth Skirt to all others—the above is offered as the most elegant form in which it has ever been produced in any country. It is made up in both white and colored hair cloth.

THE PATENT
PARAGON SKIRT.

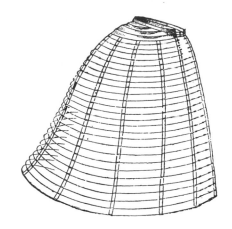

This Skirt is made by an entirely new process—by means of a double tape firmly cemented together in a secure manner. Being the sole Agents of the Patentee, we are enabled to offer these goods upon the most favorable terms.

Nos. 16, 20, 25, 30.

*Compared to the burdensome horsehair crinoline,
the metal version was sweet liberty.*

ton or linen. (The word *crinoline* derives from the Latin *crinis*, meaning hair, and the Latin *linum* for thread.)

Through the ensuing two decades, women aspired to greater and greater fullness with their crinoline petticoats, sometimes wearing as many as eight at a time. Naturally, this added not just volume but also an enormous amount of weight to their dresses. So the bell-shaped skirts could swell only to a size and weight that a woman had the physical ability to endure.

Thus, women on both sides of the Atlantic were quick to embrace the cage crinoline—an affordable new invention that relieved them of their petticoat burden while continuing to expand their physical presence.

Like the whalebone it replaced, the metallic hoop was lightweight and flexible. By modern standards of comfort, the cage crinoline may appear to be just that, a confining cage. But by mid-nineteenth-century standards, the cage crinoline was liberty itself.

This airy edifice allowed women to swell in volume without having to load their hips with stiff petticoats. "The crinoline looked solid, but actually bounced about with every step or gust of wind," Sarah Levitt tells us in *Victorians Unbuttoned*.[2] On the downside, it could be quite noisy. A Frenchman, Monsieur Hippolyte Tain, in his *Notes on England*, unfavorably compared the locomotion of a lady in a cage crinoline with the ticking of a clock—"energetic, discordant, jerking, like a piece of mechanism."[3]

Jean Philippe Worth, son of the most influential couturier of the nineteenth century, Charles Frederick Worth, who created many gowns for Empress Eugenie, recalled in his memoir that his father was quick to recognize the potential popularity of the cage crinoline soon after he established his dressmaking house at 7 rue de la Paix in Paris.

"It was seized upon with rejoicing by the overburdened women, and soon petticoats, with the exception of one or two of muslin, beautifully made, that showed as an exquisite lacy froth when their wearers stepped, were abandoned," wrote Worth fils.[4] The cage crinoline became, according to Doreen Yarwood in *The Encyclopaedia of World Costume*, "the feminine status symbol."[5]

Worth may have set the pace of fashion in Paris, but far more influential in America was the establishment of Madame Demorest, at 27 14th Street in New York City. Mme. Demorest appropriated the fashions of European royalty and then democratized them into a sort of American everywoman's couture.

In her *Demorest's Illustrated Monthly Magazine* and *Mme. Demorest's Mirror of Fashions*, she reported breathlessly on every new Worth gown that Eugenie

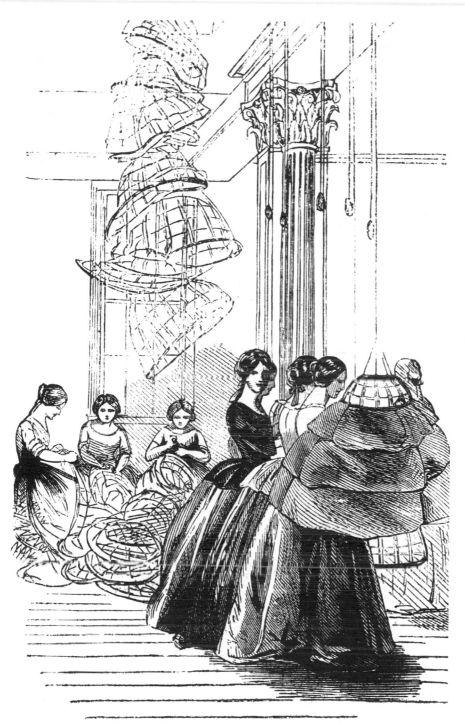

Douglas & Sherwood, based on Broadway in New York City, was one of the biggest crinoline manufacturers. It cranked out four thousand skirts a day at its peak.

THE FINISHING ROOM.

wore to a Tuileries ball. She was a hoop-skirt enthusiast, but "Madame" Demorest had a thoroughly American puritan streak as well. She prudishly condemned those who tilted their skirts flirtatiously to reveal ankles clad provocatively in red silk stockings.

Impecunious but Virtuous

The Demorests were among those stampeding not toward the gold mines of California but to the Patent Office in Washington to lay their claims on hoop-skirt innovations. Mme. Demorest was in reality the American-born and -bred Ellen Curtis Demorest. She and her husband, William Jennings Demorest, laid claim to all manner of womanly inventions, from hoop skirts to dress elevators, clever little contraptions that allowed a lady to lift her skirts up by tugging discreetly on a string.

In truth, as we shall see, they contributed little to the invention of the cage crinoline. William Demorest came up with two different hoop-skirt schemes but in both cases he was beaten to the Patent Office by earlier claimants. *Godey's Ladies' Book* in October 1861 advised that the Demorests had "the best steel skirt we have ever seen . . . though containing forty springs, it is a model of lightness & comfort."[6] *Frank Leslie's Ladies' Gazette* hailed it as the first "really excellent, cheap hoop-skirt."[7] Indeed, it was so cheap and popular that it ignited something of a crinoline price war. But it was made using technologies that had been licensed from other inventors.

A song of the era sings the praises of "Matilda Baker, the pretty little hoop-skirt maker,"[8] but the life of a seamstress was by no means a gay adventure. The Demorests treated their girls better than most. Moreover, in the heat of the Civil War, they were fervent abolitionists and defiantly hired Negro women to work alongside Caucasians. This took courage at a time when racist rhetoric was rampant. During the 1860 presidential campaign, the New York *Daily News* said that if Abraham Lincoln was elected "we shall find Negroes swarming everywhere" and warned that

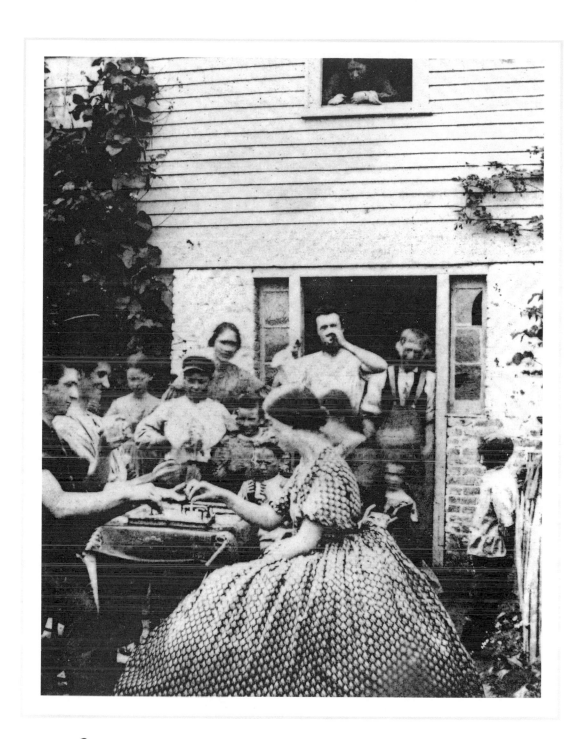

A hoop-skirted textile worker takes a break to play checkers.

(white) "working people would have to compete with the labor of 4 million emancipated Negroes."[9]

Whether she was a freed African slave or a recent Irish immigrant, a hoop-skirt maker led a virtuous if impecunious life. She was usually between seventeen and twenty-five years old and lived in a boardinghouse or at home with her family. She earned from two to three dollars a week at a time when men were paid seven dollars a week for their unskilled labor.

Many working women, in an era when respectable ladies eschewed gainful employment, preferred prostitution. A comely streetwalker could earn from ten to fifty dollars for a single trick, and business was always brisk. Walt Whitman estimated that nineteen out of twenty men, including the "best classes of men,"[10] visited brothels regularly even though the risk of contracting gonorrhea or syphilis was high. On the other hand, abortions were legal and freely available from, among others, Madame Restell, "the wickedest woman in New York."[11]

The hoop skirt was allegedly flattering on all types of feminine figures. An 1857 *Harper's Weekly* cartoon depicts two women looking into a mirror. One is tall and gaunt, the other short and thick-waisted. "These Dresses are very well in their way, but they make us all appear the same size," sniffs the stout woman, who stands admiring her reflection. "Why," she says as she glances condescendingly at her rail-thin compatriot, "a Girl might be as thin as a Whipping-post, and yet be taken for a Decent Figure."[12]

A ledger book belonging to Isabel Elliott Howell of Nashville, Tennessee, during the 1860s. A girl's hoop skirt cost 60 cents.

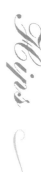

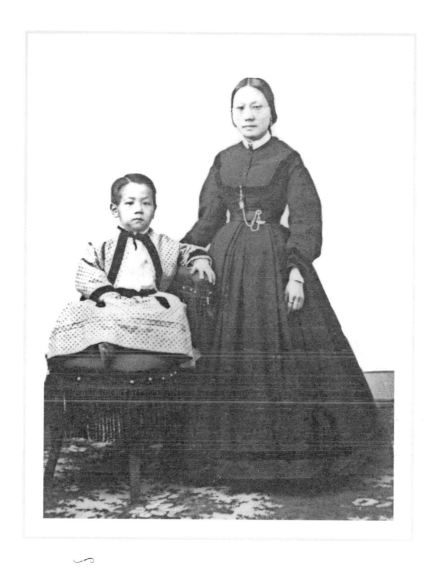

Hoop-skirted Chinese-American woman with
child in San Francisco.

Philippe Perrot, in *Fashioning the Bourgeoisie*, contends that the "metallic
cages that replaced layered petticoats were so cumbersome that they marked a distinct frontier separating the idle from the working-class populations."[13] Many women
who wore them did little more than lounge elegantly in the parlor. In fact, this new

form of clothing demanded new styles of furniture. Special armless "ladies chairs" were designed to accommodate the crinoline-imposed constraints on sitting down.

One would think that rural women and female factory workers would have seen the crinoline as an enhancement they could do without and, indeed, only the most fashionable women wore the truly gargantuan hoops. But cage crinolines ultimately would become mass produced and thus inexpensive, making them popular among all classes of women, not just the upper crust who could afford Parisian couture.

Missionary wives in Africa, peasant women in Europe, and house slaves in America are known to have worn cage crinolines. Some factory workers wore crinolines to work, as did cooks and maids, who caused no small discomfort when they blurred class lines by appropriating their mistresses' fashions.

Hoop skirts could even be seen on westward wagon trains. One member of a party on the California Trail on June 19, 1857, remarked in his diary that a young bride in the Inmann party who wore hoops soon acquired the nickname "Miss Hoopy." "We have read of hoops being worn, but they had not reached Kansas before we left so these are the first we've seen and would not recommend them for this mode of traveling," he noted. Perhaps because of winds on the high plains, the diarist observed, "the wearer has less personal privacy than the Pawnee Indian in his blanket."[14]

Beguiling Rather Than Belligerent

Clearly the metallic hoop skirt was an improvement over the heavy petticoats that previously prevailed. But if comfort was the sole driving force behind its popularity, then why did women not simply abandon skirts altogether in favor of that sensible invention that men had been sporting for centuries, namely trousers? Indeed,

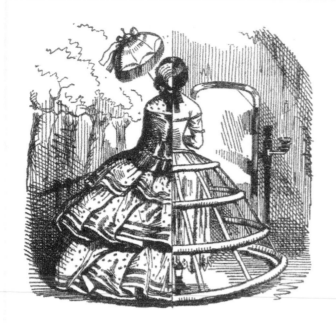

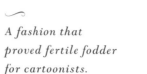

A fashion that proved fertile fodder for cartoonists.

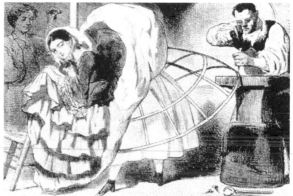

early feminists and others had advocated a form of pants for women. "Bloomers," which Elizabeth Cady Stanton and Amelia Bloomer started wearing in 1851, consisted of a knee-length woolen skirt worn over billowing Turkish trousers.

For one thing, what Bloomer wearers gained in comfort they lost in glamour. The ensemble looked ghastly on anyone plumper than the slender, pretty Mrs. Bloomer, after whom they were named.

Just as important, in a world of feme-covert, which denied a married women the right to own property or make contracts in her own name, the very wearing of trousers was an affront to the prevailing power structure. Bloomerites were "the butt of vicious caricatures and sexist jokes" and "boys pelted them with snowballs in winter and apple cores in summer," according to historians Edwin G. Burrows and Mike Wallace.[15] The hoop-skirt brigade would be ridiculed as well. But it is not insignifi-

237

cant that both Cady Stanton and Bloomer ultimately abandoned Bloomers in favor of the cage crinoline, which they proclaimed was emancipation enough as far as clothing went.

There is a subversive side to this seemingly frivolous fashion. The hoop skirt allowed women to become physically bigger than men in a way that was beguiling rather than belligerent, at a time when they were making steady inroads toward wider rights. When female shoe factory workers in Lynn, Massachusetts, went on strike for better pay on March 7, 1860, they did not wear Bloomers. Rather, they paraded through town in a snowstorm wearing the widest, sassiest hoop skirts they could find. During this same year, only twelve years after the Declaration of Sentiments was made in Seneca Falls, the New York State Legislature passed a bill drafted by Susan B. Anthony that allowed a wife to retain any property acquired by "trade, business, labor or service" as her own.[16]

The crest of the crinoline craze corresponds to other currents in society. Darwin's *Origin of Species* appeared in 1859, but perhaps more important than the idea of evolution (at least as regards the hoop skirt) was the popularity of the field of physical anthropology from which the idea of evolution had evolved.

"By the middle of the 19th century," writes Cynthia Eagle Russett in *Sexual Science: The Victorian Construction of Womanhood*, "diversity of man was strikingly apparent in reports about alien races and cultures emanating from missionaries, travelers, traders, colonialists and increasingly ethnologists in far-off lands."[17]

Sometimes those "alien" races could be found right near home. Encountering African Americans for the first time when visiting Philadelphia, Louis Agassiz, the then august and now controversial Harvard zoologist, declared that they hailed from a species separate and distinct from Caucasians.

On the European continent, in England, and in America, anthropologists were preoccupied with racial typology: the slope of the face, the color of the skin, the texture of the hair. And what was ostensibly the greatest contrast between the Caucasian and "lower" races? The pelvis.

The European woman's ample hips were supposedly evidence of both her racial and sexual superiority. As Havelock Ellis would later write, the pelvis "in some of the dark races is apelike in its narrowness and small capacity" unlike the European counterpart, which is "proof of high evolution and the promise of capable maternity."[18]

Guns and Skirts

Conventional wisdom in the history of fashion tells us that the popularity of the cage crinoline was linked to the emergence of the Bessemer steel process, which made the production of strong, flexible steel newly inexpensive. Indeed, circumstantial evidence suggests that the inventor of the very first cage crinoline worn by the Empress Eugenie was the famous British inventor Lord Bessemer.

Henry Bessemer established himself as a successful inventor early in life. While in his twenties, he devised a new type of revenue stamp that could not be reused on official documents, thus bringing an extra 100,000 pounds a year to the royal treasury.

Sometime in 1854, Bessemer approached the British war department with his latest invention: a new, powerful type of cannon shot for smooth-bore guns. Though England was embroiled in the Crimean War, the complacent British war department spurned Bessemer. He sailed off to Paris to spend some time with his friend Lord James Hay, whose daughter invited both Bessemer and Prince Napoleon, the cousin of Napoleon III, to a large dinner party.

After dinner, the men retreated to the library to smoke their cigars and talk. France, which had a reputation for ordnance innovation, was also mired in the Crimean War. When Bessemer casually mentioned his latest invention, Prince Napoleon evinced his curiosity and the inventor promptly extracted from his pocket a miniature model of the cannon shot, which he had just happened to bring along to the dinner party. (Luck, as Bessemer's contemporary Louis Pasteur would later observe, favors the prepared mind.)

Prince Napoleon arranged for Bessemer to demonstrate his invention before his cousin the emperor at the armory at Vincennes on the outskirts of Paris. Ultimately, according to Bessemer's boastful autobiography, Napoleon pledged carte blanche funding for him to return to his workshop at Baxter House in England and begin to study "the whole question of metals suitable for the construction of guns."[19]

Soon after he began his gun-metal experiments, Bessemer had a fundamental and radical revelation: Iron could be purified, and thus rendered pliable, by simply and cheaply blowing steam or air through it after it had been heated up. This was an important development because, until the mid-nineteenth century, steel was difficult and time-consuming to make on a large scale.

Bessemer was by no means the only one to have had this insight. There are perhaps a half-dozen inventors of "Bessemer" steel, most notably William Kelly, an obscure American from Eddyville, Kentucky. But Bessemer was the best businessman of the bunch, and the best connected, and as a result his name has been permanently alloyed to this method of making steel.

Alas, we have no solid evidence that Bessemer actually made Eugenie's hoops either at his foundry in England or at Vincennes in France. His autobiography, for example, mentions nothing about this. On the other hand, innovators historically have curried favor, and have thus secured financial support for their more serious endeavors, by pleasing their kings and queens and other patrons with amusing frivolities.

One must admit that the timing is propitious. After his first few feverish weeks of work, Bessemer applied for the first of his patents for "Improvements of Iron and Steel" on January 10, 1855. On April 16, Napoleon and Eugenie sailed to England to visit Victoria, and it was during this visit that the cage crinoline made its debut. Moreover, Eugenie, who was under pressure to produce an heir but had just suffered a miscarriage, was rumored to have adopted the crinoline in an effort to squelch speculation about her fertility.

Silken Skirts, Silly Flirts

Whether or not Bessemer himself actually made the empress's hoops, the perplexing fact remains that the Bessemer process was not a general working concept until ten years later, around 1865, which is just about the time the cage crinoline was losing its allure in the fashionable world.

Mass production of the hoops from Bessemer simply was not a possibility. Numerous production kinks remained to be worked out. Thus, it is a puzzling irony that this new way of making inexpensive steel had absolutely no role in the democratization of the cage crinoline.

Who then was the innovative genius who figured out how to produce them cheaply, on a large scale, for all women of all sizes and income?

To back up a bit, the cage crinoline had many antecedents. While manufacturers in New York and London and Paris would begin to turn out ready-to-wear steel crinolines, dressmakers and home seamstresses were assembling their own, inventing new hoops one at a time for personal rather than mass consumption.

These hand-crafted crinolines were made of many different materials. Initially, the preferred material, for those who could afford it, was whalebone, which was more durable than cane.[20] But in the middle of the nineteenth century the primary source of whalebone, the overhunted Greenland whale, became increasingly scarce and prices grew correspondingly dear.

Slaves in the American South fashioned hoops out of grapevines. Others used materials ranging from vulcanized rubber, which had recently been invented by Charles Goodyear, to heavy cording as this popular song from 1857 suggests:

> *Hoop! Hoop! Hoop!*
> *What a vast expansive swoop!*
>
> *Hoops of whalebone, short and crisp,*

Hoops of wire, thin as a wisp;
Hoops of brass, thirteen yards long,
Hoops of steel, confirmed and strong;
Hoops of rubber, soft and slick,
Hoops of roping, bungling thick;
Hoops of lampwick, cord and leather,
Hoops that languish in wet weather;
Hoops that spread out silken skirts,
Hanging off from silly flirts.
Sweeping off the public lands,
Turning over apple-stands;
Felling children to the ground
As they flaunt and whirl around,

Hoop! Hoop! Hoop!
What a vast, expansive hoop![21] . . .

"Cast" steel was first invented way back in 1742 by Benjamin Huntsman, a Quaker clockmaker. Huntsman's insight was that by melting "blister steel," the only kind of steel then commercially available, in a clay pot he could diffuse its carbon and by doing so make it easier to mold and shape. Moreover, Huntsman recognized how chemically tricky the production of steel was, and further enhanced its pliability by introducing different "physics."[22]

Known as Sheffield steel, since it was primarily made in Sheffield, England, it was not cheap, nor was it easy to make. But the 1850s witnessed a vast sum of numerous incremental economies and innovations in the drawing of wire as well as the manufacture of cast steel. From 1850 to 1857, the number of steel and iron patents jumped sevenfold in the United States and in France.

Sheffield steel had many applications, according to Geoffrey Tweedale in his account of the industry in America. It was used to make piano wire, scientific instruments, clock springs, clockmaker tools, surgical instruments, pen nibs, engraving plates, textile machine parts, skates, animal traps, and iron mesh for straining coal. "The small amount of crucible steel used in these industries should neither obscure its tremendous impact on the American economy nor its great importance for Sheffield," Tweedale writes.[23]

Moreover, the advent of the telegraph in the 1840s created a huge demand for telegraph wire, which was usually made of iron and soon became abundant and cheap. Many of the mass-manufactured metallic crinolines were made not of steel but of wrought iron, which, unlike pig iron, was pliable and could have easily been shaped into hoops.

A Giddy Karl Marx

So there was raw material aplenty for metallic hoop skirts. But it was not until 1857 that this material became truly inexpensive. For in 1857, world farm prices collapsed and a financial panic swept Wall Street. On October 13, stock market prices plunged, banks closed, and the crisis spread like a "malignant epidemic" to Europe and South America.[24]

Karl Marx, who at the time was formulating the capitalist critique he would lay out in *Das Kapital*, was giddy. Industry reeled. Shipbuilders, foundry mechanics, coopers, textile workers, printers, and railroad workers lost their jobs by the thousands.

Suddenly, masses of surplus steel and iron were available. Furthermore, at this same time, one of the biggest building projects in the history of America was under way: the expansion of the U.S. Capitol.

Inspired by St. Paul's in London, St. Peter's in Rome, and the Pantheon in Paris, architect Thomas Walter in 1855 designed a grand new dome for the Capitol. Because of concerns over fire—the Library of Congress had recently burned—this dome would be constructed not of wood but of iron.

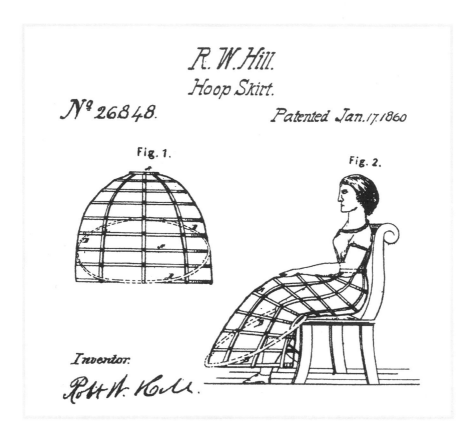

R. W. Hill.
Hoop Skirt.
Nº 26848.
Patented Jan. 17. 1860
Fig. 1.
Fig. 2.
Inventor:

Montgomery Meigs, the engineer for the new Capitol, hired a photographer for $3.50 a day to make copies of designs of the dome. "Photographic albums were sent to libraries, museums, and schools," both in the United States and abroad, "to satisfy the world's curiosity about America's great construction project," writes William C. Allen in his definitive architectural history of the Capitol.[25]

Those plans were reprinted in popular magazines and newspapers of the day who kept the public informed of the dome's progress with depictions of the "iron skirt" reinforced with "iron hoops" that were put in place just before the winter of 1857 set in.[26]

And what did the undressed iron dome look like? Exactly like a gigantic hoop skirt, hovering over the national seat of the American government.

Cage crinolines (at left, below and right) made sitting problematic for the modestly inclined, and sitability is something many inventors tried to improve.

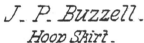

G. Mallory.
Hoop Skirt.

N° 21839

Patented Oct. 19, 1858

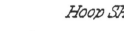

J. P. Buzzell.
Hoop Skirt.

N° 52637

Patented Feb. 13, 1866.

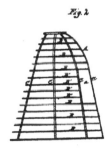

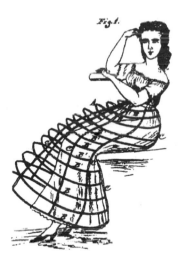

Inventor

These images of the dome seem to have triggered a similar "aha" moment in many people in many places at about the same time. The revelation was this: Could not light metal be used to replace heavy petticoats just as iron construction in buildings such as the Capitol had obviated the need for load-bearing walls?

The most fundamental idea behind the cage crinoline—the decision to make the hoops out of metal—was simply a zeitgeist idea that was rapidly and nearly simultaneously adopted by a wide number of people. By 1860 the hoops in most hoop skirts were constructed with a flat wire, about one eighth of an inch wide, made of steel or high-quality iron. This is not to say that earlier inventors had not thought of using wire. The very first American patent for wire in a skirt was granted in 1848 to Sewall Folsom of Bridgeport, Connecticut, a fertile region for clock and watch innovation. Folsom stiffened his skirt by sewing wire in a crisscross pattern. R. C. Millet, of France, anticipated the mass-produced cage crinoline with his British patent in 1856, for a skeleton petticoat made of steel springs and fastened to tape. But the idea to use metal, whether steel or iron, was an idea that belonged to no one and to everyone at the same time.

The American Dream

Different hoop-skirt inventors fought desperately to achieve a particular version of the American Dream: the ability to get rich seemingly overnight from a single, original idea.

The important ones were hotly contested and resulted in bare-knuckle lawsuits since the role of the Patent Office was (and still is) to liberally issue patents and let the alleged inventors duke it out later in the courts to determine who actually invented what. Hundreds of witnesses would be deposed, their testimony painstakingly recorded in thousands of handwritten pages. The use of metal in the cage crinoline was not the only important innovation that drove mass production of these new petticoats. A number of other inventions arose nearly simultaneously.

The two most important patent fights of the era concerned a hoop-skirt form and a hoop-skirt loom. Both of those fights took place in New York City, the place Walt Whitman described at the time as "this great, dirty, blustering, glorious, ill-lighted, aristocratic, squalid, rich, wicked, and magnificent metropolis."[27]

In October 1855, Datus E. Rugg went to the Blakeslock Hotel on Second Avenue, near 23rd Street in New York City, to fetch his wife. She was helping her good friend Sarah Maxfield put together one of those heavy crinolines designed to swell a skirt's volume by means of upholstery. Rugg was of an inventive bent, and he had recently come up with a new steam boiler gauge. He took one look at the ladies' efforts and declared that he could figure out a way, as Mrs. Maxfield would later recall, "so that we could do away with feathers and cotton."[28]

Shortly thereafter, Rugg conceived not just of a petticoat of wire but also a form on which to make it. This was important because a major hurdle on the road to mass production of cage crinolines was, of course, putting together the hoops in an efficient way.

Generally, the cage crinoline was a framework of flexible hoops held together with perpendicular bands of muslin tape. The difficulty was that each of the hoops was of a different size and had to be measured, marked, cut, and then carefully matched to the appropriate point on the muslin tapes, which themselves had to be measured and marked. This was a labor-intensive effort and as a result, early hoopskirt prices ranged from three to five dollars for what was, ultimately, a disposable consumer item.

By 1860, however, cage crinolines would be sold in such places as Nashville, Tennessee, for $1.50 apiece. This economy of scale was achieved in part by the use of a hoop-skirt form, essentially a wooden frame shaped like a hoop skirt, with slots to insert the wires and the tape. A seamstress no longer had to measure anything. Rather, she could just follow the form, which enabled her to put together the crinoline in one quarter the time it had taken her before.

At the time he came up with the idea for his form, Rugg was working for two dollars a day building hydrostats for steam engines at the Empire Works on 25th Street. Soon, however, he gave up this steady work to take the entrepreneurial plunge.

First he set up shop with an acquaintance, William A. Whitney. They had little money. Dodging landlords to avoid actual payment of rent, they moved their small operation to four different locations in four months. Along the way, Whitney lost faith in the project and disappeared. But by September of 1857, Rugg had a prototype and had ensconced himself in a workshop just around the corner from where he and his wife lived in a tenement house at First Avenue and 26th Street. That same month he applied for a patent.

The form worked well and Rugg hired a couple of seamstresses. Sarah Maxfield recalled going to the shop and seeing it in use. "The girls were putting tape on the outside and lacing on hoops, and then pinning each one as they intersected the tape," she said.[29] Rugg sold several skirts to friends of Sarah. But, alas, unbeknownst to Rugg, a large successful skirt company, Osborne & Vincent, had begun to use a very similar form.

Indeed, Osborne & Vincent put their form on display at the Crystal Palace, the glittering gallery of arts and industry, just before it burned down in October 1858. And when the company got wind that Rugg was laying claim to the hoop-skirt form, it set its legal dogs on him. As Rugg had invested everything he owned in developing his skirt form, he was unable to defend his invention claims much less feed and shelter his wife. They fled first to Missouri and then to Illinois, where Rugg went into another entrepreneurial trade quintessential to the nineteenth century: dentistry.

Rugg will return to the story. But in the meantime another important struggle over the hoop-skirt loom was getting under way.

Familial Treachery

On October 6, 1859, Ebenezer Clark opened the morning edition of the *New York Herald* to read the following notice:

TO DEALERS IN WOVEN SKIRTS

..

We hereby give notice that letters patent of the United States have just been granted resting in us the exclusive right to make, sell and use what is known in the market as the "woven skeleton skirt," whether the springs are inserted while in the looms or afterwards. It is generally known to manufacturers that this skirt is original with us; but in as much as dealers may not be aware of our rights, we hereby notify the trade that the woven skirts cannot be legally sold after this date unless they bear our stamp, or are manufactured by parties holding a license from us and the name of the manufacturer, and the date of the patent, October 4, 1859 must be stamped on each skirt. . . ."

James Draper

James Brown

William King

S. H. Doughty

22 John Street, New York City[30]

Clark was apoplectic. For he considered himself to be the true inventor of the "woven skeleton skirt"—a new iteration of the cage crinoline—and he was incensed that his brother-in-law, James Brown, with whom he had previously been on amicable terms, had usurped his rightful claim.

The patent promised to be lucrative. Thomson & Thomson, the largest skirt manufacturer in the nation, which supplied skirts not only to the United States but also England and France, had licensed it and was already paying royalties.

This was salt in the wound for Clark. His specialty was making fringe and lace on a hand loom. Yet power looms were taking more and more of such work, as they could churn out feminine frills much faster and more cheaply than any master weaver working by hand. Moreover, he was in ill health. Clark and his wife, who were childless, would soon lose their house in East New York to a bank foreclosure.

Clark had fashioned his invention in the cold, dark cellar of that house. There, he had modified a part of the loom, known as a lay, especially for a skeleton skirt. His was an ingenious idea: He was able to weave the muslin tape used to hold the hoops so that they could either be inserted later into gaps in the tape or woven directly into the tape.

Clever as his idea was, Clark had no capital of his own to apply for a patent. He importuned several business associates for funds but they all demurred.

Meanwhile James Brown, Clark's brother-in-law, had been working on a similar idea. While Clark foundered, Brown prospered. Brown specialized in weaving horsenets, a commodity not yet produced by power looms and one that seemed recession proof. Moreover, Brown had money behind him.

Brown and Clark were related by marriage, their wives being sisters. However, the first Mrs. Brown, who had borne a son and a daughter, both now grown, died in 1852. Brown had remarried and his new father-in-law, James Draper, himself a weaver, provided him with both capital and expertise, as did William King, another weaver who was related to both Brown and Clark by marriage.

Brown set up a shop on 35th Street and carefully whitewashed the windows so that rival skirt makers could not peer in. His new wife, as well as his seventeen-year-old daughter, helped fashion the skeleton skirts. Mr. Brown and Mr. Draper would weave the tapes in their shop. Then, working in the dimly lit kitchen of their house, Mrs. Brown would tie the hoops and Elizabeth Brown would sew the waistbands.

Realizing the predicament he was in, Clark quelled his fury long enough to approach his brothers-in-law about licensing their patent. But they spurned him. Thus Clark went searching for investors again, and this time he found several willing to back him in a challenge to the Brown patent—all of them hoop-skirt makers who were not inclined to pay the Brown consortium royalties.

The Brown consortium marshaled an impressive phalanx of witnesses to tell their side of the story. John Brown, James's twenty-five-year-old son and Clark's nephew, recollected that his father and Draper, his new grandfather, first showed him their loom on a fine June day in 1856. He remembered the day particularly, he said, because the whole family had taken a steamboat across the river to Fort Lee, New Jersey, to have a picnic.

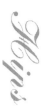

Charles Thomson, the skirt mogul, also testified on Brown's behalf. The scion of a moneyed New England family, the Yale-educated twenty-three-year-old Thomson imperiously denied that he had made a journey to see Clark's machine to steal trade secrets. Rather, he said, he had gone to confirm that Clark had no valid claim to the woven skirt invention.

Support for Brown also came from a salesman at Morton's, a store selling hosiery and fancy goods along a fashionable stretch of Broadway near the newly opened St. Nicholas Hotel. The store had been purchasing small numbers of the skirts and displaying them in the shop window, the salesman said, ever since October 1857.

But Clark mustered a strong defense of his claims. Several witnesses dated Clark's invention to the spring of 1856, a good two months before the Brown and Draper invention.

Yet, apparently, Clark's lawyer and backers felt this was not enough. Thus, at the last minute, they called in Henry McKennee, whom they deposed from seven P.M. to after midnight shortly before the proceedings were to close.

McKennee offered a story gaudy in detail. He said that he had accidentally bumped into Clark at the Crystal Palace one day in 1853 at the northwest entrance, near the daguerreotype exhibit. McKennee further contended that Clark pulled from his pocket a sketch of a skeleton skirt. He wanted to exhibit it, McKennee said, but "his model was a clumsy looking affair and I advised him not to exhibit it but to go home and make an application for a patent."[31]

Two years later, McKennee went on to say, Clark showed him an actual model, not just a drawing. They met at a seaman's hotel called the Hope and Anchor, which was run by an Irishman. "He showed it to me on the first floor in a small room at the back where seaman's luggage was kept," McKennee recollected.[32]

This story was too much for Thomas Stetson, Brown and Draper's lawyer, who earlier that year had cowed a Boston inventor into submission on behalf of the skirt-making dynamo of Douglass and Sherwood.

"As if in a fit of mad despair," Stetson fairly snorted, Clark is "endeavoring through this adaptable sailor McKennee to shift to the date of invention from the fall of 1856 to the fall of 1853 and then through this nocturnal fiction boost this imaginary invention back through a period of three years and into a period of time where no body had ever heard of, or thought of, skeleton skirts."[33]

Such a foolish attempt, he thundered, "places the finish before the beginning . . . the wrought sculpture before the quarried marble."[34]

The patent examiner in charge of the case soberly avoided comment on the McKennee testimony. Instead, he tersely found that while Clark was the first to invent, he had "neglected" and "slumbered" on his invention while Draper and Brown had brought theirs to the marketplace.[35] Thus, on October 2, 1860, the examiner ruled in favor of James Draper, ensuring him of hefty royalties and catapulting his family out of the drudgery of the working class. Clark, on the other hand, surrendered all hope of escaping poverty.

Fraud, Deception, and Bribes

Datus Rugg, still in Illinois and removed from the turmoil of the Civil War, feebly tried to defend his invention claims from afar. He had managed to convince the Patent Office to give him a second patent after Osborne & Vincent had caused the first one to be overturned in court. But now Osborne & Vincent was attacking his new patent.

One day in 1862, Rugg received a curious letter from Frederick Otis, yet another New York City skirt maker. Out of the blue, Otis offered to back Rugg in his struggle to maintain his patent in the face of Osborne & Vincent's deep-pocketed offense. His inventive fires rekindled, Rugg left his wife behind and set out for New York.

Soon after Rugg arrived in the city, however, the court overruled his second patent. Otis informed Rugg that he would not back any further appeals. Twice chastened and doubly impoverished, Rugg did not have enough money even to make his way home to Illinois. So he went to his rival, L. A. Osborne—a man fifteen years his junior who, Rugg felt, had robbed him of both the glory and the riches of his invention—and begged him for a job. Osborne gave him one. Rugg was to procure patent licenses for the company's well-defended hoop-skirt form patent, the very patent that Rugg felt was rightfully his.

The day before Rugg was supposed to start his new job, however, Otis paid Rugg a call and delivered extraordinary news. If only Rugg would take on two more backers, a certain J. O. West and a J. Wilcox, the promise of riches was once again his.

"He told me they would petition Congress," Rugg would later say. Otis said "he had a friend who was a senator and they would go to Washington and get the law altered."[36]

Buoyed by this development, Rugg returned to Illinois. He wrote his backers every day, but received little news in return. In the summer of 1863, having been kept in suspense for five months, he returned to New York, taking a menial job in a skirt factory to support himself. He earned barely enough to survive and he had to ask his backers, who really cannot be called investors as they never gave Rugg any money, for a loan so he could send money back home to his long-suffering wife. West grudgingly gave him ten dollars. Rugg asked Otis for the same amount. He got seven dollars.

In the meantime, unbeknownst to Rugg, Otis and his compatriots were offering a handsome bribe of a thousand dollars to the shop foreman of Osborne & Vincent if he would denounce the company's claim to inventorship. The foreman, however, refused the scurrilous offer.

By 1864, Rugg was destitute. Buffeted by the gales of capitalism for eight long years as he pursued the dream of his invention, Rugg abandoned hope. He wrote out an oath: Otis and the others, he finally realized, "did not expect and never had expected to get a patent and that they had only combined under a pretense of getting a patent on my invention as a means of protecting themselves against the Osborne Patent." He charged them with "fraud and deception" and, swearing that he had received no money from Osborne & Vincent, dramatically renounced any and all patent claims that he had previously made.[37]

Whether Rugg ultimately took that job with Osborne or whether he returned to his dentistry practice in Illinois is not known. One thing is for certain, however: Rugg never again applied for another patent.

Back to the Beginning

Oblivious to these dog-eat-dog fights between inventors, ladies of normally modest size and proportion by the mid-1860s had swelled to the size of a hot-air balloon. As a song of the time went,

> *What gallant ships! What swelling sails!*
> *How they resist opposing gales!*
> *With what a full relentless waft,*
> *They overwhelm each smaller craft!*[38]

"It was soon understood that the more voluminous the crinoline the more elegant the effect," wrote Jean Philippe Worth. "At last the ultimate in smartness was to have a crinoline so huge that one could not pass through a doorway."[39]

Magazines like the British *Punch* or the American *Harper's Weekly* made ferocious fun of ladies' vanity, especially as the cage puffed up to its maximum circumference. "The swinging of the crinoline imparted a new, flirtatious aspect to women's dress, although it was the size that attracted most attention—most of it unfavorable," according to fashion historian Valerie Steele.[40]

Justin McCarthy in his *Portraits of the Sixties*, cautioned that even "with all the undeniable cleverness and humour of *Punch*'s best caricatures, the younger generation can never fully realize what extraordinary exhibitions their polite ancestresses made of themselves during the terrible reign of the crinoline." The crinoline defied caricature, he argued, "for the actual reality was more full of unpicturesque and burlesque effects than any satirical pencil could realize on a flat outspread sheet of paper."[41]

L. Fellheimer.

Hoop Skirt.

Nº 63234   Patented Mar.26,1867.

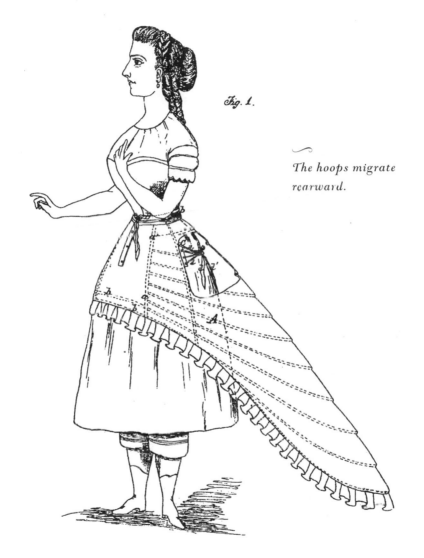

Fig. 1.

The hoops migrate
rearward.

Witnesses.   Inventor.

Gustave Dieterich   Louis Fellheimer

Charles Nash

Nov. 7, 1950 | M. C. CLAYTON | 2,528,639

COLLAPSIBLE HOOP SKIRT

Filed Aug. 12, 1948 | 2 Sheets-Sheet 1

FIG. 2

FIG. 1

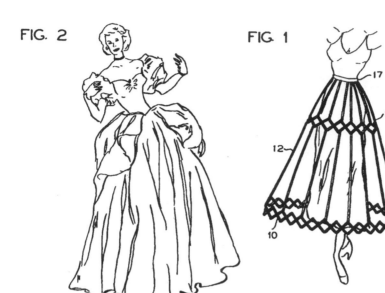

The first and only hoop skirt patent ever granted to a Southerner. It was plastic.

FIG. 3

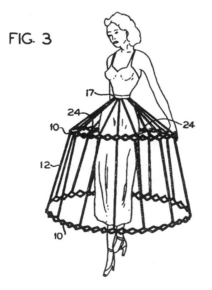

FIG. 4

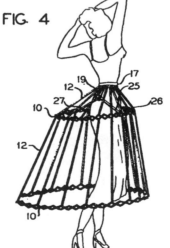

INVENTOR.
MARY C. CLAYTON

BY

ATTORNEY

The cage crinoline has not proved an enduring monument to (wo)man's aspirations to the geometrical sublime. As it grew increasingly larger, it required more and more material fabric to cover it. "When the formal crinoline was in its most ample phase, it attained diameters of more than three yards and required thirty yards of cloth," Philippe Perrot tells us.[42]

Once bedecked with ribbon and lace and velvet ruches it was no lighter than the eight or nine petticoats it had earlier displaced.

To accommodate the reacquired weight, the cage at first migrated to the rear, which we might imagine proved better ballasting for forward movement. Ultimately, however, it went into eclipse, giving rise to the reinvention of that old invention, the bustle, which swiveled attention away from the hips and toward the buttocks.

In 1876, *The Manufacturer and Builder,* an American trade journal, published an article entitled "New Use for Old Hoop-Skirts." It serves as an ignominious epitaph for the crinoline.

"As hoop-skirts have suddenly gone out of fashion," the article noted, "manufacturers have on hand immense quantities of crinoline steel which they do not know what to do with." The author advises that Berthold, a company in Dresden, Germany, had discovered a new use for the now superannuated material: When cut up, it could be turned into wire brushes. Such crinoline brushes, the journal said, stayed sharper longer than other wire brushes, were superior to coarse files, and were "the very best tool to remove slag and iron oxid [sic] from iron castings."[43] Destiny had returned the crinoline to the humble industrial origins from which it came.

The cage crinoline has not proved an enduring monument to (wo)man's aspirations to the geometrical sublime. As it grew increasingly larger, it required more and more material fabric to cover it. "When the formal crinoline was in its most ample phase, it attained diameters of more than three yards and required thirty yards of cloth," Philippe Perrot tells us.[42]

Once bedecked with ribbon and lace and velvet ruches it was no lighter than the eight or nine petticoats it had earlier displaced.

To accommodate the reacquired weight, the cage at first migrated to the rear, which we might imagine proved better ballasting for forward movement. Ultimately, however, it went into eclipse, giving rise to the reinvention of that old invention, the bustle, which swiveled attention away from the hips and toward the buttocks.

In 1876, *The Manufacturer and Builder,* an American trade journal, published an article entitled "New Use for Old Hoop-Skirts." It serves as an ignominious epitaph for the crinoline.

"As hoop-skirts have suddenly gone out of fashion," the article noted, "manufacturers have on hand immense quantities of crinoline steel which they do not know what to do with." The author advises that Berthold, a company in Dresden, Germany, had discovered a new use for the now superannuated material: When cut up, it could be turned into wire brushes. Such crinoline brushes, the journal said, stayed sharper longer than other wire brushes, were superior to coarse files, and were "the very best tool to remove slag and iron oxid [sic] from iron castings."[43] Destiny had returned the crinoline to the humble industrial origins from which it came.

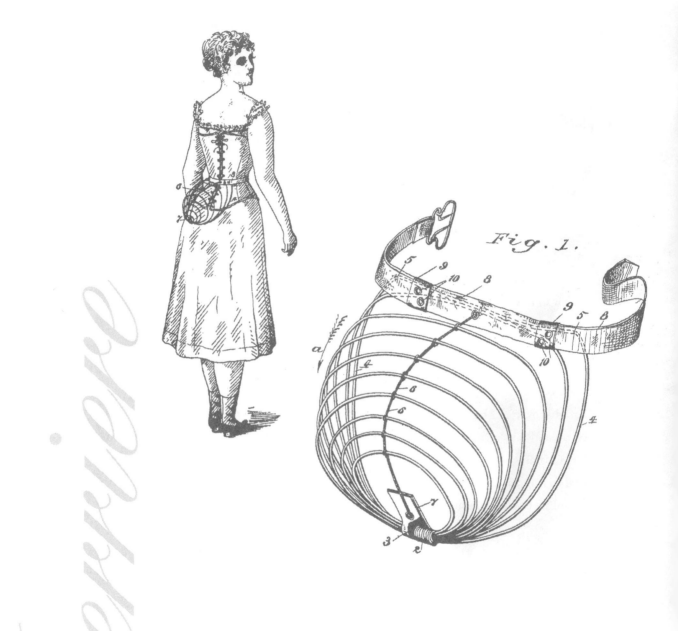

Fig. 1.

CHAPTER 9

Derriere

It must not be forgotten that often what is concealed is just that which is most wished to be displayed.

— Charles Blanc, *Art and Ornament in Dress*, 1877

bustle is often thought of as a muta-tion of the hoop skirt. But when examined carefully, it is clearly a unique invention. For the hoop skirt can be appreciated in three dimensions, while the bustle, much like the buttocks themselves, can be viewed only in profile or from the rear. Indeed, in terms of sexual ornament, the buttocks are the flip side of the breasts.

How is it that proper Victorian ladies, who would have considered it uncivi-lized to powder their noses in public, did not give a second thought to strapping on large prosthetic buttocks under layers of ribbon and braid? If, according to Balzac, dress is a revelation of a woman's "most secret thoughts, a language and a symbol," we can only wonder: What *were* they thinking?

Bustles have come in and out of fashion over the past several centuries. In eighteenth century caricatures they are frankly called "false bums." When they reap-

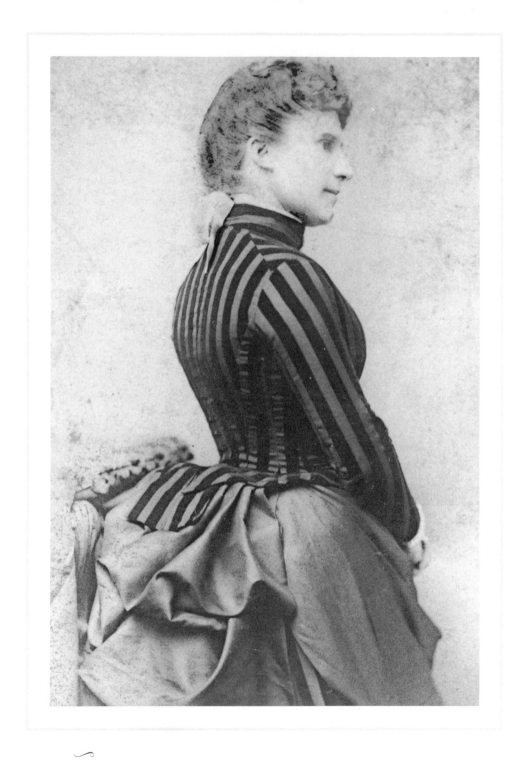

Like the women who wore them, bustles came in all shapes and sizes.

peared in the nineteenth century, they were more genteelly referred to as bustles, although even this term was too evocative; many an American lady Frenchified this into "tournure" or "pannier" or euphemized it into a "dress improver."

Fashion historians usually date the reappearance of bustles to the late 1860s or early 1870s. Ruth E. Finley, in her biography of the legendary magazine editor Sarah Josepha Hale, states that this latest incarnation of the bustle appeared as cage crinolines became excessively robust and fell of their own weight.

"These had become so large and required so much drapery to cover them— twenty-five yards of material was meager for the making of a dress—that the eighteen inches of waist permitted a woman scarcely had the strength to carry her skirt's weight," she wrote. "To relieve the strain on the back, supporting pads were worn in the hope of throwing a little of the tonnage on the rear hips. Gradually the gathers of the skirt were pushed backward, until, just before hoops were discarded, what was known as a 'back pannier' bunched the skirt over the rear of the hoops. And when the hoops finally did go, the back pannier remained to evolve into the bustle, most hideous style in all the history of dress."[1]

Finley was not alone in her animosity for the bustle. Oscar Wilde fumed that it was a "modern monstrosity," and declared that reformation of dress was of far greater importance than reformation of religion.[2]

The invention of the sewing machine and of aniline dyes wrought new, strange collisions of materials and colors: pleatings, kiltings, flounces, ruchings, and fringe came in olive and chartreuse, dark blue and cardinal red, magenta and pink. Cascading off the bustle down to the floor was a waterfall of fabric that pooled onto the ground in kaleidoscopic ripples.

"The train was intended to convey the impression that the wearer kept a carriage, but women who were not of the 'carriage class' trailed their appendages in the street," Alison Gernsheim writes in her witty photographic survey of Victorian and Edwardian fashion.[3]

Now that the crinoline was gone, humorists found new inspiration in the bustle. A writer for *Punchinello* delivered his mockery in a Huck Finn–esque colloquial dialect: "A full-dressed Girl of the period, as she sails out for an afternoon airin, looks somethin as I imagine the north pole would, with a ½ dozen rainbows rapt about it . . . there's more flummy-diddles and mushroom attachments to a woman's toggery nowadays than there is honest men in Wall Street. Durin the past season, overskirts and pannears have been looped up, makin the fair secks look as if she was gettin her garments in trin to leap over some frog-pond. . . . Long trailin dresses are comin into fashin, to the great detriment of the legitimate okerpshion of street-sweepin."[4]

Paper, Suspenders, and Hog Wire

Attached to the waist with a cloth belt, the bustle itself was not terribly restrictive to movement. "The discomforts of a bustle dress are more apparent than real, as the tournure is partly collapsible and easily moves to one side when the wearer sits down," writes Doris Langley Moore.[5] Which is not to say that sitting and bending did not become more difficult as the front of the dress became tighter and tighter. Around 1876 the humor magazine *Punch* featured a series of cartoons lampooning ladies whose dresses were so restrictive that they could neither sit down nor climb stairs. *The Queen*, a fashion magazine, editorialized that "it would be impossible to make closer drapery; the limit has been reached. The modern gown shews the figure in a way which is certainly most unsuitable for the ordinary British matron."[6]

The hair during this period was a visual echo of the bustle. Extravagant chignons of plaits or curls tripped down the back of the head. Hair pads, much like bustles, gave the illusion of volume. "If we consider that even a moderate-sized 'plait' contains as much hair as grows altogether on the head of an ordinary Englishwoman, and is probably half as long again, we may very reasonably be allowed to wonder whence the supply comes," mused Dr. Andrew Wyhnter, in his 1874 *Peeps into the Human Hive.*[7]

During the 1870s, the bustle supported "loosely gathered balloons of fabric" that were "volumetric and buoyant in effect," according to Harold Koda in *Extreme*

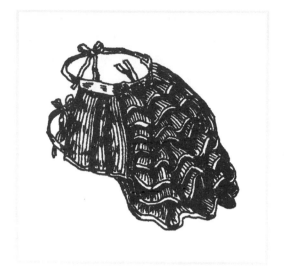

Horsehair bustle.

Beauty. At this point the bustle was for the most part a simple reincarnation of bustles before—either a half cage crinoline or an old-fashioned bustle of horsehair or stiffened gauze and net.

Festooned though it was, the bustle was limited in size by technology. Bustles stuffed with animal hair could grow only to a certain point before they became too hot and heavy to bear. Those made of metal wire could support only so much upholstery, given that they easily bent out of shape or broke under the stress of the fabric load or from being squashed when the lady sat down. (This, as one might imagine, created a serious safety hazard.)

Not that inventors of the period did not try to improve the bustle structure. Benjamin F. Moore's inflatable india-rubber bustle, he explained, was "in a crescent shape, with projecting hollow points or nipples of such a length that the compressed air within shall act to give a more gentle sweep to the dress and keep it farther away from the person."[8] Fashionable ladies, perhaps already expected to be owners of pneumatic bust pads, were to inflate the bustle by blowing into a nozzle.

In 1873, nearly a century before the paper dresses of the 1960s, James Wehl of New York invented the disposable bustle, made of pasteboard that had been

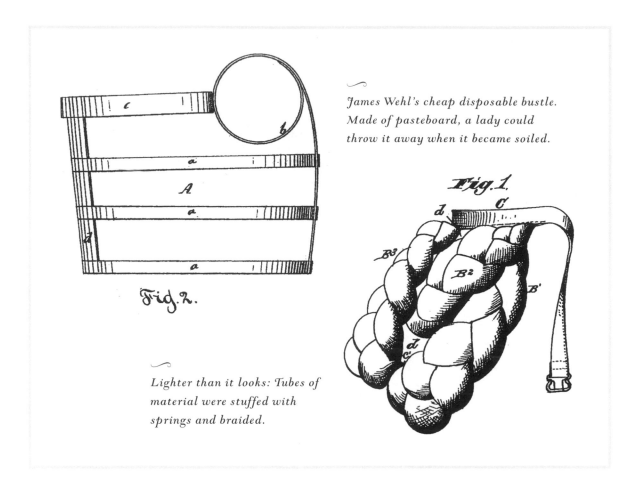

James Wehl's cheap disposable bustle. Made of pasteboard, a lady could throw it away when it became soiled.

Lighter than it looks: Tubes of material were stuffed with springs and braided.

strengthened with metal wire. "It is entirely free from danger," wrote Wehl, "for if one of my paper bustles is exposed to some external pressure the worst that may happen is to spoil its shape, while an ordinary bustle when hard pressed is liable to break, and the broken metal rings or wires may produce injury to the person wearing the bustle. My paper bustle is also very cheap, so that when it becomes soiled it can be thrown away and replaced by a new one at less expense than it costs to clean one of the ordinary bustles."[9]

In 1874 an inventor in Oshkosh, Wisconsin, came up with an improvement that thus far had eluded eastern inventors: a bustle with suspenders. Three years later, in Shelbyville, Illinois, Alwilda Swallow designed a floor-length bustle covered with hog wire.

None of these ideas, however, appears to have been a great commercial success. By 1876, bold fashion leaders were swelling at points lower and lower down the back, until the back-side focal point, punctuated sometimes by a large bow, was just below the back of the knees. The bustle had become an afterthought, deflating into a mere soupçon of its former self. Within less than a decade, however, it would swell again with renewed, gravity-defying vigor.

Aaron M. Weber of Oshkosh, Wisconsin, came up with a practical bustle: one with suspenders.

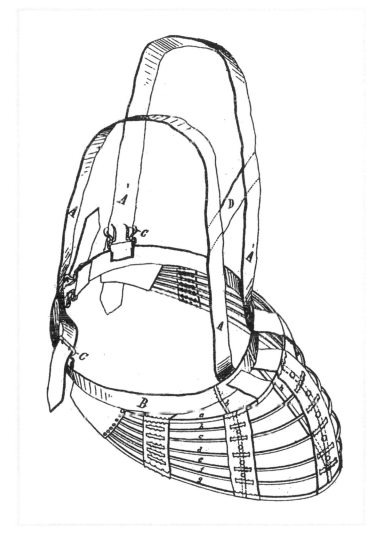

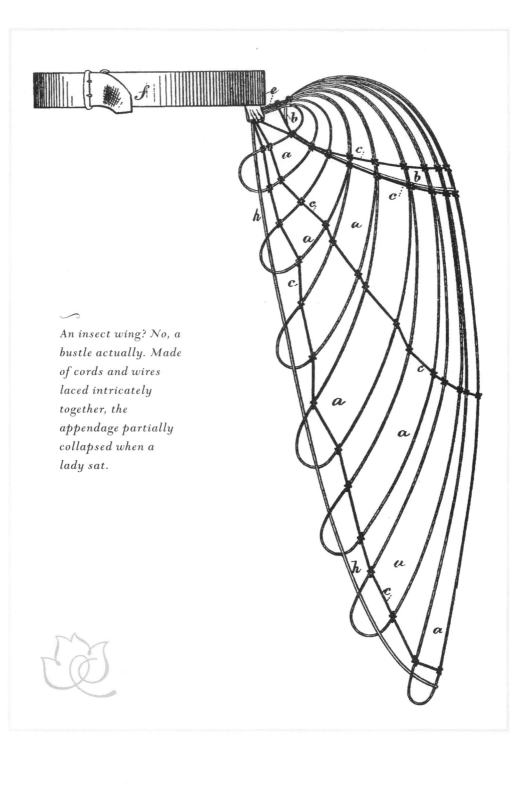

An insect wing? No, a bustle actually. Made of cords and wires laced intricately together, the appendage partially collapsed when a lady sat.

Ladies were shifting the focal point elsewhere as well. The pate of the ultra fashionable late Victorian woman was a study in excess. Her hat brimmed with naturalistic themes: iridescent beetles, baby bear cubs, miniature squirrels, carrots, turnips, beets, plums, pears, peaches, and all manner of stuffed birds—whole parrots, lovebirds, finches, blackbirds, pigeons, owls, and seagulls.

By 1883, the bustle had returned with a vengeance and the proper lady in silhouette looked as if she had the rump of a mature mare. "It was a popular conceit that the cantilevers of these bustles," writes Harold Koda, "could support an entire tea service."[10] Indeed, judging from some photographs of the times, in some cases this may not have been a conceit but a reality.

These heavily upholstered derrieres, so different from the airy affairs of just a few years before, were made possible by newly invented, more robust constructions underneath.

Wired for Beauty

This was the age of wire: telephone wire, piano wire, barbed wire, wire-brim hats, ribbon wire, spark screens for locomotive engines, and electrical wire. It was also the age of cheap iron. Ironmasters were not even bothering any more to manufacture new iron; they just recycled scrap from old railways, bridges, and cannons. Corset makers and other innovators were busy figuring out new ways to fashion light, flexible, strong bustles out of this widely available, cheap material.

During the 1880s and 1890s nearly two hundred different kinds of bustles were patented. Surely, some of this was innovation-as-marketing, with bustle makers catching the fickle eye of consumers with new models. But it is also true that the bustle was still an imperfect invention. By contrast, the bra and the hoop skirt, after a period of frenetic innovation in which dozens of widely divergent designs competed for acceptance, evolved into a basic elegant structural design that could in turn be adapted to achieve different looks.

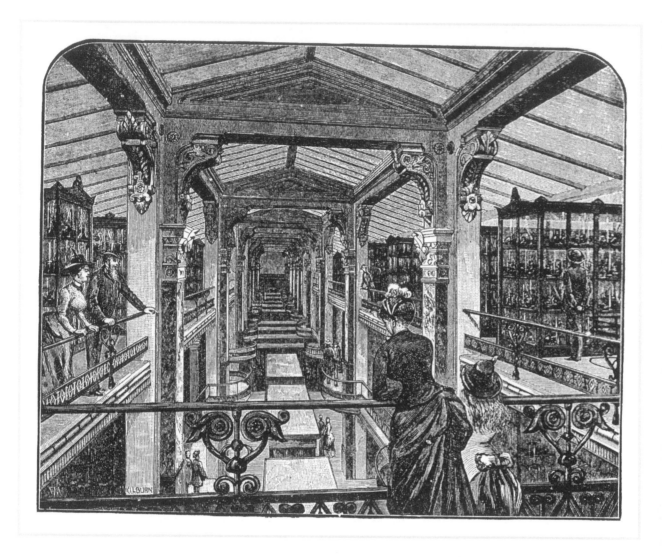

An 1880s engraving of the Great Hall of the Patent
Office, which displayed models of inventions and was a
popular tourist site. The ladies in the engraving may
well have been wearing bust forms or bustles that were
displayed in miniature form in the glass cases.

Not so the bustle, and it was not for lack of trying.

For example, the wonderfully named James R. Rheubottom and Frank M. Mack of Weedsport, New York, patented "a bustle capable of retaining the form of its arch under the various strains, thrusts, and pressure to which it is subjected while being worn and to avoid the common radical defects of 'hitching up' or 'sagging down.' "[11] After that, bustle invention swiftly sashayed west. Patents were soon granted to Keness Rice of Eureka Springs, Arkansas; Patrick O'Connor of Atlanta, Georgia; Alice Randall of Milwaukee, Wisconsin; Nevada Florence Ardeny of New Cumberland, Indiana; Olive J. Decker of Keokak, Iowa; George Eckles of Eyota, Minnesota; and May Leaman of San Jose, California.

The bustle was a democratic fashion, one celebrated and mocked in many popular songs of the day. Harry Gibbs penned "O Susan Wears a Bustle" in 1883:

> *Some fellows they are very rude,*
> *I hardly think it's fair,*
> *They're always making some remark*
> *About the clothes I wear,*
> *Whenever I go out to skate,*
> *To exercise my muscle*
> *I hear them calling after me:*
> *O Susan wears a bustle!*[12]

Two basic commercially successful designs did quickly emerge, but they were widely divergent in their design.

One was a volume of woven wire mesh that looks something like a fisherman's pot from that era for catching crabs or lobsters. The Weston & Wells Manufacturing Company in Philadelphia and the American Braided Wire Company in London appear to have cornered the market on these. Advertisements boasted that these models would "yield to the slightest pressure, yet immediately return to their proper shape after the severest usage," and "properly sustain the heaviest drapery," so that "the wearers are never mortified by their being crushed or bent into ridiculous shapes."[13]

This construction was made possible by new machines that could weave the wire three-dimensionally. Nicholas Jenkins, an inventor in Waterbury, Connecticut, was a pioneer in the field. He patented his "elastic metal," as a "fabric stiffener" in 1880. Jenkins envisioned that it would not only be used for clothing but also to make

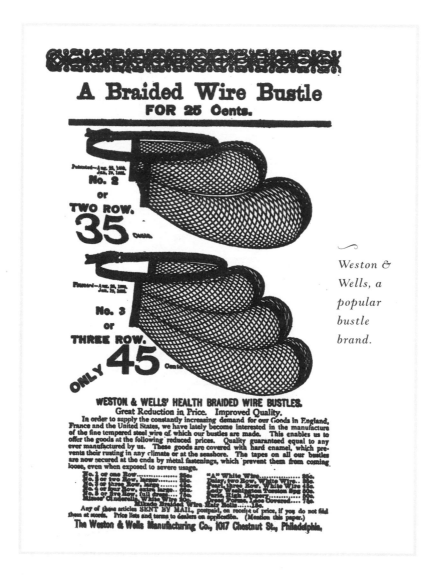

Weston & Wells, a popular bustle brand.

H. O. CANFIELD.
BUSTLE.

No. 375,923.   Patented Jan. 3, 1888.

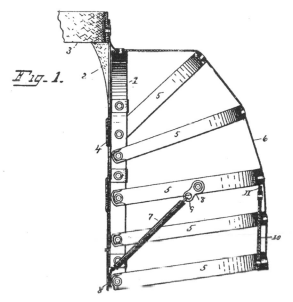

Fig. 1.

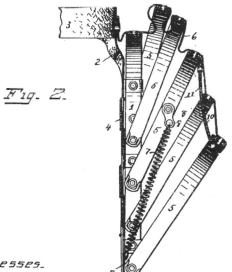

Fig. 2.

Another popular model, invented by Henry O. Canfield of Bridgeport, Connecticut.

Witnesses.
E. D. Smith
B. E. Lee.

Inventor-
Henry O. Canfield
By A. M. Wooster
Atty.

whip handles, jewelry, or as a material for suspending birdcages. "In such case it will allow the cage to teeter or dance with the motions of the bird," he wrote.[14]

These structurally impressive, wire-woven bustles could in turn support smaller, lightweight bustles of cane or stiffened fabric. Bianca Blenker of New York City patented stackable bustles in 1885. These miniature bustles were "superimposed on the lower bustle"—and one could add as many, one on top of the other, as necessary.

The second major design that supported the unprecedented satyrlike hump was a series of strong curved metal bands. Covered in fabric (to prevent rusting through the dress on rainy days), the spring-loaded bands were anchored by pivot hinges to side supports. A lady could raise the bustle when sitting; when she stood up it sprang back automatically into place. "One of the most extraordinary inventions in the whole history of fashion," exclaimed James Laver, the dean of fashion historians.[15]

Lillie Langtry, the nineteenth-century British actress who also proved a shrewd businesswoman, gave this product her celebrity imprimatur and it became known as the Langtry bustle. It actually appears to have been invented by Henry O. Canfield of Bridgeport, Connecticut, who received nine patents on his idea in as many months. Like the woven-wire bustle, it, too, could support smaller bustles above.

The Arc of Fashion

As bustle inflation reached the limits of credulity, however, and as the human body reached the limits of its ability to support such an appendage, fashionable women abruptly let their bustles drop to the ground. Other women quickly did the same. With nimble sleight of hand, they drew attention to a new zone of visual interest: the arms. "There was apparently still a deep-rooted desire for a bulge somewhere, and no sooner had it disappeared behind, than it began to grow on the upper arm," Al-

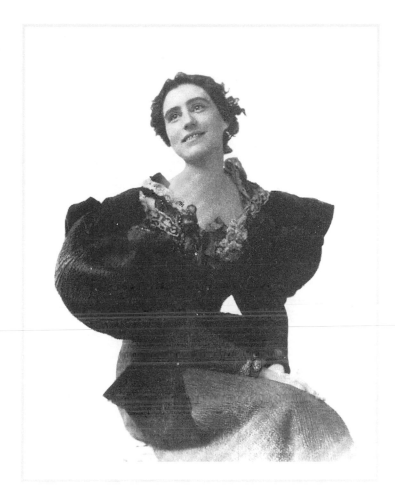

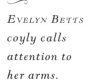

EVELYN BETTS coyly calls attention to her arms.

ison Gernsheim writes. Sleeves inflated so that by the mid-1890s "the ultra-fashionable had to sidle through doors like a crab."[16]

Thus, the bustle followed the familiar arc of fashionability traveled by virtu-ally every other beauty innovation, from blue eye shadow to stiletto heels. In the arms race of beauty competition, the bustle became increasingly exaggerated until that tenuous point where the woman sporting it looked as if she was not quite human but, rather, of a different species altogether. It is at this point of ultimate exaggeration

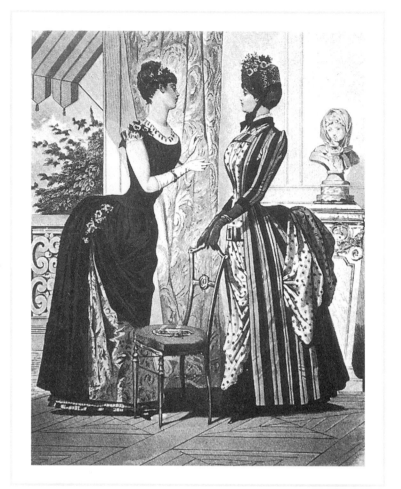

Bustles big enough to cantilever a tea service.

that a beauty innovation is abandoned in favor of a new novelty, one that highlights another part of the body—usually in a modest way that, as the innovation is adopted by many women, becomes increasingly outrageous. And so the cycle begins again.

"If every one were cast in the same mold there would be no such thing as beauty," Charles Darwin wrote in *The Descent of Man.* "If all our women were to become as beautiful as the Venus de Medici we should for a time be charmed, but we should soon wish for variety; and, as soon as we had obtained variety, we should wish to see certain [characteristics] a little exaggerated beyond the then existing common standard."[17]

What of the bustle? It remained an object of fun for a while. A rodeo show in the late nineteenth century featured "the oldest woman rider from the San Angelo Country" riding the wildest bronc in Fort Worth. She held a U.S. flag in each hand, balancing on the bronc as it reared up, bucking back and forth and pawing the air. After a rip-roaring ride the "old woman" got off the bronc, discarding her "rustles and bustles." To everyone's surprise the fashionable old lady was old Booger Red, known as "the ugliest and toughest man of the west."[18] Thomas Edison also had his fun with this fashion. One of his early experimental silent film clips from the turn of the century is called "Aunt Sallie's Wonderful Bustle" and it features a woman who flips over a railing, exposing the underside of her bustle.

Did the bustle go extinct before it could further evolve? It has not yet enjoyed a real revival, even though, as the history of breast enhancement attests, naturalistic foam-rubber prosthetics, or even Hottentot-like surgical implants are technologically possible. The 1902 Sears catalog, perhaps hoping for a bustle revival so that it could sell off excess stock, offered for sale four different models of bustles, forlornly nestled among more modern offerings such as the Edison kinetoscope, electric belts, zithers, and cast-iron pig troughs.

The advertising copy for one of these, however, suggests that the bustle had not gone extinct but simply gone incognito. The Lenox Glove Fitting Hip Bustle "rounds out the figure," extends "over the hips very lightly and gracefully." Nor, the Sears catalog assured, "can it be detected."[19]

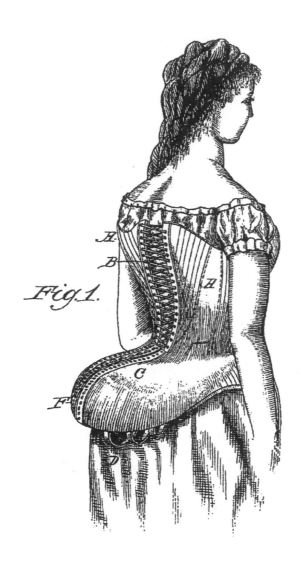

Fig. 1.

conclusion

Some of the beauty inventions you have just read about are obsolete. Others have endured and continue to evolve. Many more remain yet to be imagined.

If we can trust the prognostications of futurists like Ray Kurzweil, the pace of technological change is quickening at a geometric, perhaps even exponential, rate. This change will transform human intelligence and culture but also will roil our definition of human beauty.

As I sit here writing, I am trolling online through new patent applications. I find a technique for growing virgin skin to replace wrinkled human hides, a body-scanning device for custom-fitting form-clinging clothing, and a method for growing breast tissue from stem cells. I don't see a patent for genetically engineering periwinkle eyes and lime-green hair. But can such possibilities really be far away?

As innovation gallops forward, trends are transmitted at Internet speed. Thus we are witnessing a phenomenon that might be called the Law of Accelerating Beauty. At some point women will be able to so easily and safely transform their physical beings that the congenitally pretty will no longer have a survival advantage over the congenitally average. I don't think we have reached that point yet. But we will.

The corollary to the Law of Accelerating Beauty might be called the Principle of Age Deceleration. Is forty the new twenty? It is if you are Elle Macpherson, W magazine quipped recently. If antiwrinkle technology innovation persists at the current rate, however, forty may well become the new twenty for mere mortal women as well. Decay will remain inevitable. But we will become ever more nimble at staving off that moment when, like the society matrons in the futuristic film *Brazil*, we dissolve into the tapestry.

Certain self-improvements or adornments are folded into our culture with little controversy or debate. Dental work has quietly become as much about vanity as health. All we really "need" is a stub to chew with, not a porcelain crown that looks even better than our real teeth and certainly not a topping of pure white bleach strips. Yet the dentally improved rarely attract the ire and accusations of vanity that breast implantees do.

Exercise, too, is seen as a virtuous pursuit. To be healthy, all people need to do is walk briskly several times a week and do a little stretching, as Gina Kolata has pointed out in her book *Ultimate Fitness*. Yet we tend to think of someone who spends two hours a day body sculpting at the gym as virtuous. In fact, she is not any less vain than someone who achieves the same effect with liposuction. (Though working out, at least today, is far safer than plastic surgery.)

Mary Tannen, beauty editor of the *New York Times*, recently fretted that we could be "on our way toward evolving into a race of supermodels." Others worry that the current obsession with plastic surgery, this season's spectator sport on television, has turned Beauty into a kind of physiological sameness. They are right. Yet this trend is not unique to plastic surgery; nor is it a new phenomenon. Virtually every beauty invention that has taken flight—from corsets to cosmetics—has tended to mold Woman into a collective, ideal form. It is just that the technology has gotten a lot more effective.

Given the emphasis that humans place on appearance, it seems to me that Beauty inventions can be considered, for many, tools of empowerment. And it is not just about blending in. Invention has also allowed those who dare to innovate to synthesize a unique kind of attractiveness when they themselves may not have been born to Beauty.

The only constant in beauty innovation is change itself. What is standard today will not be standard tomorrow. My sister-in-law was mocked during her adolescence for having naturally full lips. Today actresses and others require regular surgical upkeep to maintain the Angelina Jolie pout that my sister-in-law owns naturally.

Only a few are bold enough to innovate, but innovate they will, just as surely as others will follow. As the masses adopted the bikini wax, rock stars and fashion elite began to opt for a totally nude pubis, studded with fake gems. One day in the coming century, a handful of fashion mavens will turn up sporting novel crystal exoskeletons that change hue according to the wearer's mood. As the price dips and everywoman can afford knock-off models, the mavens will shed their exoskeletons and don something else. What exactly is anybody's guess. Woman's impulse to reinvent herself is age old. The relentless parade of invention merely changes what is possible.

notes

For full citations, please consult the bibiliography.

Introduction

1. Steven Pinker, *How the Mind Works*, pp. 471–472.
2. Recounted in Donald Symons, *The Evolution of Human Sexuality*, p. 211.
3. Dorothy Parker, "General Review of the Sex Situation" from *The Portable Dorothy Parker*, Copyright 1926, 1954 by Dorothy Parker. Reprinted by permission of The Viking Press.
4. Isak Dinesen, in "The Old Chevalier," *Seven Gothic Tales*, p. 63, Penguin paperback edition.
5. Nancy Etcoff, *Survival of the Prettiest*, p. 242.
6. Ruth Schwartz Cowan, *More Work for Mother: The Ironies of Household Technology from the Open Hearth to the Microwave*, p. 127.

Chapter 1: Eyes

1. See David Buss, *The Evolution of Desire*, p. 119. "Initiating visual contact also proves to be a highly effective tactic for women who seek to attract a sex partner. Looking intensely into a man's eyes and allowing a man to see her staring are judged to be among the top 15 percent of effective tactics women can use to attract short-term sex partners."
2. Autumn Stanley, *Mothers and Daughters of Invention*, p. 451.
3. Quoted in ibid., p. 451.
4. Ibid., pp. 451–452.
5. Harriet Hubbard Ayer, *Harriet Hubbard Ayer's Book: A Complete and Authentic Treatise on the Laws of Health and Beauty*, pp. 434–435.
6. Ibid.
7. Ibid.

8. Quoted in Kathy Peiss, *Hope in a Jar: The Making of America's Beauty Culture*, p. 47.
9. Quoted in Daniel Boorstin, *The Americans: The Democratic Experience*, p. 176.
10. Peiss, p. 47.
11. Quoted in ibid., p. 47.
12. Lois W. Banner, *American Beauty*, p. 119.
13. Sarah Jane Pierce, *Homely Girls*, p. 81.
14. Helena Rubinstein, *My Life for Beauty*, p. 48.
15. Ibid., p. 41.
16. Ibid., p. 61.
17. Document #5 from the Max Factor Archives of Procter & Gamble.
18. Barry Paris, *Garbo: A Biography*, p. 230.
19. Ibid., p. 229.
20. Ibid., p. 229.
21. Quoted in ibid., p. 230.
22. Fenja Gunn, *The Artificial Face*, p. 156.
23. Maria Riva, *Marlene Dietrich*, pp. 124–125.
24. Quoted in Gwen Kay, "Regulating Beauty: Cosmetics in American Culture from the 1906 Pure Food and Drugs Act to the 1938 Food, Drug and Cosmetic Act," p. 49–50. [*New Republic* 65 (9 September 1925): 65].
25. Mark Pendergrast, *Mirror Mirror*, p. 247.
26. Frederick Lewis Allen, *Only Yesterday*, p. 264.
27. Richard Corson, *Fashions in Makeup*, p. 22.
28. *Toilette of Health*, p. 133.
29. Ibid.
30. http://www.maybelline.com/us/beginnings.html.
31. Quoted in Kay, p. 67 ["Gentlemen Prefer—," *Reader's Digest* 28 (April 1936): 18 (condensed from an article in *Vogue*)].
32. Frederick Lewis Allen, *Since Yesterday*, p. 35.
33. Quoted in Kay, p. 66 [G. W. Vanden, "It's Cosmetic

Time in America," *American Hairdresser* 55, no. 7 (July 1932): 60].

34. Ruth deForest Lamb, *American Chamber of Horrors*, p. 18.

35. Carolyn Thomas de la Pena, *The Body Electric*, pp. 209–210.

36. Neville Williams, *Powder and Paint*, pp. 146–147.

37. Ibid.

38. *Breakfast at Tiffany's*, directed by Blake Edwards, 1961.

Chapter 2: Lips

1. Kathy Peiss, *Hope in a Jar*, p. 14.

2. Gilbert Vail, *A History of Cosmetics in America*, p. 95.

3. U.S. patent 29,944.

4. U.S. patent 67,182.

5. Lois W. Banner, *American Beauty*, p. 49.

6. Ibid.

7. M. S. Balsam, ed., *Cosmetics: Science and Techology*, p. 365.

8. Quoted in Jeffrey L. Meikle, *Twentieth Century Limited: Industrial Design in America, 1925–1939*, p. 12.

9. Quoted in Neville Williams, *Powder and Paint: A History of the Englishwoman's Toilet*, p. 136.

10. Ibid., pp. 129–130.

11. Nancy Milford, *Zelda: A Biography*, p. 77.

12. Ibid., p. 60.

13. *Watkins Timely Suggestions*, p. 20.

14. Quoted in Fenja Gunn, *The Artificial Face*, p. 149.

15. See Peiss, pp. 188–189.

16. *Vogue's Book of Beauty*, p. 22.

17. Clare Booth Luce, *The Women*, p. 84.

18. Peiss, pp. 3–4.

19. Library of Congress American Memory Collection. Accession #WI1063, 10/10/1940.

20. Richard Corson, *Fashions in Makeup*, p. 469.

21. Jennifer H. Miller, "Casting Race: A History of Makeup Technology in the U.S. Film Industry, 1890–1940," pp. 182–183.

22. Margaret Allen, *Selling Dreams*, p. 45.

23. Hazel Bishop, Unpublished Memoirs, Schlesinger Library on the History of Women in America, Carton 4.

24. Ibid., p. 10.

25. *The New Jersey Journal*, December 21, 1963. Clipping at Schlesinger. No page number.

26. Bishop's memoirs, p. 10.

27. Ibid.

28. Ibid., p. 11

29. Ibid., p. 13.

30. A&S sold an average of 300 lipsticks a day for "an extended period of time," according to Bishop's memoir, p. 18.

31. Advertisement in Hazel Bishop collection, Schlesinger Library.

32. *Advertising Age*, February 7, 1955, p. 1.

33. *Mayfair*, summer 1951 issue, p. 3.

34. *Business Week*, 17 March 1951, pp 42–45.

35. *Advertising Age*, 22 February 1954.

36. *Consumer Reports*, August 1951, pp. 349–352.

37. Bishop memoir, p. 12.

38. Unidentified newspaper clipping in Hazel Bishop collection, Schlesinger Library.

Chapter 3: Breasts

1. Of course, sometimes this amounts to false advertising. Women with androgen insensitivity syndrome, for example, have full breasts (and clear skin and luxurious hair) but no uterus. See *Eve's Rib* by Robert Pool or *Woman: An Intimate Geography* by Natalie Angier.

2. Thank you, Mata Dova, for this reference.

3. Caresse Crosby, *The Passionate Years*.

4. Jane Farrell-Beck and Colleen Gau, *Uplift: The Bra in America*, p. 199.

5. Ibid., p 25.

6. Quoted in ibid.

7. Ibid., p. 14.

8. U.S. Patent 719,075.

9. U.S. Patent classifications searched for devices meant to artificially augment the bust include: 2/463; 128/890; 450/17; 450/38; 450/42–5; 450/55; 450/57; 450/84; 623/7. During the period from 1850 to 1950 I found sixty-nine patents for breast augmentation devices (I am including here exclusively inventions that were unequivocally *not* postsurgery breast replacements). Forty-three of the sixty-nine (63 percent) were granted to women. Those women inventors were Anne McLean (1858, 1866, 1867); Elizabeth Marshall (1864); Clementine Rutherford (1866); Mary Tilton (1870);

Helen Millar (1873); Elisabeth Stowell (1874); Susanna E. Burns (1875); Harriet May (1876); Elisabeth S. Weldon (1876); Julia Bates (1876); Julia Banfield (1877); Hariet Chapman (1877); Charlotte McGee (1877); Anna Pike (1877); Imogen E. Banker (1881); Zénone Ledochowski (1884); Elizabeth Leetch (1885); Sarah Warren (1887); Elizabeth Case (1887); Dora Harrison (1897, 1898, 1907); Lucy James (1889); Mary Williams (1889); Emma Foley (1891); Marguerete M. Farrell (1893); Ida M. Rew (1895); Minnie Widup Comly (1899); Jessamine Quigley (1899); Célina Jullien-Binard (1900); Katherine Stenhouse (1904); Chrisie Launer (1906); Anna Coleman (1908); Lydia Martell (1912); Mabel Harrington (1914); Mabel V. Heuchan (1917); Lillian M. Bender (1924); Elsie B. Meadows (1934); Ruth Gerst (1946); Josephine Peliser (1947); Flora Wilkenfeld (1948).

10. U.S. Patent 22,443.

11. U.S. Patent 43,321.

12. C. Willett Cunnington and Phillis Cunnington, *The History of Underclothes,* p. 198.

13. Lola Montez, *The Arts of Beauty; or, Secrets of a Lady's Toilet, with hints to Gentlemen on the Art of Fascinating,* p. 52.

14. Susan C. Power, *The Ugly-Girl Papers: or, Hints for the Toilet,* p. 234.

15. National Museum of American History archives, accession number 219034 c. 1867–68.

16. U.S. Patent 173,698.

17. U.S. Patent 212,184.

18. U.S. Patent 579,824 (1897); U.S. Patent 599,180 (1898); and U.S. Patent 861,115 (1907).

19. U.S. Patent 1,033,788.

20. T. S. Eliot, "Whispers of Immortality."

21. Marilyn Yalom, *A History of the Breast,* p. 69.

22. Letter dated May 16, 1901, in Warshaw Collection, in Aurum Folder, National Museum of American History archives.

23. American Medical Association, *Nostrums and Quackery.*

24. Power, p. 235.

25. Zoe Hamilton, *Boudoir Manual,* p. 9 Folder 1–40, Warshaw Collection, National Museum of American History archives.

26. Sears Roebuck catalog, 1897, 1968 reprint.

27. Sears Roebuck catalog, 1902, 1969 reprint.

28. Health-Culture Company of New York City, *Womanly Beauty.*

29. Quoted in Gerald Jonas's history, "Dancing: The Pleasure, Power, and Art of Movement," p. 174.

30. Ibid.

31. Ibid.

32. Ibid., p. 175.

33. *It,* directed by Clarence Badger and Josef von Sternberg, filmed in 1926 and released in 1927.

34. Frank Westmore, *The Westmores of Hollywood,* pp. 48–49.

35. Robert S. Lynd and Helen Merrell Lynd, *Middletown: A Study in Modern American Culture,* p. 266.

36. Ibid., p. 267.

37. Quoted in William E. Leuchtenberg, *The Perils of Prosperity,* p. 161.

38. Ibid., p. 168.

39. Quoted in ibid., p. 171.

40. James Joyce letter quoted in Barbara Maddox, *Nora: The Real Life of Molly Bloom.*

41. Lynd and Lynd, p. 258.

42. Farrell-Beck and Gau, p. 26.

43. Ibid., pp. 58–81.

44. Ibid., pp. 53–54 for the total count. I came up with the Kops count after examining patent classes 450/85; 450/28; 450/41. However, bra-type inventions have about twenty different classifications and it is nearly impossible to know whether any search has been exhaustive.

45. This observation thanks to Jane Farrell-Beck, phone interview in November 2002.

46. Quoted in Jill Susan Fields, "The Production of Glamour: A Social History of Intimate Apparel, 1909–1952," p. 97.

47. Quoted in Farrell-Beck and Gau, p. 73.

48. Ibid., p. 63.

49. Quoted in ibid.

50. Fields, pp. 142–143.

51. U.S. Patent 1,087,579.

52. Quoted in Fields, p. 144 [*Corsets & Brassieres,* February 1938, pp. 48–49].

53. Jane Russell, *An Autobiography: My Path and My Detours,* p. 58.

54. Ibid.

55. Quoted in Farrell-Beck and Gau, p. 88.

56. Ibid. [*CUR,* March 1943, p. 77].

57. Letter, 8 January 1944, to Maiden Form Brassiere, Inc. from Louis Landaw, M.D., Paterson, New Jersey. In Maidenform Collection, National Museum of American History.

58. Frederick Lewis Allen, *Since Yesterday: The 1930s in America*, p. 137.

59. Ibid.

60. Quoted in ibid., pp. 151–152.

61. See ibid., p. 152.

62. Quoted in ibid.

63. Quoted in Elizabeth Haiken, *Venus Envy: A History of Cosmetic Surgery*, pp. 233–234 [Lois Mattox Miller, "Surgery's Cinderella," *Independent Woman*, July 1939, p. 201].

64. Marilyn Yalom, *A History of the Breast*, p. 177.

65. Quoted in ibid.

66. Vardis Fisher, "Women's Fashions," *Weiser American*, 6 September 1954.

67. Undated copy of advertising material, author's collection.

68. Yalom, p. 178.

69. Ibid.

70. *Maidenform at 40*. In Maidenform Collection at the National Museum of American History archives.

71. Farrell-Beck and Gau, p. 156.

72. "Hurrah for The Bra," *Life* magazine, June 1989.

73. Haiken, p. 236.

74. Quoted in ibid., p. 243.

75. Ibid., p. 244.

76. Ibid., p. 249.

77. Ibid., pp. 228–284.

78. See *Ann Plast Surg*. 35, no. 5 (November 1995): 505–509; discussion 509–510; *Plast Reconstr Surg*. 91, no. 2 (February 1993): 352–361; *J Urol*. 110, no. 2 (August 1973): 210; *Urology*. 8, no. 1 (July 1976): 68–72; *Plast Reconstr Surg*. 57, no. 4 (April 1976): 517–519.

79. Mimi Swartz, "Silicone City: The Rise and Fall of the Implant—or How Houston Went From an Oil-Based Economy to a Breast-Based Economy," *Texas Monthly* 23, no. 8 (August 1995): 64.

80. Quoted in Haiken, p. 258.

Chapter 4: Hair

1. A. F. Niemoeller, *Superfluous Hair and Its Removal*, p. 14.

2. Bill Severn, *The Long and Short of It: Five Thousand Years of Fun and Fury over Hair*, p. 92.

3. Ibid., p. 94.

4. Ibid., p. 100.

5. Ibid., p. 105.

6. Cynthia Eagle Russett, *Darwin in America: The Intellectual Response 1865–1912*, pp. 91–92.

7. Knight Dunlap, *Personal Beauty and Racial Betterment*, pp. 38–39.

8. Severn, p. 102.

9. George Henry Fox, *The Use of Electricity in the Removal of Facial Hair and the Treatment of Various Facial Blemishes*, p. 8.

10. Ibid., pp. 8–10.

11. Ibid.

12. Henrietta P. Johnson, "Facial Blemishes" in *An International System of Electro-Therapeutics*, Horatio R. Bigelow, editor, pp. H-1–H-8.

13. Ibid., p. H-3.

14. Lola Montez, *The Arts of Beauty; or, Secrets of a Lady's Toilet*, pp. 91–92.

15. Ibid., p. 92.

16. Arthur Ralph Hinkel and Richard W. Lind, *Electrolysis, Thermolysis and the Blend: The Principles and Practice of Permanent Hair Removal*, p. 150.

17. M. C. Phillips, *Skin Deep: The Truth About Beauty Aids*, p. 302.

18. Montez, pp. 91–92.

19. Johnson, p. H-5.

20. Fox, pp. 14–15.

21. Ibid.

22. Ibid., p. 18.

23. A. Dale Covey, M.D., *Profitable Office Specialties*, p. 262.

24. Hinkel and Lind, p. 170.

25. Everett G. McDonough, *Truth About Cosmetics*.

26. deForest Lamb, p. 29.

27. Ibid.

28. Excerpt from a letter written to Eleanor Roosevelt in May 1934, quoted in Gwen Elizabeth Kay, "Regulating Beauty: Cosmetics in American Culture from the

1906 Pure Food and Drugs Act to the 1938 Food, Drug and Cosmetic Act," p. I.

29. Bob McCoy. *Quack: Museum of Questionable Medical Devices*, p. 199.

30. Ruth deForest Lamb, *American Chamber of Horrors*, p. 83.

31. Rebecca Herzig, "Removing Roots: 'North American Hiroshima Maidens' and the X Ray." *Technology and Culture*, October 1999, p. 732.

32. Bettyann Holtzmann Kevles, *Naked to the Bone: Medical Imaging in the Twentieth Century*, p. 47.

33. Ruth Brecher and Edward Brecher, *The Rays: A History of Radiology in the United States and Canada*, p. 82.

34. Kevles, p. 69.

35. Ibid., p. 47.

36. Ibid., p. 48.

37. Ibid., p. 76.

38. Ibid., p. 80.

39. Herzig, p. 739.

40. M. J. Rush, "Hypertrichosis: The Marton Method, a Triumph of Chemstry," *Medical Practice*, March 1924. Reprint in folder 0317–01, American Medical Association historical files.

41. Albert C. Geyser, "Truth and Fallacy Concerning the Roentgen Ray in Hypertrichosis." Reprint from *Scientific Therapy and Practical Research*, New York, 1926. Tricho System brochure, AMA, HHF, Hair Removal, Folder 0317–17.

42. AMA, HHF, Hair Removal, Folder 0317–01.

43. Herzig, p. 729.

44. AMA, HHF Tricho Hair Removal, Folder 0318–02.

45. AMA, HHF, Hair Removal, Folder 0317–02.

46. Letter, AMA, HHF, Tricho Hair Removal, Folder 0318–01.

47. Geyser, in Tricho brochure.

48. AMA, HHF, Hair Removal Jarton, Julet, Marcell, Correspondence 0317–01.

49. Hinkel and Lind, p. 201.

50. Quoted in Christine Hope, "Caucasian Female Body Hair and American Culture," *Journal of American Culture*, 5 (1982): 93–99.

51. Ibid.

52. Russell Adams, *King Gillette: The Man and His Wonderful Shaving Device*, p. 92.

53. Ibid.

54. Ibid.

55. Ibid., p. 49.

56. Hope, pp. 93–99.

57. Quoted in ibid., p. 96.

58. Ibid., pp. 93–99.

59. Ibid.

Chapter 5: Skin

1. Gilbert Vail, *A History of Cosmetics in America*, p. 88.

2. Mary Lisa Gavenas, *Color Stories*, p. 133.

3. Ibid., p. 134.

4. Ibid., p. 135.

5. "Pond's Extract," 1905 advertisement in Duke University digital Scriptorium Collection.

6. "Pond's Extract," 1907 advertisement in Duke University digital Scriptorium Collection.

7. Pond's advertisements in Duke University digital Scriptorium Collection.

8. Fenja Gunn, *The Artificial Face*, p. 11.

9. Vail, pp. 119–120.

10. Margaret Allen, *Selling Dreams: Inside the Beauty Business*, pp. 55–56.

11. Ibid., p. 23.

12. Alfred Allan Lewis and Constance Woodworth, *Miss Elizabeth Arden*, p. 76.

13. Patrick O'Higgins, *Madame: An Intimate Biography of Helena Rubinstein*, pp. 12–13.

14. Rachel P. Maines, *The Technology of Orgasm: "Hysteria," the Vibrator, and Women's Sexual Satisfaction*, p. 67.

15. Ibid.

16. Ibid., p. 3.

17. A. Dale Covey, M.D., *Profitable Office Specialties*, p. 232.

18. Ibid.

19. *The Marvel Violet Ray Book of Instructions* (New York: Eastern Laboratories, Inc., n.d.), p. 5.

20. Marinello Company, *The Science of Beautistry: Official Textbook*, p. 28.

21. *The Science of Beautistry: Official Textbook Approved for Use in All the National Schools of Cosmeticians Affiliated with Marinello* (New York: National School of Cosmeticians, 1932), pp. 205–206.

22. *The Cosmetiste: A Textbook on Cosmetology with Special Reference to the Employment of Electricity in the*

Care of the Hair, Scalp, Face, and Hands, also Permanent Waving and Hair Curling, p. 170.

23. *Vogue's Book of Beauty*, p. 14.

24. Ibid.

25. Joan Kron, *Lift: Wanting, Fearing, and Having a Face-Lift*, p. 145.

26. Quoted in ibid., p. 145.

27. Covey, p. 216.

28. Kron, pp. 147–148.

29. Ibid., p. 148.

30. Ibid., p. 147.

31. Ibid., p. 106.

32. Ibid., p 41.

33. Ibid., p. 42.

34. Quoted in Elizabeth Haiken, *Venus Envy: A History of Cosmetic Surgery*, p. 77.

35. Quoted in ibid., p. 77.

36. Covey, p. 237.

37. Haiken, p. 147.

38. Kron, p. 45.

39. U.S. Patent 2,896,613, granted 28 July 1959 to A. M. Brown.

40. U.S. Patent 550,492, granted 26 November 1895 to E. Ent.

41. U.S. Patent 1,062,399, granted 20 May 1913 to A. M. Hess and A. L. Tibbals.

42. Quoted in Haiken, p. 139.

43. Kron, p. 47.

44. Haiken, p. 47.

45. Quoted in Kron, p. 47.

Chapter 6: Waist

1. Marilyn Yalom. *A History of the Breast*, p. 162.

2. Beatrice Fontanel, *Support and Seduction: A History of Corsets and Bras*, p. 30.

3. Quoted in Cunnington, *The History of Underclothes*, p. 132.

4. Quoted in Norah Waugh, *Corsets and Crinolines*, p. 104.

5. Madame Caplin had become quite the national institution by the time she died. She is perhaps the only corsetiere to have been eulogized in a national poem. James Torrington Spence Lidstone, in his epic *Londoniad*, sang her glories thusly, stuffing doggerel into a stanza as one would an overly plump woman into a corset:

    How shall the poet, in a single lay,
    the glory of her age and tie portray?
    Suffice it for the wondering world to mark
    She tooke from beside the medal in Hyde Park;
    The only prize that for corsets given
    to any manufacturer under heaven.
    [Quoted in Sarah Levitt, *Victorians Unbuttoned*, p. 29.]

6. Quoted in "New Science" by Paul F. Boller, in *The Gilded Age*, edited by H. Wayne Morgan, p. 257.

7. Judy Crichton, *America 1900*, p. 114.

8. Fenja Gunn, *The Artificial Face*.

9. Amy Friedlander. *Natural Monopoly and Universal Service: Telephones and Telegraphs in the U.S. Communications Infrastructure, 1837–1940*, p. 43.

10. Wiebe Bjiker, lecture at National Museum of American History, 2000.

11. Letter from Mrs. Alexander Graham Bell to Dr. Alexander Graham Bell, May 24, 1895. Alexander Graham Bell Papers, Library of Congress.

12. Teresa Dean, *How to Be Beautiful*, p. 155.

13. Maxine James Johns, "Women's functional swimwear, 1860–1920," pp. 139–140.

14. *Chicago Tribune*, 8 July 1877, p. 11.

15. Johns, pp. 139–140.

16. Nancy Milford, *Zelda: A Biography*, p. 17.

17. Waugh, p. 91.

18. Valerie Steele, *The Corset: A Cultural History*, p. 67.

19. Quoted in Valerie Steele, *Fashion and Eroticism: Ideals of Feminine Beauty from the Victorian Era to the Jazz Age*, p. 167.

20. Thorstein Veblen, "The Economic Theory of Woman's Dress," *Popular Science Monthly*.

21. Steele, *The Corset*, p. 67.

22. Colleen Ruby Gau, "Historic medical perspectives of corseting and two physiologic studies with reenactors," pp. 108–109.

23. Dean, p. 145.

24. Quoted in Jill Susan Fields, "The Production of Glamour: A Social History of Intimate Apparel, 1909–1952," p. 74.

25. Quoted in Gau, "Historic medical perspectives," p. 111 [Jennette C. Lauer, *Fashion Power*].

26. See ibid.

27. Quoted in ibid., p. 111 [John W. Field and Bernard

Smith, *Fig Leaves and Fortunes: A Fashion Company Named Warnaco* (West Kennebunk, Mass.: Phoenix, 1990), p. 18].

28. "Colleen Gau, in her 1998 doctoral thesis at Iowa State University, p. 79, states that "[T]he studies I performed indicated [Gaches-Sarraute's] corset did not allow enhanced physical performance; rather, it restricted the subjects more severely. In every category of testing, the straight-front [which created the S-shaped silhouette] corset actually created more troubles for the wearers than did the hourglass corset style when laced to the same degree. The pelvis was pushed down in front, creating a severe lumbar curvature (sway-back) and this posture changed the center of gravity which caused stress to be placed differently on joints and muscles."

29. C. Willett Cunnington and Phillis Cunnington, *The History of Underclothes*, p. 201.

30. Karen Brown-Larimore, "The changing line of the corset from 1820 to 1915," p. 16.

31. U.S. Patent 67,250.

32. Advertisements from ephemera file at the Bakken Library.

33. From *Harper's Weekly*, ca. 1880s, Bakken ephemera file.

34. From *The Graphic* (London) April 17, 1886.

35. Bakken ephemera file.

36. Paul Poiret, *My First 50 Years*, pp. 72–73.

37. Quoted in Fields, p. 69 [CUR in the November 1921 issue, p. 30].

38. Ibid.

39. Quoted in ibid., p. 99 ["Adjustment and Care of the Corset: A Corset Rightly Laced and Rightly Worn Insures Poise and Grace to the Figure," *Good Housekeeping*, October 1921, p. 45]. The industry even successfully lobbied Congress to declare one week in September National Corset Month.

40. *Vogue*, August 1917, pp. 67, 80.

Chapter 7: Hands

1. Leo Tolstoy, *Anna Karenina*.

2. Andrew Tobias, *Fire and Ice*, p. 59.

3. Quoted in Jeffrey L. Meikle, *Twentieth Century Limited*, p. 12.

4. *Ladies' Home Journal*, February 1929.

5. Gilbert Vail, *A History of Cosmetics in America*, pp. 136–141.

6. I owe this observation to Kate Forde's article "Celluloid Dreams: The Marketing of Cutex in America, 1916–1935," *Journal of Design History*.

7. Quoted in Richard Corson, *Fashions in Makeup*, pp. 482–483.

8. Neville Williams, *Powder and Paint: A History of the Englishwoman's Toilet*, p. 145.

9. Ibid.

10. Tobias, p. 68.

11. Revlon press release, 1950.

12. Tobias, p. 52.

13. U.S. patent 1,878,103. The inventor is Theodore F. Bradley of Westfield, New Jersey.

14. U.S. Patent 1,878,477. Also see a subsequent patent, 1,878,103, granted in 1932 to Theodore F. Bradley and assigned to Ellis-Foster.

15. U.S. Patent 2,173,755.

16. Tobias, p. 53.

17. Quoted in ibid., p. 69.

18. Ibid., p. 67.

19. Ibid., p. 69.

20. Ibid., p. 117.

21. U.S. patent 2,195,971, granted to Richard C. Peter and U.S. Patent 2,261,622, granted to Robert Tucks.

22. Tobias, p. 70.

23. E-mail correspondence from Gwen E. Kay, 4 June 2003.

24. Clare Booth Luce, *The Women*, p. 79.

25. Ibid., p. 85.

26. Annelore Harrell, Lowcountry Now, posted Tuesday, 18 March 2003.http://www.lowcountrynow.com/stories/031803/LOCannelore.

27. M. C. Phillips, *Skin Deep: The Truth About Beauty Aids*, pp. 37–38.

28. Vail, pp. 136–141.

29. Notebooks quoted in Alison J. Clarke, *Tupperware: The Promise of Plastic in 1950s America*, pp. 31–32.

30. See "History of Nail Care" in *Nails Magazine*, February 1993, pp. 30–46.

Chapter 8: Hips

1. Quoted in Theo Aronson, *Queen Victoria and the Bonapartes*, p. 32.

2. Ibid., p. 36.

3. Quoted in Ashelford, *The Art of Dress*, p. 99.

4. Jean Philippe Worth, *A Century of Fashion*, pp. 50–51.

5. Doreen Yarwood, *The Encyclopaedia of World Costume: Ordinary Americans & Fashions, 1840–1900*, p. 125.

6. Quoted in Joan Severa, *Dressed for the Photographer*, p. 201.

7. Quoted in Nora Waugh, *Corsets and Crinolines*, p. 31.

8. "Matilda Baker," H. De Marsan, Publisher., No. 60 Chatham Street, New York. [n.d.] digital American Memory Collection of the Library of Congress.

9. Quoted in Edwin G. Burrows and Mike Wallace, *Gotham: A History of New York City to 1898*, p. 865.

10. Quoted in ibid., p. 805.

11. Ibid., pp. 807–812.

12. Quoted in Hillel Schwartz, *Never Satisfied*, pp. 57–58.

13. Philippe Perrot, *Fashioning the Bourgeoisie*, p. 72.

14. Quoted in Severa, p. 98.

15. Burrows and Wallace, p. 814.

16. Ibid., p. 820.

17. Cynthia Eagle Russett, *Sexual Science: The Victorian Construction of Womanhood*, pp. 24–25.

18. Quoted in ibid., p. 29.

19. Henry Bessemer, *Sir Henry Bessemer, F.R.S., An Autobiography*, p. 137.

20. It wasn't actually bone but rather the upper palate of a whale's mouth. After removal of the hairy fringe that hangs from the top of the mouth, which allows the whale to sift ocean water for tasty prey, the palate was boiled for half a day until soft enough to cut into the narrow, flexible, fibrous strips known as whalebone.

21. This song appeared in the October 1857 issue of *Graham's Illustrated Magazine* and in the August 1857 *Harper's New Monthly Magazine*.

22. Geoffrey Tweedale, *Sheffield Steel and America: A Century of Commercial and Technological Interdependence 1830–1930*, p. 8.

23. Tweedale, p. 8.

24. Burrows and Wallace, p. 843.

25. William C. Allen, *History of the United States Capitol: A Chronicle of Design, Construction, and Politics* (Washington, D.C.: U.S. Government Printing Office, 2001), p. 258.

26. Ibid., p. 259.

27. Burrows and Wallace, p. 706.

28. See patent interference case *Mann v. Rugg* 1862 at the National Archives 241/650/74, Compartment 24, Shelf 4. Also see patent interference case *Mann V. Rugg* 1865 241/650/74, Compartment 27, Shelf 1, Box 367. For this chapter, I also drew on transcripts, documents, and even actual hoop skirts contained in the following patent interference case files at the National Archives: *Samuel S. Sherwood v. Sylvester J. Sherman* (1860); *David Hawkins v. Thomas S. Gilbert* (1864); *Leopold Sanders v. Thomas S. Gilbert* (1864); *Phillippe Lippman v. Joseph W. Bradley* (1865); *Alfred R. Stanley v. Chas D. Wrightington* (1868); *Geo. Ramsay v. Edward F. Woodward v. Edwin Larcher* (1857); *Samuel Guernsey v. A. Smart* (1859); *Stillman Houghton v. T. S. Sperry v. Theodore Day* (1866); and *D. B. Hale v. Henry F. Brown* (1859).

29. See transcript, *Mann v. Rugg* 1862 and 1865.

30. See patent interference case *James Draper v. Ebenezer Clark* (1859–1860), National Archives, 241/650/74, Compartment 22, Shelf 6. Boxes 161 and 161A.

31. See *Draper v. Clark* deposition transcripts.

32. Ibid.

33. *Draper v. Clark*, 1860.

34. Ibid.

35. Ibid.

36. *Mann v. Rugg*, 1865.

37. Ibid.

38. This song appeared in the October 1857 issue of *Graham's Illustrated Magazine* and in the August 1857 *Harper's New Monthly Magazine*.

39. Worth, p. 50.

40. Valerie Steele, *Fashion and Eroticism: Ideals of Feminine Beauty from the Victorian Era to the Jazz Age*, p. 59.

41. Quoted in Elisabeth McClellan *Historic Dress in America*, pp. 265–66.

42. Perrot, p. 108.
43. 1876, *The Manufacturer and Builder*, digital Making of America collection, Cornell University Library.

Chapter 9: Derriere

1. Ruth E. Finley, *Sarah Josepha Hale.*
2. Alison Gernsheim, *Victorian & Edwardian Fashion: A Photographic Survey*, p. 70.
3. Ibid., pp. 63–64.
4. *Punchinello* 2, no. 187 (December 17, 1870), quoted in Frank Luther Mott, *A History of American Magazines*, vol. 3.
5. Doreen Yarwood, *The Encyclopaedia of World Costume*, p. 167.
6. From *The Queen*, 1877, quoted in C. Willett Cunnington, and Phillis Cunnington, *The History of Underclothes*, p. 170.
7. Quoted in Gernsheim, p. 61.
8. U.S. Patent 25,211.
9. U.S. Patent 130,345.
10. Harold Koda, *Extreme Beauty: The Body Transformed*, p. 133.
11. U.S. Patent 275,710.
12. "O Susan Wears a Bustle," music by Harry Gibbs, words by George R. Jackson. Sheet music in the digital American Memory Collection, Library of Congress.
13. Quoted in Julie Wosk, *Women and the Machine*, p. 65.
14. U.S. Patent 225,754.
15. James Laver, *Costume and Fashion: A Concise History*, p. 198.
16. Gernsheim, p. 798.
17. Charles Darwin, *The Descent of Man*, p. 295.
18. Ruby Mosley, Sangelo, Texas, oral history digital American Memory Collection, the Library of Congress.
19. 1902 Edition of the Sears, Roebuck Catalog, 1969 reprint.

bibliography

Adams, Russell. *King Gillette: The Man and His Wonder-ful Shaving Device.* Boston and Toronto: Little, Brown and Company, 1978.

Allen, Frederick Lewis. *Only Yesterday: An Informal His-tory of the 1920's.* 1931. Reprint, New York: Harper & Row, 1964.

———. *Since Yesterday: The 1930s in America.* 1939. Reprint, New York: Harper & Row, 1986.

Allen, Margaret. *Selling Dreams: Inside the Beauty Busi-ness.* New York: Simon & Schuster, 1981.

Allen, William C. *History of the United States Capitol: A Chronicle of Design, Construction, and Politics.* Wash-ington, D.C.: U.S. Government Printing Office, 2001.

Angeloglou, Maggie. *A History of Makeup.* London: The Macmillan Company, 1970.

Angier, Natalie. *Woman: An Intimate Geography.* Boston: Houghton Mifflin, 1999.

Aronson, Theo. *Queen Victoria and the Buonapartes.* Lon-don: Cassell, 1972.

Ashelford, Jane. *The Art of Dress: Clothes and Society, 1500–1914.* New York: Abrams, 1996.

Ayer, Harriet Hubbard. *Harriet Hubbard Ayer's Book: A Complete and Authentic Treatise on the Laws of Health and Beauty.* 1899. Reprint, New York: Arno Press, 1974.

Ayer, Margaret Hubbard, and Isabella Taves. *The Three Lives of Harriet Hubbard Ayer.* Philadelphia: J.B. Lip-pincott Company, 1957.

Baker, Jean H. *Mary Todd Lincoln: A Biography.* New York and London: W.W. Norton & Company, 1987.

Baker, Robert, ed. *A Stress Analysis of a Strapless Evening Gown.* Englewood Cliffs, N.J.: Prentice-Hall, 1963.

Baldwin, Deborah. "Caresse Crosby and the Bra." www.discovery.com, 1998.

Balsam, M. S., ed. *Cosmetics: Science and Techology.* 3 vols. New York: Wiley-Interscience, 1972–74.

Banner, Lois W. *American Beauty.* Chicago: University of Chicago Press, 1983.

Basalla, George. *The Evolution of Technology.* New York: Cambridge University Press, 1988.

Basten, Fred; Robert A. Salvatore; and Paul A. Kaufman. *Max Factor's Hollywood.* Los Angeles: General Pub-lishing Group, 1995.

Baxter, Annette Kar. *To Be a Woman in America, 1850–1930.* New York: Times Books, 1978.

Beauty Is Power. New York: G.W., Carleton & Co.; Lon-don: Tinsley Brothers, 1871.

Beauty Secrets. Good Houskeeping Consumer Panel Re-port. New York, 1959.

Bedi, Joyce E. "Exploring the History of Women Inven-tors." From Lemelson Innovative Lives Series. Wash-ington, D.C.: Smithsonian Institution, 2002. www.si.edu/lemelson/centerpieces/ilives/womenin-ventors.html.

Bell, Mrs. Alexander Graham. Letter to Dr. Alexander Graham Bell, 24 May 1895. Library of Congress, digi-tal American Memory Collection.

Berney, Adrienne. "Streamlining Breasts: The Exaltation of Form and Disguise of Function in 1930s' Ideals." *Journal of Design History* 14, no. 4 (2001):327–342.

Bessemer, Henry. *Sir Henry Bessemer, F.R.S., An Autobi-ography.* London: Offices of "Engineering," 1905.

Bigelow, Horatio R. *An International System of Electro-Therapeutics.* With illustrations furnished by Geo. H. Fox, M.D. F.A. Davis Company, Publishers. London: F.J. Rebman, 1895.

Bishop, Hazel. "A Method for the SemiQuantitative Analysis of Lipstick." Reprint from the *Journal of the Society of Cosmetic Chemists* 5, no. 1 (March 1954).

———. Unpublished autobiography. Harvard's Schlesinger Library on the History of Women in Amer-ica.

Bishop, Philip W. "The Beginnings of Cheap Steel." From

Contributions from the Museum of History and Technology. Paper 3, United States National Museum Bulletin 218, 27–47. Washington, D.C.: Smithsonian Institution, 1959.

Blum, Stella, ed. *Victorian Fashions & Costumes from Harper's Bazaar 1867–1898.* Mineola, N.Y.: Dover Books, 1974.

Boehlke, Heidi L. "Ruth M. Kapinas, Munsingwear's Forgotten 'Foundettes' Designer." *Dress* 20 (1993): 45–52.

Bogardus, Ralph F. "The Reorientation of Paradise: Modern Mass Media and Narratives of Desire in the Making of American Consumer Culture." *American Literary History* 10, no. 3 (Fall 1998).

Boorstin, Daniel. *The Americans: The Democratic Experience.* New York: Random House, 1973.

Bowman's Corset and Brassiere Trade: A Compilations of the Manufacturers of Corsets, Brassieres, Corset Waists, Girdles, etc. in the United States. New York: Bowman Publishing Co., 1920.

Brecher, Ruth, and Edward Brecher. *The Rays: A History of Radiology in the United States and Canada.* Baltimore: Williams and Wilkins, 1969.

Breward, Christopher. *The Culture of Fashion.* Manchester, Eng.: Manchester University Press, 1995.

Brown-Larimore, Karen. "The changing line of the corset from 1820 to 1915." Unpublished master's thesis. University of Wisconsin-Madison, 1984.

Bryson, Charles Lee. *Health and How to Get It.* Racine, Wis.: Hamilton Beach Manufacturing Company, circa 1900.

Bundles, A'Lelia. *On Her Own Ground: The Life and Times of Madam C. J. Walker.* New York: Washington Square Press, 2002.

Burrows, Edwin G., and Mike Wallace. *Gotham: A History of New York City to 1898.* Oxford, Eng.: Oxford University Press, 1999.

Buss, David M. *The Evolution of Desire.* New York: Basic Books, 1994.

Buyers' Guide 1905–1906: Thomas' Register of American Manufacturers. New York: Thomas Publishing Co., 1905.

Capretz, Marilyn M. "Women's dresses (1850–1879) from selected south Louisiana costume collections." Unpublished master's thesis. University of Southwestern Louisiana, 1994.

Carter, Alison. *Underwear: The Fashion History.* London: B. T. Batsford, 1992.

Clarke, Alison J. *Tupperware: The Promise of Plastic in 1950s America.* Washington, D.C.: Smithsonian Institution Press, 1999.

Cohn, David Lewis. *The Good Old Days.* New York: Simon and Schuster, 1940.

Colburn, Carol Ann. "The dress of the James J. Hill family 1863–1916." Unpublished Ph.D. dissertation. University of Minnesota, 1989.

Consumer Reports. "Lipsticks." August 1951, pp. 349–352.

"Corset and the Lungs." *Shafts* 7, no. 7 (September 1893).

Corson, Richard. *Fashions in Makeup.* London: Peter Owen, 1957.

———. *Stage Makeup.* 1942. Reprint, New York: Appleton-Century-Crofts, 1960.

Cosbey, Sarah Louise. "Diversity in fashion and women's roles from 1873 to 1912." Unpublished Ph.D. dissertation. Iowa State University, 1997.

Cosmetiste: A Textbook on Cosmetology with Special Reference to the Employment of Electricity in the Care of the Hair, Scalp, Face, and Hands, also Permanent Waving and Hair Curling. Chicago: The Wm. Meyer Co., 1936.

Covey, A. Dale, M.D. *Profitable Office Specialties.* Detroit, Mich.: Physicians Supply Company, 1912.

Crawford, Morris De Camp, and Elizabeth A. Guernsey. *The History of Corsets in Pictures.* New York: Fairchild Publications, 1951.

Crichton, Judy. *America 1900.* New York: Henry Holt, 1998.

Crosby, Caresse. *The Passionate Years.* New York: Dial Press, 1953.

Crown Skirts. Promotional pamphlet for hoop skirts. National Archives. New York: W.S. & C.H. Thomson & Co., 1859.

Cunningham, Patricia A., and Susan Voso Lab. *Dress in American Culture.* Bowling Green, Ohio: Bowling Green State University Popular Press, 1993.

Cunnington, C. Willett, and Phillis Cunnington. *The History of Underclothes.* 1951. Reprint, New York: Dover Publications, 1992.

Cutcliffe, Stephen, and Robert Post. *In Context: History and the History of Technology.* Bethlehem, Pa.: Lehigh University Press, 1989.

Dalrymple, Priscilla Harris. *American Victorian Costume in Early Photographs*. Mineola, N.Y.: Dover Publications, 1991.

Darwin, Charles. *The Descent of Man and Selection in Relation to Sex*. 1871. Reprint, New York: The Heritage Press, 1972.

Davis, Kathy. *Reshaping the Female Body: The Dilemma of Cosmetic Surgery*. New York and London: Routledge, 1995.

Dawkins, Richard. *The Selfish Gene*. Oxford, Eng.: Oxford University Press, 1976.

Dayagi-Mendeles, Mikhal. *Perfumes and Cosmetics in the Ancient World*. Jerusalem: Israel Museum, 1989.

Dean, Teresa H. *How to Be Beautiful*. Chicago: Donohue & Henneberry, 1889.

De Castelbajac, Kate. *The Face of the Century: 100 Years of Makeup and Style*. New York: Rizzoli, 1995.

deForest Lamb, Ruth. *American Chamber of Horrors*. New York: Farrar & Rinehart, 1936.

de Gencé, Comtesse. *Le Cabinet de Toilette d'une Honnête Femme*. Paris: Bibliothèque des Ouvrages Pratiques, 1909.

de la Pena, Carolyn Thomas. *The Body Electric: How Strange Machines Built the Modern American*. New York: New York University Press, 2003.

de Marly, Diana. *Worth: Father of Haute Couture*. New York: Holmes & Meier, 1990.

DeNavarre, Maison G. *The Chemistry and Manufacture of Cosmetics*. Vols. 3 and 4. Orlando, Fla.: Continental Press, 1975.

Dinesen, Isak. *Seven Gothic Tales*. New York: Penguin paperback edition.

Dixon, Marion. "Feminine Form." *Hygeia*. August 1942, pp. 581–624.

Drachman, Virginia G. *Enterprising Women: 250 Years of American Business*. Chapel Hill: University of North Carolina Press, 2002.

Dugatkin, Lee Alan. *The Imitation Factor: Evolution Beyond the Gene*. New York: The Free Press, 2000.

Dunlap, Knight. *Personal Beauty and Racial Betterment*. St. Louis, Mo.: C.V. Mosby Company, 1920.

Etcoff, Nancy. *Survival of the Prettiest: The Science of Beauty*. New York: Anchor Books, 2000.

Ewing, Elizabeth. *Fashion in Underwear*. London: B. T. Batsford, 1971.

———. *History of Twentieth Century Fashion*. Revised and Updated by Alice Mackrell. Lanham, Md.: Barnes & Noble Books, 1992.

Farrell-Beck, Jane, and Colleen Gau. *Uplift: The Bra in America*. Philadelphia: University of Pennsylvania Press, 2002.

Fernandez, Nancy Page. " 'If a woman had taste . . .' Home Sewing and the Making of Fashion, 1850–1910." University of California-Irvine, 1987.

Fields, Jill Susan. "The production of glamour: a social history of intimate apparel, 1909–1952." Unpublished Ph.D. dissertation. University of Southern California, 1997.

Finley, Ruth E. *Sarah Josepha Hale*. Philadelphia: J.B. Lippincott, 1931.

First Annual Report of the Convex Weaving Company. New York: Convex Weaving Company, 1866.

Fitzgerald, F. Scott. *The Great Gatsby*. 1925. Reprint, New York: Charles Scribner's Sons, 1953.

Flügel, John Carl. *The Psychology of Clothes*. 1930. Reprint, New York: International Universities Press, 1971.

Fontanel, Béatrice. *Support and Seduction: A History of Corsets and Bras*. Willard Wood, trans. New York: Harry N. Abrams, 1997.

Foote, Shelley. "Bloomers." *Dress* 5 (1980):1–12.

Forde, Kate. "Celluloid Dreams: The Marketing of Cutex in America, 1916–1935." *Journal of Design History* 15, no. 3 (2002): 175–189.

Forty, Adrian. *Objects of Desire*. New York: Pantheon Books, 1986.

Fox, George Henry. *The Use of Electricity in the Removal of Facial Hair and the Treatment of Various Facial Blemishes*. Detroit, Mich.: George S. Davis, 1886.

Friedel, Robert. *Pioneer Plastic: The Making and Selling of Celluloid*. Madison: University of Wisconsin Press, 1983.

Friedlander, Amy. *Natural Monopoly and Universal Service: Telephones and Telegraphs in the U.S. Communications Infrastructure, 1837–1940*. Reston, Va.: Corporation for National Research Initiatives, 1995.

Galvanized Iron Wire as Employed in the Telegraph and Telephone. Worcester, Mass.: Washburn and Moen Manufacturing Co., 1881.

Gardner, Kirsten. Unpublished paper on artificial breasts for breast-cancer patients. Presented 26 May 1999 at the Hagley Museum Spring Conference on Beauty and Business (Wilmington, Delaware).

Gau, Colleen Ruby. "Historic medical perspectives of corseting and two physiologic studies with reenactors." Unpublished Ph.D dissertation. Iowa State University, 1998.

Gavenas, Mary Lisa. *Color Stories*. New York: Simon & Schuster, 2002.

"General Guide to Max Factor Information in the P&G Archives." Cincinnati: Procter & Gamble, no date.

Gernsheim, Alison. *Victorian & Edwardian Fashion: A Photographic Survey*. 1963. Reprint, Mineola, N.Y.: Dover Publications, 1981.

Giedion, Siegfried. *Mechanization Takes Command: a Contribution to Anonymous History*. New York: Oxford University Press, 1948.

Gilman, Sander L. *Making the Body Beautiful: A Cultural History of Aesthetic Surgery*. Princeton, N.J.: Princeton University Press, 1999.

Gladwell, Malcolm. *The Tipping Point: How Little Things Can Make a Big Difference*. Boston: Little, Brown and Company, 2000.

Goodman, Walter. *The Clowns of Commerce*. New York: Sagamore Press, 1954.

Goodyear, Charles. *Gum-Elastic and Its Varieties, with a Detailed Account of Its Applications and Uses, and of the Discovery of Vulcanization*. Vols. 1 and 2. 1853. Reprint, London: Maclaren and Sons, Ltd., 1937.

Gordon, Beverly. "Meanings in Mid-Nineteenth Century Dress: Images from New England Women's Writings." *Clothing and Textiles Research Journal*. 10, no. 3 (Spring 1992): 44–53.

Gordon, Jane. *Technique for Beauty*. London: Faber and Faber, 1940.

Gordon, Robert B. *American Iron: 1607–1900*. Baltimore: The Johns Hopkins University Press, 1996.

Gould, James L., and Carol Grant Gould. *Sexual Selection: Mate Choice and Courtship in Nature*. 1989. New York: Reprint, Scientific American Library, 1997.

Griggs, Claudine. *S/he: Changing Sex and Changing Clothes*. Oxford: Berg, 1998.

Griscom, George. *The Telegraph Cable: Historical View of the Art of Electro-Magnetic Telegraphing . . . An Argument Addressed to the U.S. Senate Committee on Patents*. Philadelphia: King & Baird, Printers, 1867.

Gunn, Fenja. *The Artificial Face*. Newton Abbot, David & Charles, 1973.

Haiken, Elizabeth. *Venus Envy: A History of Cosmetic Surgery*. Baltimore: The Johns Hopkins University Press, 1997.

Harry, Ralph Gordon. *Harry's Cosmeticology*. 6th edition. Revised by J. B. Wilkinson and others. London: L. Hill, 1973.

"Health-Beauty, Or Common Sense Instead of Drugs." New York: Health-Beauty Publishing, circa 1900. Bakken Library ephemera collection.

Helvensten, Sally. "Popular Advice for the Well-Dressed Woman in the 19th Century." *Dress* 5 (1980): 31–47.

Herzig, Rebecca. "Removing Roots: 'North American Hiroshima Maidens' and the X Ray." *Technology and Culture* 40, no. 4 (October 1999): 723–745.

Hinkel, Arthur Ralph, and Richard W. Lind. *Electrolysis, Thermolysis and the Blend: The Principles and Practice of Permanent Hair Removal*. 1968. Reprint, Los Angeles, Calif.: Arroway Publishers, 1979.

Hollander, Anne. *Seeing Through Clothes*. New York: Viking Press, 1978.

————. *Sex and Suits: The Evolution of Modern Dress*. New York: Alfred A. Knopf, 1994.

Hope, Christine. "Caucasian Female Body Hair and American Culture." *Journal of American Culture* 5 (1982): 93–99.

Horn, Marilyn J. *The Second Skin: An Interdisciplinary Study of Clothing*. 1968. Reprint, Boston: Houghton Mifflin, 1975.

Horowitz, Roger, and Arwen Mohun, eds. *His and Hers: Gender, Consumption, and Technology*. Charlottesville: University of Virginia Press, 1998.

Hounshell, David, and John Kenly Smith Jr. *Science & Corporate Strategy: Du Pont R&D, 1902–1980*. Cambridge, Eng.: Cambridge University Press, 1988.

"How to Massage at Home." Vibrator manual. Bakken Library ephemera collection. Dayton, Ohio: National Vacuum Machinery Co., circa 1900.

Howes, Francis Williams. *The Chemistry of Cosmetic Practice*. Chicago, 1936.

Hrdy, Sarah Blaffer. *The Woman That Never Evolved*. Cambridge, Mass.: Harvard University Press, 1981.

"Hurrah for the Bra: It's 100 Years Old This Month." *Life*, June 1989.

Johns, Maxine James. "Women's functional swimwear, 1860–1920." Unpublished Ph.D. dissertation. Iowa State University, 1997.

Johnson, Henrietta P. "Facial Blemishes." In *An Interna-*

tional System of Electro-Therapeutics. Edited by Horatio R. Bigelow. London: F.J. Rebman, 1895.

Johnston, Patricia. *Real Fantasies: Edward Steichen's Advertising Photography*. Berkeley: University of California Press, 1997.

Jonas, Gerald. *Dancing: The Pleasure, Power, and Art of Movement*. New York: Harry N. Abrams, 1992.

Kay, Gwen Elizabeth. "Regulating beauty: Cosmetics in American culture from the 1906 Pure Food and Drugs Act to the 1938 Food, Drug and Cosmetic Act." Unpublished Ph.D. dissertation. Yale University, 1997.

Kevles, Bettyann Holtzmann. *Females of the Species*. Cambridge, Mass.: Harvard University Press, 1986.

———. *Naked to the Bone: Medical Imaging in the Twentieth Century*. New Brunswick, N.J.: Rutgers University Press, 1997.

Kidwell, Claudia B., and Margaret C. Christman. *Suiting Everyone: The Democratization of Clothing in America*. Washington, D.C.: Smithsonian Institution Press, 1974.

Koda, Harold. *Extreme Beauty: The Body Transformed*. New Haven, Conn.: Yale University Press, 2001.

Koontz, Marcy L. "The Costume collection at the Goodwood Plantation, Tallahassee, Florida: One hundred and fifty years of the most intimate possessions of Margaret Wilson Hodges Hood and her family, 1823–1975." Unpublished dissertation. Florida State University, 1995.

Kron, Joan. *Lift: Wanting, Fearing, and Having a Face-Lift*. New York: Viking, 1998.

Kunzle, David. *Fashion and Fetishism: A Social History of the Corset, Tight-Lacing and Other Forms of Body-Sculpture in the West*. Totowa, N.J.: Rowman and Littlefield, 1982.

Kushner, Rose. *Breast Cancer: A Personal History and an Investigative Report*. New York and London: Harcourt Brace Jovanovich, 1975.

Larson, Joyce Marie. "Clothing of pioneer women of Dakota Territory, 1861–1889." Unpublished master's thesis. South Dakota State University, 1978.

Lauer, Jennette C. *Fashion Power*. Englewood Cliffs, N.J.: Prentice-Hall, 1981.

Laver, James. *Clothes*. London: Burke, 1952.

———. *Costume and Fashion: A Concise History*. London: Thames and Hudson, 1985.

Lears, T. J. Jackson. *Fables of Abundance: A Cultural History of Advertising in America*. New York: Basic Books, 1994.

Lee, Michelle. *Fashion Victim: Our Love-Hate Relationship with Dressing, Shopping, and the Cost of Style*. New York: Broadway Books, 2003.

Lehrman, Karen. *The Lipstick Proviso*. New York: Doubleday, 1997.

Leuchtenberg, William E. *The Perils of Prosperity*. Chicago: University of Chicago Press, 1958. Paperback.

Levins, Hoag. *American Sex Machines*. Holbrook, Mass.: Adams Media Corporation, 1996.

Levitt, Sarah. *Victorians Unbuttoned*. London: George Allen & Unwin, 1986.

Lewis, Alfred Allan, and Constance Woodworth. *Miss Elizabeth Arden*. New York: Coward, McCann & Geoghegan, 1972.

Luce, Clare Boothe. *The Women*. 1937. Reprint. New York: Random House, 1964.

Lucey, Donna M. *Photographing Montana 1894–1928: The Life and Work of Evelyn Cameron*. New York: Alfred A. Knopf, 1991.

Lurie, Alison. *The Language of Clothes*. New York: Random House, 1981.

Lynd, Robert S., and Helen Merrell Lynd. *Middletown: A Study in Modern American Culture*. 1929. Reprint, New York: Harvest, 1956.

Maddox, Barbara. *Nora: The Real Life of Molly Bloom*. Boston: Houghton-Mifflin, 2000.

Maidenform Mirror. Maidenform Collection. National Museum of American History, Washington, D.C., 1944–1965.

Maines, Rachel P. *The Technology of Orgasm: "Hysteria," the Vibrator, and Women's Sexual Satisfaction*. Baltimore: The Johns Hopkins University Press, 1999.

Manchester, William. *The Glory and the Dream: A Narrative History of America 1932–1972*. New York: Bantam Books, 1975.

Marinello Company. *The Science of Beautistry: Official Textbook Approved for Use in All the National Schools of Cosmeticians Affiliated with Marinello*. New York: National School of Cosmeticians, 1932.

Mayham, Stephen L. *Marketing Cosmetics*. New York and London: McGraw-Hill Book Company, 1938.

McClellan, Elisabeth. *Historic Dress in America 1607–1870*. 1904. Reprint, New York: Arno Press, 1977.

McCoy, Bob. *Quack: Museum of Questionable Medical*

Devices. Santa Monica, Calif.: Santa Monica Press, 2000.

McDonough, Everett Goodrich. *Truth About Cosmetics.* New York: Drug and Cosmetic Industry, 1937.

McHugh, Jeanne. *Alexander Holley and the Makers of Steel.* Baltimore: The Johns Hopkins University Press, 1980.

McLeod, Edyth Thornton. *How to Sell Cosmetics.* New York: The Drug and Cosmetic Industry, 1937.

Meikle, Jeffrey L. *American Plastic: A Cultural History.* New Brunswick, N.J.: Rutgers University Press, 1997.

————. *Twentieth Century Limited: Industrial Design in America, 1925–1939.* Philadelphia: Temple University Press, 1979.

Mendes, Valerie, and Amy de la Haye. *20th Century Fashion.* London: Thames & Hudson, 1999.

Milford, Nancy. *Zelda: A Biography.* New York: Harper & Row, 1970.

Miller, Geoffrey. *The Mating Mind: How Sexual Choice Shaped the Evolution of Human Nature.* New York: Vintage, 2001.

Miller, Jennifer Heather. "Casting race: a history of makeup technology in the United States film industry, 1890–1940." Unpublished Ph.D. dissertation. University of Rochester, 1999.

Misa, Thomas J. *A Nation of Steel: The Making of Modern America, 1865–1925.* Baltimore: The Johns Hopkins University Press, 1995.

Montez, Lola. *The Arts of Beauty; or, Secrets of a Lady's Toilet, with hints to Gentlemen on the Art of Fascinating.* New York: Dick & Fitzgerald, 1858.

Moore, Doris Langley. *The Woman in Fashion.* London: Batsford, 1949.

Morgan, H. Wayne, ed. *The Gilded Age.* Syracuse, N.Y.: Syracuse University Press, 1970.

Morgan, Marabel. *The Total Woman.* New York: Pocket Books, 1975.

Mosley, Ruby. "Range-Lore." Oral history, American Life Histories: Manuscripts from the Federal Writers' Project, 1936–1940. Library of Congress digital American Memory project. [Interviewer: W.H. Martin.]

Mott, Frank Luther. *A History of American Magazines,* Cambridge, Mass.: Harvard University Press, 1938. Volume 3.

"New Use for Old Hoop Skirts." *The Manufacturer and Builder,* p. 189. Cornell University Library's Making of America digital collection.

Niemoeller, A. F. *The Complete Guide to Bust Culture.* New York: Harvest House, 1939.

————. *Superfluous Hair and Its Removal.* New York: Harvest House, 1938.

Norris, Herbert, and Oswald Curtis. *Nineteenth-Century Costume and Fashion.* 1933. Reprint, N.Y.: Mineola, Dover Publications, 1998.

Nye, David E. *American Technological Sublime.* Cambridge, Mass.: MIT Press, 1994.

O'Donohue, Mrs. Power. *Riding for Ladies.* Boston: Roberts Brothers, 1887.

O'Higgins, Patrick. *Madame: An Intimate Biography of Helena Rubinstein.* New York: Viking Press, 1971.

Olian, Joanne, ed. *Victorian and Edwardian Fashions from "La Mode Illustrée."* Mineola, N.Y.: Dover Publications, 1998.

Paris, Barry. *Garbo: A Biography.* New York: Alfred A. Knopf, 1995.

Peiss, Kathy. *Hope in a Jar: The Making of America's Beauty Culture.* New York: Metropolitan Books, 1998.

Pendergrast, Mark. *Mirror Mirror: A History of the Human Love Affair with Reflection.* New York: Basic Books, 2003.

Perrot, Philippe. *Fashioning the Bourgeoisie.* Princeton, N.J.: Princeton University Press, 1994.

Perutz, Kathrin. *Beyond the Looking Glass: America's Beauty Culture.* New York: William Morrow and Company, 1970.

Petroski, Henry. *The Evolution of Useful Things.* New York: Alfred A. Knopf, 1992.

Pfister, Harold Francis. *Facing the Light: Historic American Portrait Daguerreotypes.* Washington, D.C.: Smithsonian Institution Press, 1978.

Phillips, M. C. *Skin Deep: The Truth About Beauty Aids.* New York: Garden City Publishing Co., 1934.

Pierce, Mrs. Sarah Jane. *Homely Girls: A Lady's Book Containing Nearly a Thousand Recipes and Hints as Aids to the Toilet, Representing the Labor of 25 Years.* Tiffin, Ohio: W.H. Keppel, 1890.

Pinker, Steven. *How the Mind Works.* New York: W.W. Norton, 1997.

Plessis, Alain. *The Rise & Fall of the Second Empire: 1852–1871.* Cambridge, Eng.: Cambridge University Press, 1987. Paperback edition of English translation.

Poiret, Paul. *My First 50 Years.* Translated by Stephen Haden Guest. London: V. Gollancz, 1931.

Pool, Robert. *Eve's Rib: Searching for the Biological Roots of Sex Differences.* New York: Crown Publishers, 1994.

Postrel, Virginia. *The Substance of Style: How the Rise of Aesthetic Value Is Remaking Commerce, Culture, and Consciousness.* New York: Harper Collins, 2003.

Potter, David M. *People of Plenty.* Chicago: University of Chicago Press, 1954.

Power, Susan C. *The Ugly-Girl Papers: or, Hints for the Toilet.* New York: Harper & Brothers, 1874.

Reyburn, Wallace. *Bust-Up: The Uplifting Tale of Otto Titzling and the Development of the Bra.* American edition. New York: Prentice-Hall, Inc., 1972.

Rhodes, Richard. *The Making of the Atomic Bomb.* New York: Simon & Schuster, 1986.

Ridley, Matt. *The Red Queen: Sex and the Evolution of Human Nature.* New York: Macmillan Publishing, 1993.

Riva, Maria. *Marlene Dietrich.* New York: Alfred A. Knopf, 1993.

Rooks, Noliwe M. *Hair Raising: Beauty, Culture, and African American Women.* New Brunswick, N.J.: Rutgers University Press, 1996.

Ross, Ishbel. *Crusades and Crinolines: The Life and Times of Ellen Curtis Demorest and William Jennings Demorest.* New York: Harper & Row, 1963.

———. *Taste in America: An Illustrated History of the Evolution of Architecture, Furnishings, Fashions, and Customs of the American People.* New York: Thomas Y. Crowell Company, 1967.

Rubinstein, Helena. *My Life for Beauty.* 1964. Reprint, New York: Paperback Library, 1972.

———. *The Art of Feminine Beauty.* New York: H. Liverwright, 1930.

Rudnick, Lois Palken. *Mabel Dodge Luhan: New Woman, New Worlds.* Albuquerque: University of New Mexico Press, 1984.

Rudofsky, Bernard. *The Unfashionable Human Body.* London: Hart-Davis, 1972.

Rush, M. J. "Hypertrichosis: The Marton Method, a Triumph of Chemstry." *Medical Practice,* March 1924. Reprint in folder 0317–01, American Medical Association.

Russell, Jane. *An Autobiography: My Path and My Detours.* New York: Jove Books, 1986.

Russett, Cynthia Eagle. *Darwin in America: The Intellectual Response 1865–1912.* San Francisco: W.H. Freeman and Company, 1976.

———. *Sexual Science: The Victorian Construction of Womanhood.* Cambridge, Mass.: Harvard University Press, 1989.

Ruthstein, S. *Manual of Toilet and Cosmetic Formulas.* Chicago: Berry Printer, 1915.

Schirmer, Lothar, ed. *Women Seeing Women: A Pictorial History of Women's Photography from Julia Margaret Cameron to Annie Leibovitz.* New York: W.W. Norton, 2001.

Schwartz, Hillel. *Never Satisfied.* New York: Anchor Books, 1990.

Schwartz, Lynell. *Vintage Compacts & Beauty Accessories.* Atglen, Pa.: Schiffer Publishing Ltd., 1997.

Schwartz Cowan, Ruth. *A History of American Technology.* Oxford, Eng.: Oxford University Press, 1997.

———. *More Work for Mother: The Ironies of Household Technology, from the Open Hearth to the Microwave.* New York: Basic Books, 1983.

Sears Roebuck Catalogue, 1897. Edited by Fred L. Israel. Introduction by S. J. Perelman and Richard Rovere. New York: Chelsea House Publishers, 1968.

Sears Roebuck Catalogue, 1902. Introduction by Cleveland Amory. New York: Bounty Books, 1969.

Sears Roebuck Catalogue, 1927. Edited by Alan Mirken. New York: Bounty Books, 1970.

Severa, Joan. *Dressed for the Photographer: Ordinary Americans & Fashion, 1840–1900.* Kent, Ohio: Kent State University Press, 1995.

Severn, Bill. *The Long and Short of It: Five Thousand Years of Fun and Fury Over Hair.* New York: David McKay Company, 1971.

Shorter, Edward. *A History of Women's Bodies.* New York: Basic Books, 1982.

Shulman, Irving. *Harlow: An Intimate Biography.* New York: Bernard Geis Associates, 1964.

Sims, Naomi. *All About Health and Beauty for the Black Woman.* Garden City, N.Y.: Doubleday & Company, 1982.

Smith, George Hand. *Cast Steel: Process of Manufacture Direct from the Ore.* New York: Benton & Andrews, 1864.

Smith, Merritt Roe, and Leo Marx. *Does Technology Drive History?* Cambridge, Mass.: MIT Press, 1994.

Spitz, Peter H. *Petrochemicals: The Rise of an Industry.* New York: John Wiley & Sons, 1988.

Stabile, Toni. *Cosmetics: Trick or Treat?* New York: Arco Publishing Company, 1967.

Stanley, Autumn. *Mothers and Daughters of Invention: Notes for a Revised History of Technology.* Metuchen, N.J., and London: Scarecrow Press, Inc., 1993.

Steele, Valerie. *The Corset: A Cultural History.* New Haven, Conn.: Yale University Press, 2001.

———. *Fashion and Eroticism: Ideals of Feminine Beauty from the Victorian Era to the Jazz Age.* New York: Oxford University Press, 1985.

Strasser, Susan. *Satisfaction Guaranteed: The Making of the American Mass Market.* New York: Pantheon Books, 1989.

Sullivan, Mark. *Our Times: The United States 1900–1925.* Vol. 1. New York and London: Charles Scribner's Sons, 1926.

Summers, Leigh. *Bound to Please: A History of the Victorian Corset.* Oxford, Eng.: Berg, 2001.

Susman, Warren I. *Culture as History: The Transformation of American Society in the Twentieth Century.* New York: Pantheon Books, 1984.

Swartz, Mimi. "Silicone City: The Rise and Fall of the Implant or How Houston Went From an Oil-Based Economy to a Breast-Based Economy." *Texas Monthly* 23, no. 8 (August 1995):64–79.

Symons, Donald. *The Evolution of Human Sexuality.* New York: Oxford University Press, 1979.

Temin, Peter. *Iron and Steel in Nineteenth Century America.* Cambridge, Mass.: MIT Press, 1964.

Tenner, Edward. *Our Own Devices: The Past and Future of Body Technology.* New York: Alfred A. Knopf, 2003.

Tobias, Andrew. *Fire and Ice.* New York: Warner Books. Paperback edition. [1976]

Toilette of Health, Beauty, and Fashion: Embracing the Economy of the Beard, Breath, Complexion, Ears, Eyes, Eye-Brows, Eye-Lashes, Feet, Forehead, Gums, Hair, Head, Hands, Lips, Mouth, Mustachios, Nails of the Toes, Nails of the Fingers, Nose, Skin, Teeth, Tongue &c. &c. No author listed. Boston: Allen and Ticknor, 1834.

Tolstoy, Leo. *Anna Karenina.* Boston: Harvard Classics, 1917.

Tone, Andrea. *Devices & Desires: A History of Contraceptives in America.* New York: Hill and Wang, 2001.

Turner, Albert. *The Attainment of Womanly Beauty of Form and Features.* New York: Health-Culture Company, 1900.

Tweedale, Geoffrey. *Sheffield Steel and America: A Century of Commercial and Technological Interdependence 1830–1930.* Cambridge, Eng.: Cambridge University Press, 1987.

Umbach, Wilfried. *Cosmetics and Toiletries: Development, Production and Use.* Translated by Brian K. Gore. New York: Simon & Schuster, 1990.

Vail, Gilbert. *A History of Cosmetics in America.* New York: Toilet Goods Association, 1947.

Van Dulken, Stephen. *Inventing the 19th Century: 100 Inventions that Shaped the Victorian Age.* New York: New York University Press, 2001.

Veblen, Thorstein. "The Economic Theory of Woman's Dress," *Popular Science Monthly,* December 1894, p. 203.

Venkataraman, K. *The Analytical Chemistry of Synthetic Dyes.* New York: John Wiley & Sons, 1977.

Vinikas, Vincent. *Soft Soap, Hard Sell: American Hygiene in an Age of Advertisement.* Ames, Iowa: Iowa State University Press, 1992.

Vogue's Book of Beauty. New York: Condé Nast Publications, Inc., 1933.

Walkley, Christina, and Vanda Foster. *Crinolines and Crimping Irons, Victorian Clothes: How They Were Cleaned and Cared For.* London: Peter Owen, 1978.

Wall, Florence Emeline. *Opportunities in Beauty Culture.* New York: Vocational Guidance Manuals, 1952.

———. *Principles and Practice of Beauty Culture.* New York: Keystone Publications, 1946.

Wares, Lydia Jean. "Dress of the African American woman in slavery and freedom: 1500 to 1935." Unpublished Ph.D. dissertation. Purdue University, 1981.

Warner, Deborah J. "Women Inventors at the Centennial." In *Dynamos and Virgins Revisited: Women and Technological Change in History.* Edited by Martha Moore Trescott. Metchen, N.J. and London: Scarecrow Press, 1979.

Watkins Timely Suggestions. Winona, Minn.: J.R. Watkins Company, circa 1920. Smithsonian Institution's Warshaw Collection.

Waugh, Nora. *Corsets and Crinolines.* 1954. Reprint, New York: Routledge/Theatre Arts Books, 1995.

Westmore, Frank. *The Westmores of Hollywood.* New York: Berkley Medallian Edition, 1977.

Willett, Julie A. *Permanent Waves: The Making of the American Beauty Shop.* New York: New York University Press, 2000.

Williams, Neville. *Powder and Paint: A History of the Englishwoman's Toilet.* London: Longmans, Green and Co., 1957.

Wilson, Donald L. *Natural Bust Enlargement with Total Mind Power: How to Use the Other 90% of Your Mind to Increase the Size of Your Breasts.* Larkspur, Calif.: Total Mind Power Institute, 1979.

Wilson, Edward O. *Sociobiology.* Cambridge, Mass.: Belknap Press, 1975.

Wilson, Elizabeth. *Adorned in Dreams: Fashion and Modernity.* Berkeley: University of California Press, 1985.

Wilson, Elizabeth, and Lou Taylor. *Through the Looking Glass: A History of Dress from 1860 to the Present Day.* London: BBC Books, 1991.

Winchester, James H. "A Lift for Milady's Spirits." *Petroleum Today.* Spring 1963, pp. 10–12.

Worden, Edward Chauncey Worden. *Nitrocellulose Industry.* New York: D. Van Nostrand Company, 1911.

Worth, Jean Philippe. *A Century of Fashion.* Translated by Ruth Scott Miller. Boston: Little, Brown and Company, 1928.

Wosk, Julie. *Women and the Machine.* Baltimore: The Johns Hopkins University Press, 2001.

Wright, Robert. *The Moral Animal: The New Science of Evolutionary Psychology.* New York: Pantheon Books, 1994.

Yalom, Marilyn. *A History of the Breast.* New York: Ballantine, 1998.

Yarwood, Doreen. *The Encyclopaedia of World Costume.* London: B. T. Batsford, 1978.

Zimmer, Fritz. *Nitrocellulose Ester Lacquers.* London: Chapman & Hall, Ltd., 1934.

illustration credits

Patent Drawings
No small amount of folk art lies hidden in the patent archives, as Siegfried Giedion once observed. I am indebted to the anonymous illustrators who created the drawings reproduced here. They were taken from the patents listed below, which are identified by inventor, date, and patent number.

p. xvi
Helen A. Ballard
Judith Hart
1933
1,907,476

p. 10
Julius Ehmann
1931
1,795,482

p. 14
Charles Nessler
1923
1,450,259

p. 20
Alexandre Gimonet
1935
2,007,245

p. 21
Sarah E. Bohner
1932
1,873,928

p. 22
Helen Payes et al.
1936
2,035,667

p. 23
Hortense C. Erickson
1932
1,850,540

p. 25
Tosca Wagner
1933
1,905,399

p. 25
Leslie Edward Pithie
1942
2,271,034I9

p. 26
Stephen S. Newton
1876
185,693

p. 27
Frank L. Engel Jr.
1939
2,148,736

p. 29
Ira Joss et al.
1962
3,033,213

p. 32
Dan Seman
1926
1,592,907

p. 37
J. B. Mason Jr.
1923
1,470,994

p. 38
Gordon W. Nelson
1926
1,611,937

p. 38
Gordon W. Nelson
1930
1,782,365

p. 39
Edwin H. Kostler
1931
1,810,249

p. 40
Maurice Levy
1932
1,862,271

p. 43
Hazel M. Montealegre
1924
1,497,342

p. 47
Winifred T. Parkin
1934
1,953,910

p. 47
Ottomar Voelk
1934
1,965,327

p. 48
Marie L. Helehan
1938
2,117,061

p. 52
Herman C. Schlicker
1940
2,219,909

p. 53
Josephine A. Rountree
1926
1,583,316

p. 62
Peggy Brown
1931
1,795,073

p. 67
Mortimer Clarke
1884
298,067

p. 68
L. Lendry
1893
507,373

p. 68
Marie Tucek
1893
494,397

p. 70
Hugo Schindler
1893
504,054

p. 71
Ebenezer Murray
1899
623,413

p. 73
Anne S. McLean
1858
22,443

p. 74
Eleanor Marshall
1864
43,321

p. 76
Mary P. R. Tilton
1870
110,310

p. 77
Sherwood B. Ferris
1877
188,007

p. 77
Sherwood B. Ferris
1876
181,781

p. 78
Zénone de Lpedòchowski
1884
301,451

p. 79
John Tallman
1875
162,869

p. 88
Edgar Guggenheim
1916
1,167,992

p. 89
Louise A. Sherry
1922
1,434,231

p. 89
Francis H. Morrison
1928
1,667,796

p. 90
Caroline Gudeman
1933
1,923,821

p. 93
Kaletae Hadley
1921
1,400,056

p. 94
Waldemar Kops
1917
1,237,059

p. 114
Hugo Gernsback
1927
1,620,539

p. 125
Mary E. Hall
1921
1,394,171

p. 138
Chin Leong Li
S. Quisling
1926
1,588,387

p. 139
Gerd Wosse
1931
1,812,425

p. 139
Vincent J. Moir
1938
2,113,962

p. 141
T. C. Di Giovanna
1955
2,714,788

p. 144
M. J. Pinault
1893
495,265

p. 162
Louis W. G. Flynt
1916
1,175,513

p. 168
Evangeline I. Gilbert
1926
1,572,891

p. 169
Eugenie Haagen
1964
3,154,071

p. 172
Imogene E. Banker
1881
241,589

p. 181
Moses K. Bortree
1875
165,534

p. 181
Elizabeth Stowell Weldon
1877
189,672

p. 188
Seligman Gutman
1878
210,025

p. 202
Anna Hamberg
1934
1,942,332

p. 208
Telemachus G. Christopoulos
1952
2,595,640

p. 216
J. W. Boughton
1885
48,508

p. 216
Joseph Revson
1937
2,096,975

p. 217
Juliette Perras
1940
2,218,296

p. 219
Louis Halk
1929
1,715,914

p. 219
Arthur Earl Austin
George Allen Austin
1940
2,220,363

p. 221
Thomas Lee
Teresa Lee
1971
3,598,685

p. 224
C. Neumann
1863
40,355

p. 244
R. W. Hill
1860
26,848

p. 245
J. P. Buzzell
1866
52,637

p. 245
G. Mallory
1858
21,839

p. 255
Louis Fellheimer
1867
63,234

p. 256
Mary C. Clayton
1950
2,528,639

p. 264
Charles C. Carpenter
1885
324,226

p. 271
Henry O. Canfield
1888
375,923

p. 258
Ed Fraser
1887
371,135

p. 265
Aaron M. Weber
1874
155,480

p. 276
Mark A. Waterhouse
1883
290,505

p. 264
James Wehl
1872
130,345

p. 266
Albert Carter
1875
170,710

Other Illustrations

Allyn & Bacon: 6, 42.

Association for the Study of the Afro-American Life and History, King-Tisdell Cottage: 182.

Athena Images: xvi, xix, 8, 13, 30, 46, 49, 81, 85, 87, 97, 98, 105, 112, 117, 127, 129, 157, 160, 162, 178, 179, 185, 191, 195, 199, 220, 222, 229, 234, 235, 237, 264, 268, 270, 274.

Bakken Library: 82, 124, 136, 159.

Bob McCoy, Museum of Questionable Medical Devices: 106.

Richard Chenoweth: 132.

Chesebrough-Pond USA: 164.

Cutex/Medtech Inc.: 206.

Denver Public Library, Western History Department: 142 (photo by Harry Rhoads); 185 (photo by D. F. Barry); 186 (photo by Harry Rhoads).

Ft. Pulaski National Monument: 227.

Priscilla Harris Dalrymple and Dover Books: 273.

Joan Gerhart and Janice Mary Riordan: 45.

Library of Congress: 116 (LC-USF33–30509-HM5); 218 (US262–20742–301972); 231 (US262–053519–301972).

Lisette Model Estate (photo by Lisette Model): 61.

Maybelline Corporation: 10, 18.

Museum of American Textile History (Pl. 58): 233.

National Archives (111-B-1599; photo by Mathew Brady): 191.

Proctor & Gamble Corporation: 41.

Valentine Museum C68.89.F.: 260.

Warshaw Collection, American History Archives, Smithsonian Institution: 3.

index

Note: Page numbers in *italics* refer to illustrations.

Abunda, 107
acrylic polymers, 223
Adair, Eleanor, 153
Adamson, Percy, 99
alkanet, 34, 35
Allen, Margaret, 50, 153
alum, 146
Alvarez, Walter C., 170–71
American, Sampson, 35
American Beauty (Banner), 36
American Chemical Society, 60
American Dream, 246
American System of Dressmaking, The (Merwin), 69
amplifiers, 104
anhydrous methanol, 211
aniline dyes, 22–24, 261
Anthony, Susan B., 238
anthropology, 118–20, 238–39
antibiotics, 170
Arden, Elizabeth, 7, 152–54, 158, 159–60, 163
Ardena Bath, *160*, 161, 163
Ardena skin tonic, 152, 154
arsenic, 122
Arts of Beauty (Montez), 75
Asther, Nils, 11
atomic bomb, 134
Attraction wafers, 83–84
Aurum company, Chicago, 82–83
automobiles:
    and lacquers, 205, 214
    and sex, 91–92
Avedon, Richard, 58

back panniers, 261
Bailey Beauty Supply Company, 215
Bainbridge, John, 11
Baker, Josephine, 8
baldness, 128–29
Ball, Lucille, 50, 170
banana oil, 211
Bankhead, Tallulah, 11
Banner, Lois, 36
Bannerman, Margaret, 48
Bara, Theda, 8–9
bathhouses, 186–87
Beal, Joseph H., 197
Bearded Lady, *117*, 119
beards, 117–19, 120–21
Beaton, Cecil, 11
Beautee-Fit Brassiere Company, 100
beauty, changing standards of, xvii–xviii
Beauty Book (Strauss), 44–45
Beecher, Catherine, xviii
Beeman, Phosa D., 69
Beerbohm, Max, 5–6
bee-stung mouth, 35–36
Bell, Alexander Graham, 72
Bell, Mrs. Alexander Graham, 185
Belmont, Mrs. Alva, 151
Berg, Alfred, 51–55, 60
Bernhardt, Sarah, 36, 166
Bessemer steel, 239–40, 241
Bestform bras, 97
betel, 34
Betts, Evelyn, *273*
bicycles, 183, 185–86, *185*
Bishop, Hazel, 50–57, 59–60
Bishop, Henry, 51
Bishop, Mabel Billington, 51–53
Bissett, Enid, 95
Bliven, Bruce, 12
Bloomer, Amelia, 237, 238
Bloomers, 237–38
Bohner, Sarah E., 21

Booger Red, 275
Borah, Mrs. William, 151
borax, 146
boric acid, 154
Bortree, Moses K., 181
Bourke-White, Margaret, 15
Bow, Clara, 9, 42, 88–90, 94
Boyshform, 66, 93
Brady, Mathew, 4, 191
bralessness, 108–9
bras:
    burning, 109
    and corsets, 66, 69–70, *70*, 72
    design elements of, 96, 100
    development of, xxiii, 64–66, 88–90, 94–96, *94*, 97, 99
    engineering of, *67*, 68, *70*, *71*, 76, *89*, 90, 93
    flapper flatteners, 65–67, 93
    "I dreamed" campaign, *98*, 108
    inflatable, *105*
    padded, 107–8
    push-up, 63
    rip-cord, 70
    rubber in, 75–76, 80, 93, 99–100, 104
    sizing systems for, 96, 99
    for teen market, 92–94
    underwire, 99–100
    use of word, 92–93
Brassiere, Philippe de, 64
breast-feeding, 176
breasts, 63–113
    cleavage of, 100
    corsets for, 66, 69, 72, 73, 74–75, 77, 78, 87
    enlargers for, 82–85
    falsies, xvii, 69, 72, 73, 74, 103–4, 107–8
    flatteners for, 65–67, 82, 86, 88, 93

hydromassage for, 107
inflatable, 75–76, 80–81, *81, 105, 106*
insurance for, 70
pads for, 76, 79–80, *79*
protective gear for, 101
rollers for, *82*
rubber, 75–76, 80, *81*
and sexuality, 89–92
silicone treatments of, 111–13
sizes of, 81–84, 96, 107
suction action on, 84–85, *85*
surgery on, 63, 104, 109–13
and war effort, 101–2
see also bras
breath, bad, 140
Brill, A. A., 91
bromo-acid, 46
Brooklyn Bridge, 66
Brooks, Louise, 11
Brown, Adolph M., 167
Brown, James, 249, 250–51
Brown-Larimore, Karen, 197
Bryson, Michael A., 79–80
buffalo cartilage, 196
busc en poire, 189
busks, 175, 178, *179, 188,* 189
bustles, 80, 257, 259–72, *260, 263,* 273–75, *274, 276*
    awkwardness with, 262, 263, 273–74
    disposable, 263–64, *264*
    engineering of, *248, 264, 265, 266, 271*
    as false bums, 249
    materials of, 263, *264,* 269–70, *270,* 272
    patents of, 269–72
    stackable, 272
    with suspenders, 264–65, *265*
    trains of, 261
Bust-Up (Reyburn), 64
Buzzell, J. P., 245
Byers, Eben M., 24

Cadolle, Herminie, 69
cakewalk, 86
calisthenics, 35, 183
Canfield, Henry O., 271, 272
Caplin, Madame Roxy Anne, 178
carbolic acid, 122, 163, 164
carmine, 35, 36

Carothers, Wallace, 143
Carroll, Madeleine, 36
Castle, Bea, 57
Castle, Vernon and Irene, 86–87
castor oil, 50
cauterization, 122
cellulose; celluloid, 205, 223
Charleston (dance), 87, *87*
chignons, 262
Chin Leong Li, 138
chin strap, *158*
Civil War, 4, 118, 180, 226, 228, 232
Clairol, 52
Clark, Ebenezer, 248–52
Clarke, Mortimer, 67
Clayton, Mary C., 256
Cleopatra look, 16
cocaine, 125
cochineal, 36
cold cream, 149–51
Complexion wafers, 83–84
conspicuous consumption, 183
conspicuous invention, 183
Coolidge Effect, xxi
cork, 76, 79, 196
corporate espionage, 59
corselets, 175
corsets, *181, 184, 191*
    "anatomique," *195*
    and bras, 66, 69–70, *70,* 72
    for breasts, 66, 69, 72, *73,* 74–75, 77, 78, 87
    busks, 175, 178, *179, 188,* 189
    colors and trimmings of, 197
    dancing, 87, 91
    decline of, 174
    development of, 174–79
    in economic theory, 190
    "electric," 198
    and girdles, 103
    lazy lacing, *178,* 179
    mechanical, 178–79
    monkeys with, 190, 192
    opponents of, 190, 192
    out of favor, 200–201
    paper, 197
    reinvention of, xxiii, 103, 174, 176, 196
    S-curve, 192, 196
    stays of, 175, 178, 189
    steel-ribbed, 99, 194, 196, 198
    straight front, 192–93, 194

synthetic materials for, 103
tightlacing, *191,* 192–93
trademarks of, 95
Corsets and Crinolines (Waugh), 189
Corson, Richard, 16
Cosmetic (Max Factor), 9, 17
Cowan, Ruth Schwartz, xxiv
Crabtree, "Lottie" Mignon, 4
Crawford, Joan, *41,* 42, 170
crinolines, 226, 228–30, *229*
    awkward size of, 229, 236, 254, 257, 261
    manufacture of, *231,* 246, 247
    materials in, 241–42, 245–46
    popularity of, 236, 238, 239
    word derivation, 229
Cronin, Thomas, 113
Crosby, Caresse, 64–66
Crouch, Franklin B., 83
Crum, J. Howard, 166, 167
Crystal Palace, 248, 251
Cueto, André A., 129
cult of the Anglo-Saxon, 119
cumin seeds, 82
"Cupid's bow" mouth, 42, 43, *43*
Curie, Marie, 131
Cutex nail polish, *206,* 207, 214, *219*

Daly, Kay, 210
dancing, 86–87, 91, 143
Daniel, John, 130
Darwin, Charles, xxi, 228, 238, 274
Davis, Bette, 12, 170
Dawn, Jack, 49
deafness, relief of, 169
Dean, Teresa, 185, 192
DeBevoise, Charles, 66
Demorest, Madame, 230, 232
Dennis, Oliver G., 80–81
deodorants, 140
depilatories, xix, 22, 116, 122, 126–29, *127,* 140, 143
Derma-Vac Facial System, 161
derriere, *see* bustles
De Ver, Ira, 194
Diaghilev, Sergei, 7
diathermy, 135–36, 159
diathermy massage, *162*
Dietrich, Marlene, 11–12, 140

Di Giovanna, Tigellia Cisco, 141
dimple producing appliance, *168*
Dinesen, Isak, xxii
Dior, Christian, 104, 107, 110
Dr. Charles Flesh Food, 83
Dr. Forest's Bust Developer, 85
Doda, Carol, 112
Dodge, Mabel, 91
douche, contraceptive, 150
Douglas & Sherwood, *231*
Draper, James, 249, 252
dress elevators, 232
Duco, 205, 207
Dudley, William L., 130
Duffey, E. B., 194
Dumoulin, Madame, 177
Dunlap, Knight, 119
Dunlop, John Boyd, 75
DuPont, 205, 207, 214
du Pont, Mrs. Nicholas R., 151

Eastman, George, 15
Eau de Veau, 146
écorchement, 164
Edison, Thomas, 72, 275
egg whites, 146
Ekberg, Anita, 104
electrolysis, 120–22, 123–26, *124*,
    125, 135–36, *136*
elephant seal, 116
Eliot, T. S., 81
Elizabeth, Queen of England, 146
Elka, 211, 212, 213
Ellis, Havelock, 192–93, 239
Eloise Rae company, 83
Empire fashions, 176, 228
enameling, 4
Engel, Frank L., Jr., 27, 28, 30
Ent, Elizabeth, 169
eosin, 46
Ephron, Nora, 107
epilatories, *see* depilatories
Ercoff, Nancy, xxiii
Eterna 27, 155
Eugenie, Empress, 225, 228
Ever-On, 215
evolution, theories of, xxi, xxiii,
    119, 238
exercise, 183, 185–86, *185*, *186*
Exquisite Form bras, *105*
Extreme Beauty (Koda), 262–63
eyebrows, plucking, *139*, 140

eyelets, metal, 177
eyes, 1–31, *6*
    artificial lashes, *14*
    eyebrow pencils, 9, 11, 39
    eyelash curlers, 9, *10*, *22*, 28
    kohl on, 4, 7, 8, 15, 28
    lampblack on, 16
    Lash Lure, 20–24
    mascara, *see* mascara
    and photography, 4–5, 15

face-lifts, 165–67, 169–71
facial "hirsuties," 121–22
facial massage, 156, 158
facial senescence, 169
Factor, Max, 9, 17, 42
falsies, xvii, 69, 72, *73*, *74*, 103–4,
    107–8
Farrell-Beck, Jane, 65, 92
farthingales, 228
Fashioning the Bourgeoisie
    (Perrot), 235
fat-roller, *162*
Faucigny-Lucinge, Princess de, 208
Fay-Miss bras, 93
Fellheimer, Louise, 255
feme-covert, 237, 238
feminists, xviii, 109
Ferris, Sherwood B., 77
Field, John, 99
Field, Mrs. Marshall, 151
"Fighting the Corsetless Evil"
    (Pulfer), 200
fingernail glossifier, 211
fingernails, artificial, *222*, 223
Fink, Marie, 133
Finley, Ruth E., 261
Fire and Ice, 57–59
Fish, Harriet M., 35
Fitzgerald, F. Scott, 44, 207
flapper flatteners, 65–67, 93
flappers, *142*, 151, 200
Flatterettes, 103–4
Flügel, John Carl, xx
Flynt, Louis W. G., 162
focus-group research, 213
Folsom, Sewall, 246
Foot-O-Scopes, 131
Ford, Henry, 91, 205
Formfit Company, 96, 103
Fox, George Henry, 120–22,
    124–25

Foy, Lavinia, 194
Francis, Connie, 60
Franklin, Benjamin, 34
Franklyn, Robert Alan, 110
Freud, Sigmund, 89–90, 91, 155
fucus, 34
Fuller, Henry C., 212

Gaches-Sarraute, Josephine Ines,
    193–94
galbanum, 123
Galen, 149
Garbo, Greta, 9, 11, 12, *13*
gargling, 140
Gau, Colleen, 65, 92
gay deceivers, xvii, 69
General Motors, 207
Gernsheim, Alison, 261, 273
Gerow, Frank, 113
Gersuny, Robert, 109
Geyser, Albert C., 132
Gibson girls, 66, 94, 196
Giedion, Siegfried, xxiv–xxv
gigantomastia, 104
Gilbert, Evangeline I., *168*
Gilded Age, 180, 183
Gillette, King, 137, 138
Gillette razor blades, 137–38
Gilman, Charlotte Perkins, 90
Givenchy look, 109
Glass of Fashion, The (Beaton), 11
Godey's Lady's Book, 146
Gooding, Ella E., 48
Goodyear, Charles, 75, 241
Gordon, Jane, 12
Grable, Betty, 143
Great Depression, 17, 19, 51, 214
great masculine renunciation, 34–35
Great Underarm Campaign, 137
Greeley, Horace, 118
Greene, Jacob W., 74
Griffin, Merv, 57
Gudeman, Caroline, 90
Guggenheim, Edgar, 88
Gunn, Fenja, 151
Gutman, Seligman, 188

Haagen, Eugenie, 169
Hadley, Kaletae, 93
Hager Medical Company, 83
Haig, Mrs. E. Huston, 83

Haiken, Elizabeth, 110, 113
Hain, Leon, 100
hair, 115–43
    excess, 119–20
    facial, 117–21
    lack of, 119, 128–29
    on legs, 140, *141*, 143
    removal of, xviii-xix, 115–18,
        120–28, 129, 131–34,
        136–43, *138*, *139*
    shaving, 122, 136–43, *141*
    underarm, 136–38, 140, 143
    volume of, 262
hair follicles, 122, 125, 135
hair-growing machine, *129*
hairlessness, 117–19, 122
hair-straightening combs, 217
Hale, Sarah Josepha, 146
Half-Way bra, 108
Hall, Mary E., 125
Hamilton, Zoe, 83
hands, 203–23
    artificial fingernails, *222*, 223
    buffed nails, 204–5
    clip-on nail guards, *219*
    manicures, 208, 219, *220*
    "moon manicure," *206*, 208
    nail appliqués, *221*
    nail extensions, 223
    nail polish, 204–9, *206*,
        211–17, 219, 221–22
    nail polish applicators, 215,
        216, 217, *219*
    nail wraps, 223
    as sexual ornaments, 203–4
"harem" skirts, 200
Harlow, Jean, 12, 36, 140
Harrell, Annelore, 219
Harris, Ella, 165
Harris brothers, 57
Harrison, Dora, 80
Hayworth, Rita, 223
Health-Culture Company, 85
Hecht and Company, 54
Helehan, Marie L., 48
Hepburn, Audrey, *30*, 31, 108–9
Hera, 63
Hess, Abbie M., 169
Hill, R. W., 244
Hinkel, Arthur Ralph, 135, 136
Hippocrates, 149
hips, 225–57
    hoop skirts, *224*, 225–48, *227*,

233, *235*, *244*, *245*,
    253–57, *255*, *256*; see also
    crinolines
    and racial typology, 238–39
    skeleton skirts, 248–52
    trousers, 236–37
History of the Breast, A (Yalom),
    108
hobble skirts, 200
Hoffman, Robert, 209, 213
Hollander, Eugen, 165
Hollywood Lift, 167, 169, *169*
Holmes, Oliver Wendell, 4
home permanent–wave kits, 57
hoop skirts, *see* hips
Hope, Christine, 137
horsehair, 196
hot combs, 217
hot-wax bath, *160*, 161, 163
hourglass figure, *182*, 192, 194
Howe, Julia Ward, 190
How to Be Beautiful (Dean), 192
Hrdy, Sarah Blaffer, xxii
"hubba hubba girl," 70
Hubbard Ayer, Harriet, 2–4,
    148–49
Hughes, Howard, 100
Huntsman, Benjamin, 242
Hussy lipstick, 47–48
Hutchinson, Pearl, *45*
Hutton, Barbara, 170
hydrocarbon solvents, 31
hydrogenated cottonseed oil, 9
hydrogen sulfide, 126
hydromassage, 107
hypertrichosis, 120–21
hypomastia, 110
hysterical paroxysm, 155–56

ideal, feminine, 151
ideal proportions, 96, 104, 173–74
Ivalon implants, 110–11

Jaeger, Gustav, 193
James, Alice, 156
James, Lucy, 70
JC Penney, 69
Jenkins, Nicholas, 270
jitterbug, 143
jock straps, 193
Johns, Maxine James, 186

Johnson, Henrietta P., 121–22,
    123–25
Josselin, Jean Julien, 178
Joyce, James, 91
Jurgovan, Edna, 170
J. Walter Thompson, 94, 151

Kama Sutra, 16
Kapinas, Ruth, 96
Kellermann, Annette, 187
Kenealy, Arabella, 190, 192
Kent, Frank, 91
Kevlar, 51
Kevles, Bettyann Holtzmann, 130
Knauth, Elma, 169–70
Koda, Harold, 262, 267
Kodak cameras, 15
kohl, 4, 7, 8, 15, 28
Kolmar Laboratories, 53
Kops Brothers, 93–95
Koremlu, xx, 22, 127–29
Kostler, Edwin H., 39
Kree, Paul M., 126
Kron, Joan, 110, 163, 165
Kurkus, Virginia, 143
Kurlash, 9
Kwolek, Stephanie, 51

Lachman, Charles, 212–13
lacquers, 205, 207, 214
Ladies' Sanitary Association, 190
Lady Bountiful, *106*, 107
Lady lipstick, 47, 48
Lady's Pocket Companion, 5
Laleek Longlash, 19
Lamarr, Hedy, 42
Lamb, Ruth deForest, 22, 24, 129
lampblack, 16
Landaw, Louis, 102
Lange, Dorothea, 15
Langtry, Lillie, 5, 272
lanolin, 154
lanugo, 123
Lash, Harvey, 113
Lash Lure, xx, 20–24
Lastex, 99
Launer, Christie, 74
Laver, James, xx
lead, 150
LeClair, F. A., 46
Lee, Thomas and Teresa, 221

Leetch, Elizabeth, 74
legs, shaving, 140, *141*, 143
Leigh, Dorian, 58
Lendry, Ludwig, 68
Levin, Oscar, 133
Levitt, Sarah, 230
Levy, Maurice, 38–39, 40
Lewis, Eleanor Custis, 34
Liebault, Jean, 82
Lift (Kron), 165
Lily of France, 103
Limner, Luke, 190
Lind, Richard W., 135, 136
Lindsey, Timmie Jean, 113
Lippmann, Walter, 91
lips, 33–61
    bee-stung mouth, 35–36
    calisthenics for, 35
    "Cupid's bow," 42, 43, *43*
    permanent smile, *53*
    rouge for, 34–35, 36–37
    shapes of, 42, *42*
    stencils for, *48*
lipstick, 44–50
    color-coordinated, 57–58
    development of, 50–60
    kissproof, 59–60
    no-smear, 54–57, *54*, 59–60
    packaging of, 37–40, *37*, *38*,
        39, *40*, 50, *52*, *54*
    and sexuality, 47–48
"Lipstick on Your Collar" (Connie
    Francis), 60–61
Lister, Joseph, 163
Lloyd's of London, 70
Lollobrigida, Gina, 104
Longworth, Mrs. Nicholas, 151
Louden, Madelon, 103
Lpedóchowski, Zénone de, 78
Lublin, Kora M., 126, 127–29
Luce, Clare Booth, 47, 217
Lynd, Robert and Helen, 91
Lysol, 150

Madison, Dolley, 34
Maiden Form/Maidenform, 95, *98*,
    99, 102, 103, 108
Maines, Rachel, 155
Making of a Beautiful Face
    (Crum), 167
Mallory, G., 245
Mammary Cell Food, 83

mammiform, 72, 74
mandrill baboon, 116
manicures, 219, *220*
Mansfield, Jayne, 104
margarine, 211
Marie, queen of Romania, 151
Marinello machine, 160–61
Mark Eden Bust Developer, 107
Marshall, Eleanor M., 72, 74
Marshall, H. L. J., 133
Martin Method, 132
Marx, Karl, 243
mascara, 1, 7, 15–16, 17–24, *18*,
    25, 27
    applicators, *3*, *18*, *20*, *25*, *26*,
        27–28, *27*, *28*, *29*, 30–31
    eyelash guards for, *21*, *23*
Mascaramatic, 28, 30
masks, *158*, 159–61, 163
Mason, James Bruce, Jr., 37, 39
Maybelline, 17, *18*, 19
McCarthy, Justin, 254
McKennec, Henry, 251
McLean, Anne S., 72, 73
medical induction coils, 160
melanoma, 150
Mencken, H. L., 91
menstrual pads, 140
mercury, 22, 150
Merwin, Pearl, 69
Michel, Charles, 123
micromastia, 110
microwaves, 135, 159–60
Miller, Lois Mattox, 104
Millet, R. C., 246
Mirault, Monsieur, 148
mirrors, 15
Miss America, 93, 173
Model Company, 95
Model T's, 91
monkeys, corsets on, 190, *192*
Monroe, Marilyn, 104, 107, 110,
    173
Montealegre, Hazel Mann, 43
Monteil, Germaine, 57
Montez, Lola, 75, 76, 122, 123
"moon manicure," *206*, 208
Moore, Benjamin F., 263
Moore, Doris Langley, 262
moose, antlers of, 116
Morgan, Marabel, xxii-xxiii
Morrow, Doretta, 28
Munsingwear, 96

Murray, Arthur, 87
Murray, Ebenezer, 71
muscle toners, 160

nails, *see* hands
Nair, 129
Napoleon III of France, 118
Neal, Roy S., 70
Neff, Elinor Guthrie, 143
Negri, Pola, 8
Nelson, Arthur, 132
Nelson, Gordon W., 38
neoprene, 103
Nessler, Charles, 14
Newell, Caroline, 69
New Look, 104, 110
Newton, Stephen S., 26
New Woman, 45, 91
nitrocellulose, 204–5, 207, 211, 212
Noël, Suzanne, 166
Nostrums and Quackery (AMA),
    82
NueDé forms, 103
nylon, 103, 143, 214

obsolescence, built-in, 99
Ogle, Charles, 35
Osborne & Vincent, 248, 252–53
"O Susan Wears a Bustle" (Gibbs),
    269

PABA (para-aminobenzoic acid), 150
packaging, 38–39, 215, 217
Palmer, Bertha, 2
Palmer, Joseph, 118
Pangman, John, 110
paper dresses, 263
paraffin injections, 109
Parker, Dorothy, xxi
Parkin, Winfred T., 47
Parrington, Vernon, 180
Pasteur, Louis, 239
Patterson, Ethel Lloyd, 167
Peeps into the Human Hive
    (Wyhnter), 262
pelvis, 238–39
Pendergrast, Mark, 15
penile implants, 113
Perelman, S. J., 59
periwigs, 34

permanent wave machines, 217, *218*
permanent waves, home kits, 57
Perrot, Philippe, 235, 257
*Personal Beauty and Racial
     Betterment* (Dunlap), 119
Petelle, Martha, 166
petroleum jelly, 17
Petroski, Henry, xxiv
petticoats, *see* hips
phenol peel, 163–65
Phillips, M. C., 221
photographic portraits, 4–5, 15
picture magazines, 15
Pierce, Sarah Jane, 5
Pill, the, 109
pine-bark extract, 154
Pinkham, Lydia E., 193
pitch plaster, 123
Pithie, Leslie E., 25
plaits, 262
plasticizers, 207, 211
plastic surgery, 110, 167, 170–71
platinum tips, 209
Poiret, Paul, 7, 200
Poix, Gabrielle M., 103
polyurethane, 110
Pond, Theron T., 150
Pond's cold cream, 149–51
Pond's Extract, 150
Pond's Vanishing Cream, *164*
Pons, Helen, 100
Portable Complection, 5
Powder and Paint (Williams), 44,
     209
Power, Susan C., 75, 76, 83
Princes Bust Developer, 84, *85*
Psychology of Clothes, The
     (Flügel), xx
Pulfer, G. B., 200
punching (hair removal), 123

quicklime, 122
Quisling, Sverre, 138

racial determinism, 118–20
racial typology, 238–39
radiation, 130–36
Radithor, 24
razors, 122, 136–43
Récamier, Juliette, 148–49
resins, 207, 211

Revlon, 57–59, 209–11, 219
Revson, Charles, 57–59, 155,
     209–11, 212–15, 217
Revson, Joseph, 215, 216
Reyburn, Wallace, 64
Rhodes, Richard, xxiv
rhythmotherapy, 156
Riva, Maria, 11
Robinson, Henry Peach, 4
rodent poison, 127
Rodgers, H. J., 4
Roentgen, William, 130
Roosevelt, Alice, 151
Rosenthal, Ida, 95
rouge, 34–35, 36–37
Rountree, Josephine A., 53
Rowland, Alexander, 119
rubber:
     bras, 75–76, 80, 93, 99–100, 104
     inflatable breasts, 75–76,
          80–81, *81*, *105*, *106*
Rubinstein, Helena, 7, 8–9, 28, 57,
     152, 154–55
Rugg, Datus E., 246–48, 252–54
Russell, Jane, 100, 110
Russett, Cynthia Eagle, 238

Sabouraud, Raymond, 126, 127,
     128, 129
safety razors, 137–38
Saint Laurent, Yves, 109
St. Pierre, Henri E., 134, 135, 136
San Francisco police inspectors, 134
Sanger, Margaret, 192–93
Sanitary Woolen System, 193
Sargent, Dudley A., 187
Sawyer, Edward J., 197
Sayre, Zelda (Fitzgerald), 44, 187,
     189
Schindler, Hugo, 70
Schmitt, Frank, 70
Scott's Electric Corset, 198
Scovill Manufacturing Company, 38
Selling Dreams (Allen), 50, 153
Severn, Bill, 118
sewing machines, 189, 261
sexual climax, 155–56
sexual display, 116
Sexual Science (Russett), 238
sexual selection, theory of, 119
Seymour, Jim, 148–49
shaving, 122, 136–43, *141*

S. H. Camp and Company, 96
Shearer, Norma, 36
Sherry, Louise Antoinette, 70, 89
silicone, 111–13
Singer, Isaac, 189
skin, 145–71
     beauty creams, 148–51
     face-lifts, 165–67, 169–71
     fat-roller, *162*
     masks, *158*, 159–61, 163
     massage, 156, 158
     phenol peel, 163–65
     soap, *157*
     tonics, 152–55
     vibrators, 155–56, 158–59
     whiteners, 22, 150
     wrinkles, 146, *147*, 148,
          152–55, 169, 171
Skin Deep (Phillips), 221
skirts, *see* hips
sleeves, inflated, 272–73, *273*
Sloan, Alfred P. Jr., 207
Smith, Charlotte, 2
Smith, Kate, 57
soap, *157*
sodium hydroxide, 123
spandex, 103
spark-gap, 135
Spector, Raymond, 54–57
Spencer Body and Breast Supports,
     199
spoon busks, *188*, 189
Stanton, Elizabeth Cady, 36, 237,
     238
steam molding, 189
steel:
     Bessemer process, 239–40, 241
     busks, 179, *179*
     cast, 242
     in corsets, 99, 194, 196, 198
     in hoop skirts, 226, 241, 246
     Sheffield, 242
     wire, 242–43
Steele, Valerie, 254
Stout, William B., 38
Straight Front Corset, 192–93,
     194
Strauss, Rita, 44–45
Surgifoam, 110
Swabach, Stanley, 54
Swallow, Alwilda, 265
Swanson, A. Fabian, 153–54
Swartz, Mimi, 113

sweater-girl profile, 107
swimming, 186–87, *186*, 189

Tabor, Baby Doe, 4
Tallman, John, 79
Tangee lipstick, 45–46, *46*
tango, 86–87
Tattoo, 19, *49*
Technique for Beauty (Gordon), 12
Technology of Orgasm, The
    (Maines), 155
Tellef, Mrs. B., 133
thallium acetate, 127, 128, 129
thermolysis, 135–36
Thomas, Marlo, 109
Thomson & Thomson, 249, 251
Three Books for the Embellishment
    of the Human Body
    (Liébault), 82
Tibbals, Alfred Lee, 169
tightlacing, *191*, 192–93
Tilton, Mary P. R., 75–76
Titzling, Otto, 64
toe-spacing device, *208*
toilet paper, 140
Toilette of Health, 16
toluenesulfonamide formaldehyde,
    215
tongue, hair on, 120
Toni home permanent, 57
Total Woman, The (Morgan), xxii–
    xxiii
Towle, H. Ledyard, 207
transsexuals, xviii-xix
Tricho System, 132–34
Trotta, Geri, 171
Truth About Cosmetics, 126
Tucek, Marie, 68
Tupper, Earl, 55, 223
Tupperware, 55, 223
turkey cartilage, 175
turkey trot, 86, 87
Turner, Lana, 42
Twain, Mark, 59
tweezers, 122, *138*
Twiggy, 111, 173

Ugly-Girl Papers, The (Power), 75,
    83

ultraviolet rays, 150
U.S. Capitol dome, 243–45
U.S. Patent Office, 268
U.S. Rubber Company, 99

vacuum pumps, *106*
vacuum tubes, 135
Vail, Gilbert, 151
van Buren, Martin, 35
Vanderbilt, Mrs. Reginald, 151
Vanderbilt, William K., 86, 180
vanishing cream, xx, 150, *164*
Veblen, Thorstein, 183, 190
Vegetable Compound (Lydia
    Pinkham), 193
Velvet Mittens, 141
Venetian Cream Amoretta,
    154
Venus de Milo, 173
Venus of Willendorf, 173
vibrators, 155–56, 158–59
Victorians Unbuttoned (Levitt),
    230
Violet Ray machines, 158–59
vulcanized rubber, 75–76, 241
vulvular massage, 156

Wagner, Tosca, 25
waist, 172–201
    corsets, *see* corsets
    empire, 176
    and exercise, 183, 185–87, *185*,
        186, 189
    hourglass figure, *182*
waist-to-hip ratio, 173–74
Wallian, Samuel Spencer, 156
war effort, 50, 101–2, 104
Warner, Lucien, 194
Warner Company, 65, 92, 93, 99,
    100
War Production Board, 101–2
Watkins Timely Suggestions,
    44
wattles, 170
Waugh, Norah, 189
waxing, 123
Weber, Aaron M., 265
Webster, Granville S., 197
Wehl, James, 263–64

Weldon, Elizabeth S., 79, 181
Weldon, Fay, 146
West, Evelyn, 70
West, Mae, 103, 163
Westmore, Mont, 89–90
Westmore, Percy, 42
whalebone stays, 175, 189, 196,
    230, 241
What Women Should Know
    (Duffey), 194
whiskers, 118–19
Wilde, Oscar, 261
Williams, Mary A., 74
Williams, Neville, 28, 44, 209
Williams, T. L., 17
Winslow, Thyra Samter, 166
Winterstein, Helene Vierthaler,
    19
wire, 242–43, 266, 267, 269–70,
    272
Wise, Brownie, 55
witch hazel, 150
women:
    "lariat-spinning sextet," 60
    property rights of, 237–38
    sources of power for, xvii
    working, 234
Women, The (Luce), 47, 217
Women's Rights Convention,
    Seneca Falls, 228, 238
Woodbury, John H., 165
Works Projects Administration
    (WPA), 46, 96
World War I, 151, 205
World War II, 49–50, 101–2,
    104
Worth gowns, 230
Wosse, Gerd, 139
Wright, Orville and Wilbur, 72
wrinkles, xx, 146, *147*, 148,
    152–55, 169, 171
Wyhnter, Andrew, 262

Xervac, 128–29
X-rays, 130–36

Yale, Madame M., 2
Yalom, Marilyn, 108
Youth Mask, *158*, 159

about the author

T ERESA R IORDAN has written a column on invention for
The New York Times business section for ten years. She has
written about invention, politics, science, and American culture
for *The Washington Post Magazine*, ABCNews.com, *Worth*,
The Washington Monthly, *The New York Times Magazine*,
Reuters, and *People*. Her web log can be found at
www.patentlyabsurd.com.

She is married to the architect Richard Chenoweth and
has three children. They live in Silver Spring, Maryland.